T0359093

Transplant-Related Infections

Editors

HANNAH IMLAY
KIMBERLY E. HANSON

INFECTIOUS DISEASE CLINICS OF NORTH AMERICA

www.id.theclinics.com

Consulting Editor
HELEN W. BOUCHER

September 2023 • Volume 37 • Number 3

ELSEVIER

1600 John F. Kennedy Boulevard ● Suite 1800 ● Philadelphia, Pennsylvania, 19103-2899.
http://www.theclinics.com

INFECTIOUS DISEASE CLINICS OF NORTH AMERICA Volume 37, Number 3
September 2023 ISSN 0891–5520, ISBN-13: 978-0-443-18378-2

Editor: Kerry Holland
Developmental Editor: Hannah Almira Lopez

© **2023 Elsevier Inc. All rights reserved.**

This periodical and the individual contributions contained in it are protected under copyright by Elsevier, and the following terms and conditions apply to their use:

Photocopying

Single photocopies of single articles may be made for personal use as allowed by national copyright laws. Permission of the Publisher and payment of a fee is required for all other photocopying, including multiple or systematic copying, copying for advertising or promotional purposes, resale, and all forms of document delivery. Special rates are available for educational institutions that wish to make photocopies for non-profit educational classroom use. For information on how to seek permission visit www.elsevier.com/permissions or call: (+44) 1865 843830 (UK)/(+1) 215 239 3804 (USA).

Derivative Works

Subscribers may reproduce tables of contents or prepare lists of articles including abstracts for internal circulation within their institutions. Permission of the Publisher is required for resale or distribution outside the institution. Permission of the Publisher is required for all other derivative works, including compilations and translations (please consult www.elsevier.com/permissions).

Electronic Storage or Usage

Permission of the Publisher is required to store or use electronically any material contained in this periodical, including any article or part of an article (please consult www.elsevier.com/permissions). Except as outlined above, no part of this publication may be reproduced, stored in a retrieval system or transmitted in any form or by any means, electronic, mechanical, photocopying, recording or otherwise, without prior written permission of the Publisher.

Notice

No responsibility is assumed by the Publisher for any injury and/or damage to persons or property as a matter of products liability, negligence or otherwise, or from any use or operation of any methods, products, instructions or ideas contained in the material herein. Because of rapid advances in the medical sciences, in particular, independent verification of diagnoses and drug dosages should be made.

Although all advertising material is expected to conform to ethical (medical) standards, inclusion in this publication does not constitute a guarantee or endorsement of the quality or value of such product or of the claims made of it by its manufacturer.

Infectious Disease Clinics of North America (ISSN 0891–5520) is published in March, June, September, and December by Elsevier Inc., 360 Park Avenue South, New York, NY 10010-1710. Periodicals postage paid at New York, NY and additional mailing offices. Subscription prices are $368.00 per year for US individuals, $806.00 per year for US institutions, $100.00 per year for US students, $420.00 per year for Canadian individuals, $1,007.00 per year for Canadian institutions, $458.00 per year for international individuals, $1,007.00 per year for international institutions, $100.00 per year for Canadian students, and $200.00 per year for international students. To receive student rate, orders must be accompanied by name of affiliated institution, date of term, and the *signature* of program/residency coordinator on institution letterhead. Orders will be billed at individual rate until proof of status is received. Foreign air speed delivery is included in all *Clinics* subscription prices. All prices are subject to change without notice. **POSTMASTER**: Send address changes to *Infectious Disease Clinics of North America,* Elsevier Health Sciences Division, Subcription Customer Service, 3251 Riverport Lane, Maryland Heights, MO 63043. **Customer Service: 1-800-654-2452 (US). From outside of the US and Canada, call 1-314-447-8871. Fax: 1-314-447-8029. E-mail: JournalsCustomerService-usa@elsevier.com (print support) or JournalsOnlineSupport-usa@elsevier.com (online support).**

Infectious Disease Clinics of North America is also published in Spanish by Editorial Inter-Médica, Junin 917, 1er A 1113, Buenos Aires, Argentina.

Reprints. For copies of 100 or more, of articles in this publication, please contact the Commercial Reprints Department, Elsevier Inc., 360 Park Avenue South, New York, New York 10010-1710. Tel. 212-633-3874, Fax: 212-633-3820, E-mail: reprints@elsevier.com.

Infectious Disease Clinics of North America is covered in *MEDLINE/PubMed (Index Medicus), Current Contents/ Clinical Medicine, Science Citation Alert, SCISEARCH,* and *Research Alert.*

Contributors

CONSULTING EDITOR

HELEN W. BOUCHER, MD, FACP, FIDSA
Dean and Professor of Medicine, Tufts University School of Medicine, Chief Academic Officer, Tufts Medicine, Boston, Massachusetts, USA

EDITORS

HANNAH IMLAY, MD, MS
Professor of Medicine and Pathology, Division of Infectious Diseases, Department of Internal Medicine, University of Utah School of Medicine, Salt Lake City, Utah, USA

KIMBERLY E. HANSON, MD, MHS
Assistant Professor of Medicine, Division of Infectious Diseases, Department of Medicine, Division of Clinical Microbiology, Department of Pathology, University of Utah School of Medicine, ARUP Laboratories,
Salt Lake City, Utah, USA

AUTHORS

MARÍA ALEJANDRA PÉREZ, MD
ICESI University, Cali, Colombia

MARWAN M. AZAR, MD, FAST, FIDSA
Assistant Professor, Department of Medicine, Section of Infectious Diseases, Department of Laboratory Medicine, Yale School of Medicine, New Haven, Connecticut, USA

HANNAH BAHAKEL, MD
Division of Infectious Diseases, Cincinnati Children's Hospital Medical Center, Cincinnati, Ohio, USA

LARA DANZIGER-ISAKOV, MD
Division of Infectious Diseases, Cincinnati Children's Hospital Medical Center, Department of Pediatrics, University of Cincinnati College of Medicine, Cincinnati, Ohio, USA

DANIEL E. DULEK, MD
Assistant Professor of Pediatrics, Division of Pediatric Infectious Diseases, Department of Pediatrics, Vanderbilt University Medical Center, Monroe Carell Jr. Children's Hospital at Vanderbilt, Nashville, Tennessee, USA

CHRISTINE M. DURAND, MD
Department of Medicine, Johns Hopkins School of Medicine, Baltimore, Maryland, USA

JAMES EVERHART, DO
Departments of Pathology and Infectious Disease, Duke University Medical Center, Durham, North Carolina, USA

AMY G. FELDMAN, MD, MSCS
Section of Pediatric Gastroenterology, Hepatology and Nutrition, Digestive Health Institute, University of Colorado School of Medicine and Children's Hospital Colorado, Aurora, Colorado, USA

DANIEL Z.P. FRIEDMAN, MD, MSc
Assistant Professor, Section of Infectious Diseases and Global Health, The University of Chicago, Chicago, Illinois, USA

MADDALENA GIANNELLA, MD, PhD
Associate Professor of Infectious Diseases, IRCCS Azienda Ospedaliero-Universitaria di Bologna, Department of Medical and Surgical Sciences, Alma Mater Studiorum University of Bologna, Bologna, Italy

CHELSEA A. GORSLINE, MD
Assistant Professor, Division of Infectious Diseases, Department of Medicine, University of Kansas Medical Center, Kansas City, Kansas, USA

GHADY HAIDAR, MD
Division of Infectious Diseases, University of Pittsburgh School of Medicine, Pittsburgh, Pennsylvania, USA

NANCY G. HENSHAW, MPH, PhD
Department of Pathology, Duke University Medical Center, Durham, North Carolina, USA

RICARDO M. LA HOZ, MD
Director, Solid Organ Transplant Infectious Diseases, Associate Professor of Internal Medicine, Division of Infectious Diseases and Geographic Medicine, The University of Texas Southwestern Medical Center, Dallas, Texas, USA

MARIA ALEJANDRA MENDOZA, MD
Division of Public Health, Infectious Diseases and Occupational Medicine, Department of Medicine, William J. von Liebig Clinic Center for Transplantation and Clinical Regeneration, Mayo Clinic, Rochester, Minnesota, USA

NIYATI NARSANA, MD
University of California Davis School of Medicine, Sacramento, California, USA

RAYMUND R. RAZONABLE, MD
Division of Public Health, Infectious Diseases and Occupational Medicine, Department of Medicine, Mayo Clinic, William J. von Liebig Clinic Center for Transplantation and Clinical Regeneration, Mayo Clinic, Rochester, Minnesota, USA

MATTEO RINALDI, MD
Infectious Diseases, IRCCS Azienda Ospedaliero-Universitaria di Bologna, Clinical Researcher of Infectious Diseases, Department of Medical and Surgical Sciences, Alma Mater Studiorum University of Bologna, Bologna, Italy

JORDAN SALAS, BS
Department of Medicine, Johns Hopkins School of Medicine, Baltimore, Maryland, USA; Department of Medicine, Oregon Health & Science University School of Medicine, Portland, Oregon, USA

ILAN S. SCHWARTZ, MD, PhD
Associate Professor, Division of Infectious Diseases, Department of Medicine, Duke University School of Medicine, Durham, North Carolina, USA

ERICA J. STOHS, MD, MPH
Assistant Professor, Division of Infectious Diseases, Department of Medicine, University of Nebraska Medical Center, Omaha, Nebraska, USA

KAITLYN STORM, BS
Department of Medicine, Johns Hopkins School of Medicine, Baltimore, Maryland, USA

ARUNA SUBRAMANIAN, MD
Stanford University School of Medicine, Stanford, California, USA

PAUL A. TRUBIN, MD
Assistant Professor, Department of Medicine, Section of Infectious Diseases, Yale School of Medicine, New Haven, Connecticut, USA

MARIA TSIKALA VAFEA, MD
Division of Internal Medicine, University of Pittsburgh School of Medicine, UPMC, Pittsburgh, Pennsylvania, USA

PIERLUIGI VIALE, MD
Infectious Diseases, IRCCS Azienda Ospedaliero-Universitaria di Bologna, Department of Medical and Surgical Sciences, Alma Mater Studiorum University of Bologna, Bologna, Italy

Contents

Immunizations are a relatively safe and cost-effective intervention to prevent morbidity and mortality associated with vaccine preventable infection (VPIs). As such, immunizations are a critical part of the care of pre and posttransplant patients and should be prioritized. New tools are needed to continue to disseminate and implement the most up-to-date vaccine recommendations for the SOT population. These tools will help both primary care providers and multi-disciplinary transplant team members taking care of transplant patients to stay abreast of evidence-based best practices regarding the immunization of the SOT patient.

Herein, we review the current knowledge of donor-derived disease and current US Organ Procurement and Transplantation Network policies to minimize the risk. During the process, we also consider actions to further mitigate the risk of donor-derived disease. The overarching goal is to provide an infectious disease perspective on the complex decision of organ acceptance for transplant programs and candidates.

Although COVID-19 vaccines are safe, most organ transplant recipients fail to mount an antibody response after two mRNA vaccines. Thus, three mRNA vaccines constitute a primary vaccine series after solid organ transplant. However, neutralizing antibodies after three or greater mRNA vaccines are lower against Omicron versus older variants. Predictors of attenuated responses include age, vaccination within 1 year from transplant, mycophenolate, and BNT162b2. Some seronegative transplant recipients exhibit durable T-cell responses. Vaccine effectiveness in transplants is lower than in the general population. Immunosuppression reduction around revaccination warrants further study. Monoclonal antibody pre-exposure prophylaxis may be protective against susceptible variants.

Solid organ transplant recipients are at high risk of severe coronavirus disease-2019 (COVID-19). If left untreated, it results in high rates of hospitalization, intensive care unit admission and death. Early diagnosis of COVID-19 is essential to ensure the early administration of therapeutics. Treatment of mild-to-moderate COVID-19 with remdesivir, ritonavir-boosted nirmatrelvir, or an anti-spike neutralizing monoclonal antibody may prevent progression to severe and critical COVID-19. Among patients with severe and critical COVID-19, treatment with intravenous remdesivir and immunomodulation is recommended. This review article discusses strategies in the management of solid organ transplant recipients with COVID-19.

Advances in molecular diagnostics have the potential to improve patient care among solid organ transplant recipients by reducing time to pathogen identification and informing directed therapy. Although cultures remain the cornerstone of traditional microbiology, advanced molecular diagnostics, such as metagenomic next-generation sequencing (mNGS), may increase detection of pathogens. This is particularly true in the settings of prior antibiotic exposure, and when causative organisms are fastidious. mNGS also offers a hypothesis-free diagnostic method of testing. This is useful in situations whereby the differential is broad or when the infectious agent is unlikely to be detected by routine methods.

The overall burden of the main clinically relevant bacterial multidrug-resistant organisms (MDROs) (eg, methicillin-resistant *Staphylococcus aureus*, vancomycin-resistant enterococci, extended-spectrum β-lactamase producing or extended-spectrum cephalosporin-resistant Enterobacterales, carbapenem-resistant or carbapenemase-producing Enterobacterales, MDR *Pseudomonas aeruginosa*, and carbapenem-resistant *Acinetobacter baumannii*) in solid organ transplant (SOT) populations is summarized showing prevalence/incidence, risk factors, and impact on graft/patient outcome according to the type of SOT. The role of such bacteria in donor-derived infections is also reviewed. As for the management, the main prevention strategies and treatment options are discussed. Finally, nonantibiotic-based strategies are considered as future directions for the management of MDRO in SOT setting.

Although antimicrobial stewardship programs have excelled over the past decade, uptake and application of these programs to special populations such as solid organ transplant recipients have lagged. Here, we review the value of antimicrobial stewardship for transplant centers and highlight data supporting interventions that are ripe for adoption. In addition, we review the design of antimicrobial stewardship initiatives, targets for both syndromic and system-based interventions.

Pediatric solid organ transplant (SOT) recipients are at risk for infection following transplantation. Data from adult SOT recipients are often used to guide prevention and treatment of infections associated with organ transplantation in children. This article highlights key recent pediatric SOT-specific publications for an array of infectious complications of organ transplantation. Attention is given to areas of need for future study.

This review describes the epidemiology and risk factors of tuberculosis (TB) in solid organ transplant recipients. We discuss the pre-transplant screening for risk of TB and management of latent TB in this population. We also discuss the challenges of management of TB and other difficult to treat mycobacteria such as *Mycobacterium abscessus* and *Mycobacterium avium complex*. The drugs for the management of these infections include rifamycins which have significant drug interactions with immunosuppressants and must be monitored closely.

Recently, there have been significant advances in the diagnosis and management of invasive fungal infections. Compared with traditional fungal diagnostics, molecular assays promise improved sensitivity and specificity, the ability to test a range of samples (including noninvasive samples, ie, blood), the detection of genetic mutations associated with antifungal resistance, and the potential for a faster turnaround time. Antifungals in late-stage clinical development include agents with novel mechanisms of action (olorofim and fosmanogepix) and new members of existing classes with distinct advantages over existing antifungals in toxicity, drug–drug interactions, and dosing convenience (oteseconazole, opelconazole, rezafungin, ibrexafungerp, encochleated amphotericin B).

Pneumocystis infection manifests predominantly as an interstitial pneumonia in immunocompromised patients. Diagnostic testing in the appropriate clinical context can be highly sensitive and specific and involves radiographic imaging, fungal biomarkers, nucleic acid amplification, histopathology, and lung fluid or tissue sampling. Trimethoprim-sulfamethoxazole remains the first-choice agent for treatment and prophylaxis. Investigation

INFECTIOUS DISEASE CLINICS OF NORTH AMERICA

THE CLINICS ARE AVAILABLE ONLINE!
Access your subscription at:
www.theclinics.com

Preface

Updates in Prevention, Diagnosis, and Management of Infections Among Solid Organ Transplant Recipients

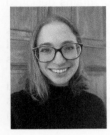
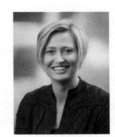

Hannah Imlay, MD, MS   Kimberly E. Hanson, MD, MHS
Editors

Solid organ transplantation (SOT) has revolutionized the management of end-stage organ disease. However, with the immunosuppressive therapy required to prevent rejection comes an increased risk of infections. Invasive infection complicates a high proportion of SOT procedures, and these infections are associated with significant morbidity and mortality.[1,2] The increasing nuances between choices of diagnostic tests, infection surveillance and prevention practices, and antimicrobial treatment options (or lack thereof for some multidrug-resistant pathogens) continue to complicate the management of SOT recipients. Dedicated infectious diseases involvement is an essential part of the multidisciplinary care of this medically complex patient population that has been demonstrated to improve patient outcomes.[1]

This issue of *Infectious Diseases Clinics of North America* is devoted to recent advances in the prevention, diagnosis, and management of infections in organ transplantation and provides valuable information with up-to-date references for providers involved in the care of SOTRs. New innovations and challenges since the last organ transplant–focused issue of Infectious Disease Clinics *of North America* include the following: the onset of the SARS-CoV-2 pandemic; new therapeutic options for Cytomegalovirus (CMV), fungal, and resistant Gram-negative infections; the growth of available molecular testing platforms; new preventive strategies; and the rise of antimicrobial stewardship programs targeted at immunocompromised patients.

The first two articles in this issue provide an update on immunization recommendations and review the current epidemiology of donor-derived infection. Immunizations that prevent common infections are more effective if timed and planned for administration before organ transplant. Similarly, the detection and mitigation of infections in the donor is essential for optimal prophylaxis in the immediate posttransplant period.

The onset of the SARS-CoV-2 pandemic in 2019 had a significant impact on SOT recipients. Two articles in this issue are devoted to topics related to SARS-CoV-2 prevention and treatment, respectively, with an emphasis on the best practice knowledge we have accrued and the important unanswered questions that remain.

Several articles discuss state-of-the art technologies and strategies used to manage suspected infection in SOT recipients, including the role of molecular diagnostic testing, new strategies for the detection, treatment, and prevention of drug-resistant organisms, and the role of antimicrobial stewardship programs designed specifically for immunocompromised hosts.

Pediatric SOT recipients experience many of the same infectious complications as do adults, but there are important differences in infection epidemiology and treatment considerations. One article in this issue is dedicated to a summary of unique aspects of pediatric transplant-associated infections.

The remaining five articles discuss recent developments in the approach to selected bacterial, fungal, and viral infections of importance for SOT recipients. These infections include Mycobacteria, fungal pathogens, *Pneumocystis jirovecii*, Human Immunodeficiency Virus, Hepatitis C, and CMV.

We are thankful to Dr Helen Boucher for inviting us to compile this issue on infections in SOT. We would also like to thank Dr Elizabeth D. Knackstedt for her expert review of the pediatric ID section and the editorial staff of *Infectious Disease Clinics of North America* for their assistance. Last, we thank the authors for sharing their immense expertise on complicated and important infectious topics.

Hannah Imlay, MD, MS
Division of Infectious Diseases
Department of Internal Medicine
University of Utah School of Medicine
30 North Mario Capecchi Drive, 3rd Floor North
Salt Lake City, UT 84132, USA

Kimberly E. Hanson, MD, MHS
Division of Infectious Diseases
Department of Medicine
Division of Clinical Microbiology
Department of Pathology
University of Utah School of Medicine
and ARUP Laboratories
500 Chipeta Way
Salt Lake City, UT 84108, USA

E-mail addresses:
Hannah.imlay@hsc.utah.edu (H. Imlay)
kim.hanson@hsc.utah.edu (K.E. Hanson)

REFERENCES

1. Hamandi B, Husain S, Humar A, et al. Impact of infectious disease consultation on the clinical and economic outcomes of solid organ transplant recipients admitted for infectious complications. Clin Infect Dis 2014;59(8):1074–82.
2. Fishman JA. Infection in organ transplantation. Am J Transplant 2017;17(4): 856–79.

Immunization of Solid Organ Transplant Candidates and Recipients: A 2022 Update

Hannah Bahakel, MD[a], Amy G. Feldman, MD, MSCS[b],
Lara Danziger-Isakov, MD[a,c,*]

KEYWORDS

• Immunization • Immunocompromised • Solid organ transplantation • Vaccine

KEY POINTS

• All age-appropriate vaccines, including accelerated live vaccines, should be administered in the pretransplant period.
• Certain nonimmune liver and kidney transplant recipients on low-dose immunosuppression can be given live vaccines posttransplant under careful medical observation.
• All medical visits should be considered opportunities to catch transplant candidates and recipients up on needed vaccines.
• Immunizations should be a prioritized part of pre and posttransplant care.

INTRODUCTION

Vaccine-preventable infections (VPIs) continue to contribute significantly to morbidity and mortality in solid organ transplant (SOT) recipients.[1] As transplant recipients are at an increased risk of complications from VPIs,[2] transplant candidates should receive all recommended age-appropriate vaccines prior to transplantation. Ideally, vaccine history should be reviewed and brought up-to-date as early as possible before transplantation (even before the formal transplant evaluation occurs), as immunologic response to vaccination decreases as organ failure progresses.[3] While antibody levels are commonly measured to assess vaccine responses as correlates of protection, vaccine responses are complex relying on both cellular and humoral immunity.[4,5] Among the vaccines discussed in this article, antibody measurements are routinely available for

[a] Division of Infectious Diseases, Cincinnati Children's Hospital Medical Center, 3333 Burnet Avenue, Cincinnati, OH 45229-3026, USA; [b] Section of Pediatric Gastroenterology, Hepatology and Nutrition, Digestive Health Institute, University of Colorado School of Medicine and Children's Hospital Colorado, 13123 East 16th Avenue, Aurora, CO 80045, USA; [c] Department of Pediatrics, University of Cincinnati College of Medicine, Cincinnati, OH, USA
* Corresponding author. Division of Infectious Disease, Cincinnati Children's Hospital Medical Center, 3333 Burnet Avenue, MLC 7017, Cincinnati, OH 45229.
E-mail address: Lara.Danziger-Isakov@cchmc.org

Infect Dis Clin N Am 37 (2023) 427–441
https://doi.org/10.1016/j.idc.2023.03.004
0891-5520/23/© 2023 Elsevier Inc. All rights reserved.

id.theclinics.com

MMR, Varicella, and pneumococcus. Family members and household contacts should also receive all recommended vaccines to help provide a cocoon of immunity around the transplant recipient. In this review article we will provide timely updates to the review article published in 2018 by Donato-Santana.[6] Specifically, we will highlight novel or changing recommendations regarding (1) live measles, mumps, rubella (MMR) and varicella zoster virus (VZV) vaccines, (2) herpes zoster (HZ) vaccine, (3) pneumococcal vaccine, (4) influenza vaccine and (5) meningococcal vaccine. Additionally, [7] we will discuss future vaccines that are on the horizon including a respiratory syncytial virus (RSV) vaccine, a cytomegalovirus (CMV) vaccine, and a pentavalent meningococcal vaccine. Finally, we will explore the ongoing problem of under-immunization of the SOT population and offer possible solutions to increase vaccine rates in this high-risk population.

LIVE, ATTENUATED MEASLES, MUMPS, RUBELLA, AND VARICELLA VIRUS VACCINES
Pretransplant Recommendations

Measles, mumps, rubella, and varicella can cause significant morbidity and mortality in transplant recipients. MMR and VZV immunization history and serologic status should be assessed during the pretransplant evaluation. The candidate should be immunized if seronegative for any of the components.[8] One dose of MMR and VZV vaccine is recommended in seronegative adults with repeat serologic testing performed at least four weeks postvaccination. An additional dose of both MMR and VZV vaccines can be repeated if seroconversion does not occur after the initial dose. Although MMR and VZV vaccines are not routinely administered in healthy children until 12 months of age when maternal antibody titers have waned, for infants approaching transplant MMR and VZV vaccines can and should be administered as early as 6 (MMR) to 9 (VZV) months of age.[3,9] A repeat dose to complete the two-dose series can be administered as soon as four weeks after the first dose if transplant is not anticipated to occur in the next 4 weeks. If transplantation has not occurred by 12 months of age, repeat vaccination is recommended. If the patient decompensates and/or an optimal organ becomes available in the 4-week period following the administration of live vaccines, administration of antiviral treatment for VZV in the form of intravenous acyclovir or ganciclovir can be considered regardless of the development of symptoms to prevent vaccine-associated disseminated infection. Unfortunately, there is no prophylaxis or treatment for measles; therefore, the likelihood of transplant within 4 weeks should be considered when deciding whether to administer MMR and VZV varicella to sick transplant candidates. Intramuscular immunoglobulin or IVIG should be given to immunocompromised hosts regardless of vaccination status within six days of exposure to an infected individual.[10] Blood products such as injectable immune globulin products, plasma products, and packed red blood cells can interfere with the immunologic response to MMR and VZV; therefore, immunization should be delayed after receipt of blood products.[7,11]

Posttransplant Recommendations

Historically, live vaccines such as MMR and VZV have not been recommended post-transplant due to concerns for inciting vaccine-strain sepsis in an immunocompromised host.[9] However, studies performed over the last decade suggest that for certain transplant recipients on low-level immunosuppression, MMR and VZV can be safe and effective.[12–17] In 2019 the American Society of Transplantation alongside proceedings from a group of international experts published recommendations that MMR and VZV vaccine can be given to nonimmune liver and kidney transplant recipients who are clinically well, greater than one year posttransplant, more than two months out from rejection episodes and on minimal immune suppression.[1,3] A recent report on 211 pediatric liver and kidney transplant recipients from 15 centers across the United States who received a total of 160 posttransplant MMR vaccines and 155 varicella vaccines demonstrated excellent safety and immunogenicity with no cases of postvaccine measles.[18] Ongoing data from this group will help further our understanding of which transplant recipients can safely receive live vaccines, and when the optimal time is to receive live vaccines posttransplant.

HERPES ZOSTER VACCINE

HZ results from the reactivation of latent VZV, and is often seen in SOT recipients, particularly those ≥ 65 years of age, those receiving intensive immunosuppression, and recipients of heart or lung transplants.[19] HZ vaccines were previously available in 2 formulations: a live-attenuated HZ vaccine and a recombinant subunit HZ vaccine. Both vaccines were shown to have efficacy in the prevention of shingles in adults ≥50 years of age in large, randomized controlled trials.[20] There are data to suggest that the use of the live-attenuated HZ vaccine in the pretransplant setting is safe and immunogenic with antibody responses similar to those seen in healthy adults.[21] However, due to the high efficacy and favorable safety profile of the recombinant HZ vaccine, administration of the live-attenuated HZ vaccine is no longer recommended, and the live attenuated vaccine is no longer available for use in the United States.[22]

The recombinant subunit HZ vaccine induces both cellular and humoral immunity and has been shown to be safe and immunogenic in immunocompromised hosts. Recent data from randomized controlled trials in adult renal transplant recipients ≥18 years of age have demonstrated that recombinant HZ vaccine was immunogenic in these patients, and that humoral and cellular immunity persisted through one-year postvaccination.[23,24] Similarly, a study administering recombinant HZ vaccine in 49 lung transplant recipients ≥50 years of age demonstrated that vaccination elicited a significant increase in VZV antibodies and induced a strong cell-mediated immune response with a favorable safety profile.[25]

In October of 2021, the Advisory Committee on Immunization Practices (ACIP) recommended 2 doses of the recombinant HZ for the prevention of herpes zoster and related complications in both immunodeficient and immunosuppressed adults ≥19 years of age regardless of prior vaccination or natural infection. However, if vaccination prior to transplantation is not possible, transplant recipients can receive the recombinant HZ vaccine 6-12 months after transplantation.[26] Two doses should be administered, with the second dose given 2-6 months after the first. The second dose can be administered as soon as 1-2 months after the first dose in circumstances where a shorter interval between doses would be advantageous. If the second dose is given prior to 4 weeks after the first dose, the second dose should be repeated at least four weeks after the most recent dose.

The recombinant HZ vaccine is approved to boost immunity and prevent the reactivation of VZV in patients who are VZV seropositive. Limited data exist regarding the HZ vaccination of varicella seronegative transplant recipients, and data regarding the duration of varicella vaccine-related antibodies following vaccination in this population is currently unavailable. A trial of 23 adult SOT recipients who were varicella seronegative and received 2 doses of recombinant HZ vaccine posttransplant showed 55% of patients developed humoral and cell-mediated immunity.[27] Limited adverse events were reported, and no episodes of rejection occurred. Although further studies are needed, this study suggests that recombinant HZ vaccination may be an option in the future to optimize protection against VZV among SOT recipients who are VZV seronegative or who were unable to receive live VZV vaccine prior to or after transplantation.

PNEUMOCOCCAL VACCINE

Pneumococcal vaccination is recommended for all adult and pediatric SOT recipients to prevent invasive pneumococcal disease.[9] There are 2 types of pneumococcal vaccines available in the United States: pneumococcal protein-conjugated vaccines, and a 23-valent polysaccharide vaccine (PPSV23). The 13-valent protein-conjugated vaccine (PCV13) has been widely available and has been shown to safe and immunogenic in SOT recipients.[28] In 2021, 15-valent PCV (PCV15) and 20-valent PCV (PCV20), which contain additional pneumococcal serotypes, were licensed for use. Phase II and Phase III randomized controlled trials to evaluate the immunogenicity of PCV15 in pediatric and adult patients demonstrated that PCV15 met noninferiority criteria compared with PCV13 for the shared serotypes and a significantly improved immunologic response for the 2 unique PCV15 serotypes.[29–31] Similarly, randomized controlled trials performed in adults to evaluate PCV20 also demonstrated noninferiority of PCV20 when compared to PCV 13.[32–34]

The optimal dosing strategy for pneumococcal vaccination in SOT recipients remains under investigation. In adult transplant recipients, vaccination with PCV13 produces a similar immune response as PPSV23.[35] In adult liver transplant patients, the immunogenicity of pneumococcal vaccination was not enhanced by the "prime boost" strategy, where PCV13 was administered 8 weeks prior to PPSV23.[36] However, a recent Phase III trial of 74 adult kidney transplant recipients who received a double dose of PCV13 followed 12 weeks later by a double dose of PPSV23 showed that a significantly higher proportion of the double dose participants developed a seroprotective response (66.7%) compared to those who received a normal dose of each vaccine (35.5%).[37]

Data are conflicting in pediatric SOT recipients on whether the prime-boost strategy is beneficial. A study of 81 pediatric SOT recipients showed that vaccination with the 7-valent pneumococcal vaccine followed by PPSV23 induced significant increases in geometric mean concentrations of pneumococcal titers.[38] However, a similar trial of 25 subjects demonstrated that although the prime-boost strategy was safe, a lower proportion of SOT recipients achieved pneumococcal antibody concentrations >1.0 µg/mL compared to control participants.[39] Regardless, the prime-boost strategy is still generally recommended in adult and pediatric SOT recipients, with the notable exception of adults who have received PCV20.[3] If PCV20 is administered, a dose of PPSV23 is not indicated. This recommendation arose from a Phase III evaluation of PCV20 in otherwise healthy adults in which PCV20 recipients had higher pneumococcal titers as compared to PPSV23 recipients.[32]

Although no data currently exist evaluating the safety and immunogenicity of PCV15 or PCV20 specifically in SOT recipients, updated recommendations for pneumococcal vaccination in immunocompromised children and adults are available and summarized in **Table 1**. Utilization of the prime-boost strategy with PCV15 and PCV20 has not yet been explored. Of note, PCV13 should not be administered at the same time as MenACWY-D due to the potential for lower pneumococcal titers when the 2 are co-administered. A minimum of four weeks should elapse between PCV13 and MenACWY-D administration. No guidance is available on the co-administration of PCV15 or PCV20 with other vaccines, and increased dose concentration of these formulations (double dosing) has not been reported.[31]

Table 1
Summary of pneumococcal vaccine recommendations in solid organ transplant recipients

Age	Previous Dose	Recommendations
<2 years of age	Unvaccinated	4 doses of PCV13 or PCV15
2–5 years of age	Unvaccinated	Two doses of PCV13 or PCV15; give 2 doses of PPSV23 after pneumococcal conjugate vaccine series is complete, first dose >8 weeks after PCV13 or PCV15, second dose >5 years later
	Incompletely vaccinated (<3 doses)	Two doses of PCV13 or PCV15, first dose >8 weeks after most recent dose, second dose >8 weeks later; give 2 doses of PPSV23 after pneumococcal conjugate vaccine series is complete, first dose >8 weeks after PCV13 or PCV15, second dose >5 years later
6–18 years of age	Unvaccinated	One dose of PCV13 or PCV15
> 19 years of age	Unvaccinated	One dose of PCV15 or PCV20; if PCV15 is used, give one dose of PPSV23 > 8 weeks later. If PCV20 is used, a dose of PPSV23 is not indicated
	Previously received one PPSV23	One dose of PCV15 or PCV20 one year later
	Previously received one PCV13 with or without PPSV23	One dose of PPSV23

INFLUENZA VACCINE

SOT recipients are at a higher risk of influenza-associated complications, including pneumonia, shock organ rejection, and death.[40] Influenza vaccination is the mainstay for the prevention of influenza disease and has been shown to decrease morbidity and mortality from influenza in transplant recipients. Currently, annual vaccination with standard-dose inactivated influenza vaccine is recommended for SOT recipients six months of age and older.[3,41]

Both humoral and cellular immunity contribute to protection following influenza immunization.[42] However, SOT recipients are known to have suboptimal immunologic response to influenza vaccination.[4,43,44] Although the Advisory Committee on Immunization Practices (ACIP) guidelines do not currently recommend alternative influenza vaccination strategies for SOT recipients, several novel strategies have been evaluated to improve immunogenicity in these hosts, including booster doses in the same season and immunizing with the high-dose influenza vaccine formulation. Other strategies such as intradermal delivery or novel adjuvants have not shown significantly better immunogenicity over the standard-dose vaccine.[43,45]

A large, randomized study evaluating a single-dose versus a two-dose booster strategy in the same season in adult SOT patients demonstrated that a booster dose given 5 weeks after initial vaccination showed higher rates of seroprotection for all 3 influenza strains compared to one vaccine dose. Although seroconversion rates at 10 weeks showed no difference, a two-dose booster strategy may be effective and induce an increased antibody response.[46]

Randomized controlled trials comparing high-dose influenza vaccine with standard-dose influenza vaccine in a single influenza season in adult SOT recipients have shown that the high-dose vaccine resulted in significantly increased seroconversion rates and antibody titers compared to standard dose.[47,48] Similarly, a pilot study in pediatric SOT recipients also showed that a higher percentage of individuals achieved seroconversion after receiving high-dose vaccine compared to standard-dose vaccine.[49] A recent randomized trial showed that the high-dose vaccine elicited a superior CD4+ and CD8+ influenza-specific T-cell response compared to standard-dose vaccine in SOT recipients.[50] These findings suggest the high-dose influenza vaccine in SOT recipients may be preferred over the standard-dose formulation in SOT recipients.

Although live, attenuated influenza vaccines have been studied in patients with HIV and malignancy and have shown to be safe in these populations, studies are lacking in SOT recipients.[51,52] Due to a theoretical risk of vaccine-derived disease, the intranasal live-attenuated influenza vaccine is not routinely recommended in the posttransplant period.

Due to the seasonal nature of influenza infection, timing of vaccination is of particular importance; however, the optimal timing of influenza vaccination relative to the transplant procedure remains unclear. The current recommendations from the Infectious Diseases Society of America suggest administering the vaccine after two months posttransplant unless a community outbreak of influenza is identified, in which case the vaccine may be administered as soon as one-month posttransplant.[9] The American Society of Transplantation guidelines recommend allowing influenza vaccination as early as one-month posttransplant, as some recent studies indicate that vaccination in this period is both safe and immunogenic.[3]

In summary, high-dose influenza vaccine is more immunogenic in SOT recipients. If standard-dose vaccine is administered, a booster dose four weeks following the initial dose in the same season should be considered. Optimal timing of vaccination relative to transplantation is not yet defined, and additional strategies to optimize immunogenicity in pediatric and adult transplant recipients require investigation.

MENINGOCOCCAL VACCINE

Currently, 3 quadrivalent meningococcal conjugate vaccines targeting serogroups A, C, W, and Y, and 2 serogroup B meningococcal (MenB) vaccines are available in the United States to prevent invasive meningococcal disease caused by these serogroups. Meningococcal conjugate (MenACWY) vaccines are recommended for all patients 11-12 years of age, as well as children and adults as young as 2 months of age who are at an increased risk for meningococcal disease. Risk factors for invasive meningococcal disease include complement component deficiencies or use of complement inhibitors such as eculizumab or ravulizumab, functional or anatomical asplenia, HIV infection, travel to countries where meningococcal disease is endemic, as well as college students and military recruits. Meningococcal B vaccination should be administered to adolescents and adults who have a complement component deficiency, functional or anatomic asplenia, or during an outbreak. Booster doses should be given one year after series completion, then every 2-3 years thereafter.[53]

SOT recipients without splenic dysfunction do not appear to be at a higher risk of invasive meningococcal disease. Similar to other attenuated vaccine responses, impaired meningococcal antibody production after vaccination has been described in adult SOT patients.[54] One study of 15 kidney and liver transplant patients analyzed the immunogenicity of meningococcal ACYW vaccines in these patients and found that immune responses to both the polysaccharide and the conjugate vaccines were suboptimal.[55] As no clinical trials to date have evaluated meningococcal B vaccination in SOT recipients, meningococcal vaccination is not routinely recommended in this population unless given for a standard, age-appropriate indication or the patient has other risk factors such as asplenia or planned travel to a high-risk area.

HUMAN PAPILLOMAVIRUS VACCINE

Compared to otherwise healthy patients, SOT recipients are at an increased risk of HPV-related disease.[56] Currently, only the 9-valent HPV vaccine is distributed in the United States and is licensed for use in both males and females 9-45 years of age.[57] The dosing schedule in SOT recipients differs slightly from the guidelines for the general and pretransplant populations. Three doses should be administered at 0, 1-2 months, and 6 months for all eligible posttransplant patients.[58] A recent study evaluated the safety and immunogenicity of the 9-valent HPV vaccine in 171 adult SOT recipients. Although the vaccine was safe and well tolerated, immunogenicity was found to be suboptimal with seroconversion rates ranging from 46 to 72% depending on the HPV type.[59] A similar study of quadrivalent HPV vaccine administered to pediatric kidney transplant recipients 9-18 years of age also showed lower titers for all the HPV serotypes and lower seroconversion rates in transplant recipients compared to subjects with chronic kidney disease without transplants.[60] Despite limited immunogenicity in this population, HPV vaccination of SOT recipients is still recommended and is believed to be beneficial given the high burden of disease.

VACCINES ON THE HORIZON
Respiratory Syncytial Virus Vaccine

RSV is a common cause of pulmonary infection in the pediatric population but is becoming increasingly recognized as an important pathogen in SOT recipients.[2] Transplant recipients are at an increased risk for complications and mortality from RSV infection, especially in the first-year posttransplant due to lymphocyte-depleting therapy.[61] As effective therapeutic options for the treatment of RSV are limited, development of a safe and immunogenic vaccine is of particular importance. No RSV vaccine is currently available, however, a maternal RSV vaccine candidate received Breakthrough Therapy Designation from the Food and Drug Administration (FDA) based on the results of phase II trials (NCT04032093) and is currently submitted to the FDA for approval. Several other trials are underway, with the majority of RSV vaccine candidates utilizing the pre-Fusion (pre-F) conformation of the RSV fusion protein to elicit neutralizing antibodies.[62,63] Nucleic acid, subunit, and vector-based vaccines that employ pre-F antigen are in Phase III trials in pregnant women and older adults. There are currently no ongoing studies to evaluate RSV vaccination in SOT recipients.

Cytomegalovirus Vaccine

CMV is a common pathogen that typically causes asymptomatic infection in otherwise healthy individuals. However, it can cause severe disease causing significant morbidity and mortality in SOT recipients.[64] Numerous candidate vaccines for CMV infection and disease have been developed and are in preclinical and clinical studies.[65] A recent Phase II trial of a DNA-based vaccine to prevent CMV infection in at-risk adult kidney transplant recipients unfortunately showed no efficacy in the prevention of CMV viremia.[66] Phase III studies of this vaccine in hematopoietic stem cell transplantation similarly did not reduce overall mortality or CMV end-organ disease.[67] A poxvirus vectored CMV vaccine to prevent CMV viremia early after hematopoietic stem cell transplantation recently showed some evidence of eliciting CMV specific immune responses.[68] This vaccine is currently undergoing additional phase I and phase II trials in pediatric and adult hematopoietic stem cell transplant recipients (NCT03354728 and NCT03560752).

Pentavalent Meningococcal Vaccine

Meningococcal vaccination is complicated by the requirement of at least 2 different vaccines each with different dosing recommendations to cover all 5 clinically relevant strains of this pathogen. To simplify this dosing schedule, pentavalent meningococcal vaccines covering serogroups A, B, C, W, and Y (MenABCWY) are currently being investigated in otherwise healthy individuals ≥10-25 years of age.[69] There are 2 new MenABCWY vaccines currently in Phase III clinical trials (NCT03135834, NCT04707391). Each vaccine is a combination of an existing MenACWY vaccine and an existing meningococcal B vaccine. Recommendations from the ACIP for the use of pentavalent meningococcal vaccine is tentatively anticipated in late 2023 if data are supportive.[70] If licensed, the pentavalent vaccine may be an option for vaccination in those currently recommended to receive both vaccines.

UNDER-IMMUNIZATION OF SOLID ORGAN TRANSPLANT CANDIDATES AND RECIPIENTS

Despite the fact that transplant candidates and recipients receive constant medical surveillance, and in spite of published recommendations that "all solid organ transplant candidates and recipients receive age-appropriate vaccines based on the CDC schedule",[9,71] many transplant candidates and recipients remain under-immunized and at increased risk for VPIs.[72] In a cross-sectional study of 362 adult kidney transplant candidates, immunization rates were as low as 55 percent for influenza, 36 percent for pneumococcus, 7 percent for HZ and 2 percent for tetanus.[73] In a study of 1800 adult kidney, liver and heart transplant recipients, only 45 percent were vaccinated against influenza during the vaccination season preceding transplant and only 52 percent received the influenza vaccine in the season posttransplant.[74] In a recent study of 281 children who underwent liver transplant across the Unites States over a one year period (excluding children transplanted for acute liver failure), only 29% were up to date on standard age-appropriate immunizations at the time of transplant.[75] A separate study utilizing the Pediatric Health Information System (PHIS) dataset revealed that sixteen percent of all pediatric SOT recipients are hospitalized in the first 5 years after transplant for a VPI (including RSV, influenza, rotavirus, varicella, pneumococcus), and that these infections resulted in significant morbidity, mortality and increased hospitalization costs.[2,76] It is concerning that safe and cost-effective vaccines are overlooked in such a high-risk population, leaving transplant recipients at risk for VPIs which negatively impact patient and graft survival.

BARRIERS TO THE IMMUNIZATION OF THE TRANSPLANT POPULATION

Barriers to vaccination exist at the individual, interpersonal, organizational, community, and societal levels.[77,78] Immunization barriers for the healthy population include concern about vaccine side effects or vaccine-induced pain, misinformation or mistrust about vaccine safety, perceived lack of necessity or efficacy, lack of access to health care, lack of insurance coverage, desire for autonomy, and moral and religious objections.[79–84] Transplant patients face all of these barriers plus additional transplant-specific immunization barriers. In a qualitative study of 82 pediatric transplant stakeholders (including parents of transplant recipients, primary care providers of transplant recipients, transplant nurses/coordinators, transplant infectious diseases specialists and transplant hepatologist, nephrologists, and cardiologists), 5 common immunization barriers were identified across organ type and transplant center. These barriers included (1) gaps in knowledge about the timing and safety of immunizations around transplant, (2) lack of communication, coordination, and follow-up between multi-disciplinary team members regarding immunizations, (3) lack of an easily accessible, centralized vaccine registry, (4) difficulty tracking when future vaccines are due and (5) subspecialty/transplant clinic functioning as the medical home for transplant patients but unable to provide all needed immunizations.[85]

MECHANISMS TO INCREASE VACCINE UTILIZATION IN THE TRANSPLANT POPULATION

VPIs continue to be a hindrance to optimal posttransplant outcome. As a transplant community, we must work to ensure that immunizations are a prioritized aspect of both pre and posttransplant care. Novel tools are needed to address and overcome all of the immunization barriers faced by transplant families and their providers. Digital health tools (including mobile-phone apps, electronic medical record-based interventions, and web-based tools) have been shown to be a successful strategy for disseminating evidence-based information, facilitating patient-provider communication, tracking when medical interventions are due, and facilitating immunization delivery.[86–89] Recently, a novel phone-app called Immunize PediatricTransplant, was developed to address transplant-specific immunization barriers and improve immunization delivery in the pretransplant period. This app provides education about vaccine use in the transplant population, stores a child's immunization records so that vaccine history is easily accessible to all providers, has a chat feature to enable communication between the family and their multiple providers, and sends automated reminders when vaccines are due based on the IDSA's accelerated immunization schedule. The app has demonstrated acceptability and usability in a pilot population and is now undergoing testing among children awaiting heart, liver, and kidney transplant across the United States.[90]

A separate intervention that would be impactful at the hospital/system level would be an effort to increase access to vaccines in subspecialty/transplant clinic. In a survey of 73 North American pediatric hepatologists representing 32 centers, only 6% reported being able to administer all needed vaccines in liver/transplant clinic.[91] Barriers to providing vaccines in liver/transplant clinic included lack of availability of vaccine in clinic, perception that it was the job of the primary care physician to give vaccines, cost of vaccines, staff training and time required to administer vaccines, and insurance coverage of vaccines.[91] Acknowledging that transplant clinic often serves as the medical home for transplant candidates and recipients, we must ensure that each visit to the transplant clinic is an opportunity to get caught up on needed vaccines.

Finally, interventions are needed at the national level through transplant and regulatory bodies to encourage the vaccination of transplant candidates and recipients with the purpose of limiting the impact of VPI on recipients of this scarce resource. Centers could be incentivized or rewarded for having high vaccine rates in their candidate and recipient populations. Ultimately, a combination of interventions at all levels will likely be needed to improve transplant immunization rates, decrease VPIs and ultimately improve posttransplant outcomes.

REFERENCES

1. Suresh S, Upton J, Green M, et al. Live vaccines after pediatric solid organ transplant: proceedings of a consensus meeting, 2018. Pediatr Transplant 2019;23(7): e13571.
2. Feldman AG, Beaty BL, Curtis D, et al. Incidence of hospitalization for vaccine-preventable infections in children following solid organ transplant and associated morbidity, mortality, and costs. JAMA Pediatr 2019;173(3):260–8.
3. Danziger-Isakov L, Kumar D, Practice AICo. Vaccination of solid organ transplant candidates and recipients: guidelines from the American society of transplantation infectious diseases community of practice. Clin Transplant 2019;33(9): e13563.
4. Candon S, Thervet E, Lebon P, et al. Humoral and cellular immune responses after influenza vaccination in kidney transplant recipients. Am J Transplant 2009; 9(10):2346–54.
5. Struijk GH, Minnee RC, Koch SD, et al. Maintenance immunosuppressive therapy with everolimus preserves humoral immune responses. Kidney Int 2010;78(9): 934–40.
6. Donato-Santana C, Theodoropoulos NM. Immunization of solid organ transplant candidates and recipients: a 2018 update. Infect Dis Clin North Am 2018; 32(3):517–33.
7. Diseases Col. Recommended timing of routine measles immunization for children who have recently received immune globulin preparations. Pediatrics 1994;93(4): 682–5.
8. Danerseau AM, Robinson JL. Efficacy and safety of measles, mumps, rubella and varicella live viral vaccines in transplant recipients receiving immunosuppressive drugs. World J Pediatr 2008;4(4):254–8.
9. Rubin L.G., Levin M.J., Ljungman P., et al., 2013 IDSA clinical practice guideline for vaccination of the immunocompromised host, Clin Infect Dis, 58 (3), 2014, e44–e100.
10. Committee on Infectious Diseases. Measles, in Red Book: 2021–2024 Report of the Committee on Infectious Diseases. American Academy of Pediatrics 2021;503–19.
11. Committee on Infectious Diseases. Active Immunization After Receipt of Immune Globulin or Other Blood Products, in Red Book: 2021–2024 Report of the Committee on Infectious Diseases. American Academy of Pediatrics 2021;40–2.
12. Weinberg A, Horslen SP, Kaufman SS, et al. Safety and immunogenicity of varicella-zoster virus vaccine in pediatric liver and intestine transplant recipients. Am J Transplant 2006;6(3):565–8.
13. Shinjoh M., Hoshino K., Takahash T., et al., Updated data on effective and safe immunizations with live-attenuated vaccines for children after living donor liver transplantation, Vaccine, 33 (5), 2015, 701–707.
14. Kawano Y, Suzuki M, Kawada J, et al. Effectiveness and safety of immunization with live-attenuated and inactivated vaccines for pediatric liver transplantation recipients. Vaccine 2015;33(12):1440–5.
15. Posfay-Barbe KM, Pittet LF, Sottas C, et al. Varicella-zoster immunization in pediatric liver transplant recipients: safe and immunogenic. Am J Transplant 2012; 12(11):2974–85.
16. Pittet L.F., Verolet C.M., McLin V.A., et al., Multimodal safety assessment of measles-mumps-rubella vaccination after pediatric liver transplantation, Am J Transplant, 2018,19(3):844-854.

17. Verolet C.M., Pittet L.F., Wildhaber B.E., et al., Long-term seroprotection of vari-cella-zoster immunization in pediatric liver transplant recipients, *Transplantation*, 103 (11), 2019, e355–e364.

18. Feldman AG, Danziger-Isakov L. Live viral vaccines after pediatric transplanta-tion. Boston, MA: American Transplant Congress; 2022.

19. Pergam S., Forsberg C.M., Boeckh M.J., et al., Herpes zoster incidence in a multicenter cohort of solid organ transplant recipients, *Transpl Infect Dis*, 13 (1), 2011, 15–23.

20. Oxman M.N., Levin M.J., Johnson G.R., et al., A vaccine to prevent herpes zoster and postherpetic neuralgia in older adults, *N Engl J Med*, 352 (22), 2005, 2271–2284.

21. Miller G., Schaefer H., Yoder S., et al., A randomized, placebo-controlled phase I trial of live, attenuated herpes zoster vaccine in subjects with end-stage renal dis-ease immunized prior to renal transplantation, *Transpl Infect Dis*, 20 (3), 2018, e12874.

22. Vaccination. 2022 1/24/22 11/11/22; Available at: https://www.cdc.gov/shingles/vaccination.html.

23. Vink P., Ramon Torrell J.M., Sanchez Fructuoso A., et al., Immunogenicity and safety of the adjuvanted recombinant zoster vaccine in chronically immunosup-pressed adults following renal transplant: a phase 3, randomized clinical trial, *Clin Infect Dis*, 70 (2), 2020, 181–190.

24. Lindemann M., Baumann C., Wilde B., et al., Prospective, longitudinal study on specific cellular immune responses after vaccination with an adjuvanted, recom-binant zoster vaccine in kidney transplant recipients, *Vaccines*, 10 (6), 2022, 844.

25. Hirzel C., L'Huillier A.G., Ferreira V.H., et al., Safety and immunogenicity of adju-vanted recombinant subunit herpes zoster vaccine in lung transplant recipients, *Am J Transplant*, 21 (6), 2021, 2246–2253.

26. Anderson T.C., Masters N.B., Guo A., et al., Use of recombinant zoster vaccine in immunocompromised adults aged$\geq$ 19 years: recommendations of the Advisory Committee on Immunization Practices—United States, 2022, *Am J Transplant*, 22 (3), 2022, 986–990.

27. L'Huillier A.G., Hirzel C., Ferreira V.H., et al., Evaluation of recombinant herpes zoster vaccine for primary immunization of varicella-seronegative transplant re-cipients, *Transplantation*, 105 (10), 2021, 2316–2323.

28. Kumar D, Rotstein C, Miyata G, et al. Randomized, double-blind, controlled trial of pneumococcal vaccination in renal transplant recipients. J Infect Dis 2003; 187(10):1639–45.

29. Platt H.L., Cardona J.F., Haranaka M., et al., A phase 3 trial of safety, tolerability, and immunogenicity of V114, 15-valent pneumococcal conjugate vaccine, compared with 13-valent pneumococcal conjugate vaccine in adults 50 years of age and older (PNEU-AGE), *Vaccine*, 40 (1), 2022, 162–172.

30. Mohapi L., Pinedo Y., Osiyemi O., et al., Safety and immunogenicity of V114, a 15-valent pneumococcal conjugate vaccine, in adults living with HIV, *AIDS (Lon-don, England)*, 36 (3), 2022, 373.

31. Kobayashi M., Farrar J.L., Gierke R., et al., Use of 15-valent pneumococcal con-jugate vaccine and 20-valent pneumococcal conjugate vaccine among US adults: updated recommendations of the Advisory Committee on Immunization Practices—United States, 2022, *MMWR Morb Mortal Wkly Rep*, 71 (4), 2022, 109–117.

32. Essink B, Sabharwal C, Cannon K, et al. 3. Phase 3 pivotal evaluation of 20-valent pneumococcal conjugate vaccine (PCV20) safety, tolerability, and immunologic noninferiority in participants 18 years and older. Clin Infect Dis 2022;75(3):390–8.

33. Klein N.P., Peyrani P., Yacisin K., et al., A phase 3, randomized, double-blind study to evaluate the immunogenicity and safety of 3 lots of 20-valent pneumococcal conjugate vaccine in pneumococcal vaccine-naive adults 18 through 49 years of age, Vaccine, 39 (38), 2021, 5428–5435.

34. Hurley D., Griffin C., Young M., et al., Safety, tolerability, and immunogenicity of a 20-valent pneumococcal conjugate vaccine (PCV20) in adults 60 to 64 years of age, Clin Infect Dis, 73 (7), 2021, e1489–e1497.

35. Eriksson M., Käyhty H., Saha H., et al., A randomized, controlled trial comparing the immunogenecity and safety of a 23-valent pneumococcal polysaccharide vaccination to a repeated dose 13-valent pneumococcal conjugate vaccination in kidney transplant recipients, Transpl Infect Dis, 22 (4), 2020, e13343.

36. Kumar D., Chen M.H., Wong G., et al., A randomized, double-blind, placebo-controlled trial to evaluate the prime-boost strategy for pneumococcal vaccination in adult liver transplant recipients, Clin Infect Dis, 47 (7), 2008, 885–892.

37. Larsen L, Bistrup C, Sørensen SS, et al. Immunogenicity and safety of double dosage of pneumococcal vaccines in adult kidney transplant recipients and waiting list patients: a non-blinded, randomized clinical trial. Vaccine 2022;40(28):3884–92.

38. Barton M, Wasfy S, Dipchand AI, et al. Seven-valent pneumococcal conjugate vaccine in pediatric solid organ transplant recipients: a prospective study of safety and immunogenicity. Pediatr Infect Dis J 2009;28(8):688–92.

39. Lin PL, Michaels MG, Green M, et al. Safety and immunogenicity of the American Academy of Pediatrics–recommended sequential pneumococcal conjugate and polysaccharide vaccine schedule in pediatric solid organ transplant recipients. Pediatrics 2005;116(1):160–7.

40. Kumar D., Ferreira V.H., Blumberg E., et al., A 5-year prospective multicenter evaluation of influenza infection in transplant recipients, Clin Infect Dis, 67 (9), 2018, 1322–1329.

41. Grohskopf LA. Prevention and control of seasonal influenza with vaccines: recommendations of the Advisory Committee on Immunization Practices—United States, 2022–23 influenza season. MMWR Recomm Rep 2022;71(1):1–28.

42. Hoft D.F., Lottenbach K.R., Blazevic A., et al., Comparisons of the humoral and cellular immune responses induced by live attenuated influenza vaccine and inactivated influenza vaccine in adults, Clin Vaccine Immunol, 24 (1), 2017, e00414–e00416.

43. Baluch A, et al. Randomized controlled trial of high-dose intradermal versus standard-dose intramuscular influenza vaccine in organ transplant recipients. Am J Transplant 2013;13(4):1026–33.

44. Kumar D, et al. Influenza vaccination in the organ transplant recipient: review and summary recommendations. Am J Transplant 2011;11(10):2020–30.

45. Kumar D, et al. Randomized controlled trial of adjuvanted versus nonadjuvanted influenza vaccine in kidney transplant recipients. Transplantation 2016;100(3):662–9.

46. Cordero E, et al. Two doses of inactivated influenza vaccine improve immune response in solid organ transplant recipients: results of TRANSGRIPE 1–2, a randomized controlled clinical trial. Clin Infect Dis 2017;64(7):829–38.

47. Natori Y, et al. A double-blind, randomized trial of high-dose vs standard-dose influenza vaccine in adult solid-organ transplant recipients. Clin Infect Dis 2018;66(11):1698–704.
48. Mombelli M, et al. Immunogenicity and safety of double versus standard dose of the seasonal influenza vaccine in solid-organ transplant recipients: a randomized controlled trial. Vaccine 2018;36(41):6163–9.
49. GiaQuinta S, et al. Randomized, double-blind comparison of standard-dose vs. high-dose trivalent inactivated influenza vaccine in pediatric solid organ transplant patients. Pediatr Transplant 2015;19(2):219–28.
50. L'huillier AG, et al. Cell-mediated immune responses after influenza vaccination of solid organ transplant recipients: secondary outcomes analyses of a randomized controlled trial. J Infect Dis 2020;221(1):53–62.
51. King JC Jr, et al. Comparison of the safety, vaccine virus shedding, and immunogenicity of influenza virus vaccine, trivalent, types A and B, live cold-adapted, administered to human immunodeficiency virus (HIV)-infected and non-HIV-infected adults. J Infect Dis 2000;181(2):725–8.
52. Halasa N, et al. Safety of live attenuated influenza vaccine in mild to moderately immunocompromised children with cancer. Vaccine 2011;29(24):4110–5.
53. Mbaeyi SA, et al. Meningococcal vaccination: recommendations of the advisory committee on immunization practices, United States, 2020. MMWR Recomm Rep (Morb Mortal Wkly Rep) 2020;69(9):1.
54. Taha M-K, et al. Risk factors for invasive meningococcal disease: a retrospective analysis of the French national public health insurance database. Hum Vaccines Immunother 2021;17(6):1858–66.
55. Wyplosz B, et al. Low immunogenicity of quadrivalent meningococcal vaccines in solid organ transplant recipients. Transpl Infect Dis 2015;17(2):322–7.
56. Grulich A, et al. Incidence of cancers in people with HIV/AIDS compared Reactivation of latent HPV infections after renal transplantation 119 with immunosuppressed transplant recipients: a meta-analysis. Lancet 2007;370(9581):59–67.
57. Markowitz LE, et al. Human papillomavirus vaccination: recommendations of the Advisory Committee on Immunization Practices (ACIP). MMWR Recomm Rep (Morb Mortal Wkly Rep) 2014;63(5):1–30.
58. Garland SM, et al. HPV vaccination of immunocompromised hosts. Papillomavirus Research 2017;4:35–8.
59. Boey L, et al. Immunogenicity and safety of the 9-valent human papillomavirus vaccine in solid organ transplant recipients and adults infected with human immunodeficiency virus (HIV). Clin Infect Dis 2021;73(3):e661–71.
60. Nailescu C, et al. Human papillomavirus vaccination in male and female adolescents before and after kidney transplantation: a pediatric nephrology research consortium study. Frontiers in Pediatrics 2020;8:46.
61. Nam HH, Ison MG. Community acquired respiratory viruses in solid organ transplant. Curr Opin Organ Transplant 2019;24(4):483.
62. Mazur NI, et al. The respiratory syncytial virus vaccine landscape: lessons from the graveyard and promising candidates. Lancet Infect Dis 2018;18(10):e295–311.
63. Mazur NI, Terstappen J, Baral R, et al. Respiratory syncytial virus prevention within reach: the vaccine and monoclonal antibody landscape. Lancet Infect Dis 2022;23(1):e2-e21.
64. Razonable RR, Humar A. Cytomegalovirus in solid organ transplant recipients—Guidelines of the American Society of Transplantation Infectious Diseases Community of Practice. Clin Transplant 2019;33(9):e13512.

65. Hellemans R, Abramowicz D. Cytomegalovirus after kidney transplantation in 2020: moving towards personalized prevention. Nephrol Dial Transplant 2022; 37(5):810–6.
66. Vincenti F, et al. A randomized, phase 2 study of ASP 0113, a DNA-based vaccine, for the prevention of CMV in CMV-seronegative kidney transplant recipients receiving a kidney from a CMV-seropositive donor. Am J Transplant 2018;18(12): 2945–54.
67. Ljungman P, et al. A randomised, placebo-controlled phase 3 study to evaluate the efficacy and safety of ASP0113, a DNA-based CMV vaccine, in seropositive allogeneic haematopoietic cell transplant recipients. EClinicalMedicine 2021;33: 100787.
68. Aldoss I, et al. Poxvirus vectored cytomegalovirus vaccine to prevent cytomegalovirus viremia in transplant recipients: a phase 2, randomized clinical trial. Ann Intern Med 2020;172(5):306–16.
69. Marshall GS, Fergie J, Presa J, et al. Rationale for the development of a pentavalent meningococcal vaccine: a US-focused review. Infect Dis Ther 2022;3: 937–51.
70. Poehling, K.A., ACIP Meningococcal Vaccines Work Group introduction. 2022. Available at: https://stacks.cdc.gov/view/cdc/118590. Accessed January 29, 2023.
71. Danziger-Isakov L, Kumar D, A.S.T.I.D.C.o. Practice, Vaccination in solid organ transplantation. Am J Transplant 2013;13(Suppl 4):311–7.
72. Burroughs M, Moscona A. Immunization of pediatric solid organ transplant candidates and recipients. Clin Infect Dis 2000;30(6):857–69.
73. Lee D.H., Boyle S.M., Malat G., et al., Low rates of vaccination in listed kidney transplant candidates, *Transpl Infect Dis*, 2015,18(1):155-159.
74. Harris K, et al. Influenza vaccination coverage among adult solid organ transplant recipients at three health maintenance organizations, 1995-2005. Vaccine 2009; 27(17):2335–41.
75. Feldman AG, et al. Immunization status at the time of liver transplant in children and adolescents. JAMA 2019;322(18):1822–4.
76. Feldman AG, et al. Hospitalizations for respiratory syncytial virus and vaccine-preventable infections in the first 2 years after pediatric liver transplant. J Pediatr 2017;182:232–238 e1.
77. Sallis JE, Owen N, Fisher EB. Ecological models of health behavior. In: Glanz K, Rimer BK, Viswanath K, editors. Health behavior and health education. 4th Edition. San Francisco: John Wiley & Sons; 2008. p. 465–85.
78. Kumar S, et al. The social ecological model as a framework for determinants of 2009 H1N1 influenza vaccine uptake in the United States. Health Educ Behav 2012;39(2):229–43.
79. Kao CM, Schneyer RJ, Bocchini JA Jr. Child and adolescent immunizations: selected review of recent US recommendations and literature. Curr Opin Pediatr 2014;26(3):383–95.
80. Temoka E. Becoming a vaccine champion: evidence-based interventions to address the challenges of vaccination. S D Med 2013;(Spec no):68–72.
81. Sharts-Hopko NC. Issues in pediatric immunization. MCN Am J Matern Child Nurs 2009;34(2):80–8 [quiz: 89-90].
82. Anderson EL. Recommended solutions to the barriers to immunization in children and adults. Mol Med 2014;111(4):344–8.
83. Esposito S, et al. Barriers to the vaccination of children and adolescents and possible solutions. Clin Microbiol Infect 2014;20(Suppl 5):25–31.

84. Lafnitzegger A, Gaviria-Agudelo C. Vaccine Hesitancy in Pediatrics. Adv Pediatr 2022;69(1):163–76.
85. Feldman AG, et al. Barriers to pretransplant immunization: a qualitative interview study of pediatric solid organ transplant stakeholders. J Pediatr 2020;227:60–8.
86. Tabi K, et al. Mobile apps for medication management: review and analysis. JMIR Mhealth Uhealth 2019;7(9):e13608.
87. Wilson K, et al. Improving vaccine registries through mobile technologies: a vision for mobile enhanced immunization information systems. J Am Med Inform Assoc 2016;23(1):207–11.
88. Wilson K, Atkinson KM, Westeinde J. Apps for immunization: Leveraging mobile devices to place the individual at the center of care. Hum Vaccin Immunother 2015;11(10):2395–9.
89. Feldman AG, et al. Underimmunization of the solid organ transplant population: an urgent problem with potential digital health solutions. Am J Transplant 2020; 20(1):34–9.
90. Feldman AG, et al. A smartphone app to increase immunizations in the pediatric solid organ transplant population: development and initial usability study. JMIR Form Res 2022;6(1):e32273.
91. Feldman AG, et al. Immunization practices among pediatric transplant hepatologists. Pediatr Transplant 2016;20(8):1038–44.

Minimizing the Risk of Donor-Derived Events and Maximizing Organ Utilization Through Education and Policy Development

Ricardo M. La Hoz, MD

KEYWORDS

- Donor-derived disease • Donor evaluation • Organ utilization • Waitlist mortality

KEY POINTS

- Reporting potential donor-derived transmission events (PDDTE) is required by Policy 15 of the Organ Procurement and Transplantation Network (OPTN). Confirmation is not required; suspicion is enough to trigger a report.
- The OPTN Ad Hoc Disease Transmission Advisory Committee reviews PDDTE with the goal of providing education and guidance to the transplant community toward preventing future disease transmission and providing input in policy development.
- In the United States, the risk of donor-derived disease in solid organ transplant recipients is 0.16%, with the majority infection related.
- In the United States, despite the advances in transplantation, pretransplant mortality rates remain high.
- At organ offer, transplant teams and the intended recipient must objectively balance the risk of pretransplant mortality and, among others, donor-derived disease.

INTRODUCTION

To adequately address the needs of the solid organ transplantation (SOT) system in the United States (US), it is essential to understand its regulatory framework. The US Congress passed the National Organ Transplant Act in 1984 to address the nation's critical organ donation shortage and improve organ allocation.[1] The act established the Organ Procurement and Transplantation Network (OPTN) to maintain a national registry for organ matching. The OPTN is a unique public–private partnership that links all US donation and transplantation professionals. The US Department of

Division of Infectious Diseases and Geographic Medicine, University of Texas Southwestern Medical Center, 5323 Harry Hines Boulevard, Dallas, TX 75390-9913, USA
E-mail address: Ricardo.LaHoz@UTSouthwestern.edu

Infect Dis Clin N Am 37 (2023) 443–458
https://doi.org/10.1016/j.idc.2023.05.002
0891-5520/23/© 2023 Elsevier Inc. All rights reserved.

id.theclinics.com

Health and Human Services implemented a regulatory framework for the structure and operations of the OPTN known as the final rule.[2] The vision and goals of the OPTN include promoting long, healthy, and productive lives for persons with organ failure by maximizing organ supply, effective and safe care, and equitable organ allocation and access to transplantation; and doing so by balancing competing goals in ways that are transparent, inclusive, and enhance public trust in the national organ donation system. The rules that govern the daily operation of all member transplant hospitals, organ procurement organizations (OPOs), and histocompatibility laboratories are the OPTN policies.[3] The OPTN Board and Committees, as well as the public and the larger donation and transplant community, play a role in policy development. Education, guidance documents, and policies promote the goals of the OPTN.

Solid organ transplantation is an accepted therapy for end-stage disease of the heart, kidneys, liver, lungs, and pancreas.[4] However, all medical interventions balance risks and benefits, and transplantation is no exception. For instance, during deceased donor evaluation, offer, and acceptance, the OPOs, transplant programs, and candidates balance, among others, pretransplant mortality with the risk of donor-derived disease. Herein, we review the current knowledge of donor-derived disease and current US OPTN policies to minimize the risk. During the process, we also consider actions to further mitigate the risk of donor-derived disease. The overarching goal is to provide an infectious disease perspective on the complex decision of organ acceptance for transplant programs and candidates.

DONOR-DERIVED DISEASE EPIDEMIOLOGY

To improve the safety of SOT, the OPTN created the Disease Transmission Advisory Group in 2005, which, later in 2007, became the Ad Hoc Disease Transmission Advisory Committee (DTAC). Notably, reporting potential donor-derived transmission events (PDDTE) is required by OPTN Policy 15 but requires vigilance and knowledge of the policy requirements by the OPOs and transplant programs. Policy 15.4 outlines the requirements for OPOs and Policy 15.5 for transplant programs.[3] Confirmation of a donor-derived event is not required prior to reporting; the concern is enough to trigger a report. DTAC reviews PDDTE reported to the OPTN to provide education and guidance to the transplant community toward preventing future disease transmission and providing input in policy development. After the report is processed by the OPTN, relevant donor and recipient information is collected from the OPO and transplant centers, respectively. Information is collected again 45 days after reporting to allow for adequate recipient follow-up. The events are reviewed and adjudicated retrospectively by the DTAC using a confidential peer review process.[5] Despite the strengths of the studies of donor-derived disease using the OPTN data, we also need to acknowledge the limitations; the main one is that the reporting system is passive, and thus the reports may not represent all PDDTE and cases of donor-derived disease. As a result, the incidence of donor-derived disease may be underestimated whereas the penetrance, graft loss, and death rates are overestimated.

Kaul and colleagues described the epidemiology of donor-derived disease in the US using data collected by the OPTN. The study used data from 2008 to 2017 and included 2185 PDDTE. Following a standardized process, the committee adjudicated 335 PDDTE (15%) as proven or probable transmissions, for an overall recipient risk of donor-derived disease of 0.18%. Of the 335 donors who transmitted disease to at least one recipient, 244 (73%) transmitted infection, 70 (21%) transmitted malignancy, and 21 (6%) transmitted noninfectious, nonmalignant diseases. In addition, most of the donor-derived events (88%) occurred within 90 days of transplantation, and the overall penetrance of donor-derived disease (proportion of recipients that developed donor-derived disease from a donor that was transmitted to at least one recipient) was 46%. Furthermore, 18% of recipients with donor-derived disease died within 45 days of the event, and 15% lost their allograft during the first year.[5]

Donor-Derived Viral Infections

The data describing the epidemiology of donor-derived disease guides the development of educational materials, guidance documents, and policies to minimize the risk of donor-derived disease and organ discard. For example, viral infections represent about a third of donor-derived infections; HCV and HBV are the most common.[5] The data derived from the OPTN contributed to the development of the 2020 Public Health Service (PHS) Guideline for assessing solid organ donors and monitoring transplant recipients for HIV, HBV, and HCV infection.[6] In particular, the analyses identified risk factors that were not associated with a risk of transmission but resulted in an increased PHS risk designation. They also provided the basis for testing all recipients for human immunodeficiency virus (HIV), hepatitis B virus (HBV), and hepatitis C virus (HCV) at 4 to 8 weeks posttransplant and 11 to 13 months after transplant in the case of HBV.[7–9] In addition, during the coronavirus disease 2019 pandemic, the OPTN Executive Committee, upon recommendation of the DTAC, approved an emergency policy that required OPOs to perform a lower respiratory tract severe acute respiratory syndrome coronavirus 2 (SARS-CoV-2) nucleic acid test (NAT) for lung donors.[10,11]

Donor-Derived Bacterial Infections

Bacteria represent about a third of donor-derived infections; Gram-positive are responsible for 20%, Gram-negative bacteria for 65%, and Mollicutes for 8%.[5] The DTAC has reviewed Gram Negative PDDTE from 2012 to 2018. There were 33 donors that transmitted to at least one recipient; 47 of the 94 exposed recipients developed infection (50% penetrance); the 45 day mortality was 14%. *Pseudomonas aeruginosa* was the most common overall etiology; the renal arterial anastomosis was commonly affected, and an allograft nephrectomy was often required with this pathogen. Six donors (18%) transmitted multi-drug resistant Gram-negative infections (4 cases of carbapenem-resistant *Klebsiella pneumoniae*, 1 *Enterobacter cloacae* with the AmpC phenotype, and 1 case of carbapenem-resistant *Acinetobacter baumannii*). This study makes us reflect on the need to identify donors at risk for multidrug-resistant organisms (MDROs), determine the appropriate timing to collect donor cultures, use adequate technique to collect samples for cultures, and decrease the turn-around time for susceptibility testing of donor isolates. It also highlights the need to study the impact of donor MDRO colonization on the organ pool and recipient outcomes and the importance of applying antimicrobial stewardship concepts to deceased donors.[12–16]

Mollicutes are a class of bacteria distinguished by the absence of a cell wall; *Mycoplasma* and *Ureaplasma* are 2 genera within the class. *Mycoplasma hominis* and *Ureaplasma spp.* colonize the urogenital tract, and the rate increases in proportion to the number of lifetime sexual partners.[17,18] Vaginal delivery increases the risk of respiratory tract colonization compared with cesarean delivery, supporting the hypothesis that exposure to vaginal secretions at birth is the mode of acquisition.[19,20] Colonization of the respiratory tract occurs in 1% to 3% of healthy adults and about 15% of those who practice orogenital sex.[21] Hyperammonemia syndrome (HS) occurs in 1% to 4% of lung transplant recipients and has a mortality rate of 58%.[22] Animal models provide evidence that the syndrome can be caused by Mollicutes.[23,24] Case reports and cohort studies provide evidence that Mollicute-induced HS is donor-derived.[25-27] Donors that tested positive were younger and were more likely to be sexually active. The mechanism of donor respiratory tract colonization is unknown; potential routes include oropharyngeal colonization during orogenital sexual activity or distant colonization after the introduction of Mollicutes in the bloodstream at the time of placement of a urinary bladder catheter in the donor. In a single-center cohort study, Roberts and colleagues screened donors for *Ureaplasma urealyticum* and *parvum* by culture and polymerase chain reaction (PCR) on an intraoperative bronchoalveolar lavage (BAL). The study included 60 donors, and 8 tested positive (13%), 5 by culture and PCR, and 3 by PCR only. Ammonia levels were used to monitor recipients. Three recipients developed HS, with a preemptive therapy strategy at a median of 7 days posttransplant; 2 died. Recipients of organs with *Ureaplasma spp.* who received empiric therapy (treatment discontinued with a negative result) did not develop HS. The authors concluded that future studies with a larger sample size are needed to determine if targeted treatment is equally effective as empiric treatment in preventing HS.[25] The cohort study by Vijayvargiya and colleagues included lung transplant recipients at a tri-site institution. Donors were tested for *M hominis* and *Ureaplasma spp* on donor bronchus swabs at the time of transplant. Of the 105 donors included, 11 (10.5%) tested positive. Recipients were monitored for hyperammonemia, tested for *M hominis* or *Ureaplasma spp* as clinically indicated, and treated with a preemptive therapy strategy. The design did not impact the development of Mollicute infection or HS. The contrasting results between these 2 studies may be the result of the study definition for HS, the screening test used (PCR with or without culture, *Ureaplasma spp* PCR without or without *M hominis* PCR), or the treatment strategy (preemptive vs empiric therapy). In a third cohort study, donors were tested for *M hominis* and *Ureaplasma spp* by culture and PCR; the treating clinicians were blinded to the results. Of the 99 donors with adequate BAL testing, 8/99 (8%) had culture-positive samples, and 15/99 (15%) had PCR-positive samples for Mollicutes. BAL culture alone (75%) had a better positive predictive value for the development of Mollicute infection compared with PCR (33%) and PCR and culture (39%); all screening methods had a high negative predictive value (>95%).[27] Collectively, these studies provide evidence for donor testing for Mollicutes coupled with either a preemptive or universal treatment strategy.

Donor-Derived Fungal Infections

Fungal infections represent about 13% of donor-derived infections; the 3 most common etiologies are invasive candidiasis (IC), cryptococcosis, and coccidioidomycosis.[5] Notably, conventional culture techniques have low sensitivity and prolonged turn-around times for diagnosing invasive fungal disease.[28-30] Candidemia is the fourth most common bloodstream infection in the intensive care unit.[31] Invasive candidiasis refers to active candidemia with or without deep-seated infection, or deep-seated infection with or without active candidemia.[32] Long-term ICU stays, central venous catheters, exposure to broad-spectrum antimicrobials, renal failure, recent surgery, and use of intravenous drugs are risk factors for IC that are often present in deceased donors.[33] Blood cultures are used to screen deceased donors for candidemia. Unfortunately, the sensitivity of this modality is only 50% compared with autopsy findings for the diagnosis of IC; thus, IC may be unrecognized in the donor.[34] The presentation of donor-derived IC includes candidemia, infected urinoma, abscess, fungus ball, or ruptured mycotic aneurysm.[35] The optimal approach to screening deceased donors for IC and the role of new diagnostic tools like PCR and T2 are unclear.[29,30] For example, for a pretest probability of IC of 0.4% in the donor, the negative predictive value of molecular testing would be greater than 99%, whereas the positive predictive value would only be 3%.[30] Further studies are required to determine the optimal strategy to decrease the risk of donor-derived IC without negatively impacting organ utilization.

Cryptococcosis is an invasive fungal infection that was classically considered a disease that occurred in patients with a predisposing factor or underlying disease such as HIV, SOT, renal disease, end-stage liver disease, sarcoidosis, or iatrogenic immunosuppression. However, it can also affect patients without a recognized immunologic defect.[36,37] In this population, the sensitivity of the serum *Cryptococcus* antigen is lower compared with patients living with HIV.[38] Most cases in SOT are because of reactivation of latent infection or *de novo* acquisition and occur at a median time of 1.5 years posttransplantation.[39] This is in contrast with the cases of donor-derived cryptococcosis reviewed by DTAC, in which the median time to presentation was 45 days.[40] Twelve donors transmitted to at least 1 recipient and exposed a total of thirty-four recipients. The penetrance of disease was 68% (23/34), and the 45 day mortality was 22% (8/23). Only 3 donors were immunocompromised, and 11 (92%) had CNS symptoms that, in retrospect, could have been a diagnostic clue for cryptococcosis. The sensitivity of blood (8%) and lower respiratory tract cultures (9%) to screen donors for active *Cryptococcus* infection was low. The sensitivity of serum *Cryptococcus* antigen was 71%, as expected for a population that was predominantly non-HIV. Collectively, this information suggests that the current screening tests (blood and lower respiratory tract culture) do not have enough sensitivity to identify donors with active cryptococcosis. Even the serum antigen does not have adequate diagnostic performance. It also reminds us that donors who died of an unexplained CNS event pose a risk of disease transmission.[41] A high index of clinical suspicion is required to identify the donor infected with *Cryptococcus*; a CSF *Cryptococcus* antigen could be the optimal test, but this may not be readily available to OPOs. Even if the results are available after transplant, prompt communication with the transplant programs could allow them to introduce preemptive therapy.[40,42]

Coccidioidomycosis is a fungal infection caused by *Coccidioides immitis* and *Coccidioides posadasii*.[43] It has classically been considered endemic to Arizona, California, New Mexico, Nevada, and Utah in the United States. Among immunocompetent patients who seroconvert to *Coccidioides*, 60% are asymptomatic, and 40% become symptomatic in 1 to 3 weeks and develop fevers, chills, night sweats, cough, pleuritic chest pain, headache, joint pain, profound fatigue, and a skin rash.[44] In SOT, the risk of posttransplant coccidioidomycosis is associated with a history of prior infection and positive serologies (ID IgM, ID IgG, CF, or EIA) at the time of transplant, treatment of rejection, and use of antithymoglobulin.[45] Most posttransplant coccidioidomycosis cases result from reactivation or de novo infection. In endemic areas, targeted screening using EIA or immunodiffusion (IgM, ID IgG) and complement fixation, coupled with prophylactic fluconazole in seropositive candidates, was associated with a lower incidence in an observational study.[46] The DTAC has reviewed cases of donor-derived coccidioidomycosis; most of the affected recipients became symptomatic within 1 month posttransplant, and the 45 day mortality was 29%.[47] This case series and case reports describe that the donors that transmitted often had retrospectively positive serologies and either a history of prior infection or long-term residency/travel to an endemic area.[48–55] Although some have advocated for serological testing for donors' with epidemiological risk factors, the DTAC analysis concluded that implementing such an approach is onerous. It is unrealistic to believe that OPOs would be able to get a reliable history of prior infection, residency, or travel to an endemic area from deceased donors. In addition, identifying donors at risk is challenging given that the geographic distribution of this dimorphic mycosis is expanding.[16,35,56]

Donor-Derived Parasitic Infections

Parasites account for 12% of donor-derived infections.[5] Strongyloidiasis, toxoplasmosis, and *Trypanosoma cruzi* are the 3 most common etiologies.[5] Strongyloides infects 370 million people worldwide and is endemic to the tropics and subtropics.[57] In the United States, the disease is endemic to the Appalachian area, although recent studies have raised the concern that the parasite may be endemic in other areas.[57–62] *Strongyloides stercoralis* can complete its life cycle in the environment and in the human host. Therefore, the parasite has an autoinfection cycle that produces long-term persistent infections.[63] From 2009 to 2013, the CDC investigated 7 clusters with at least 1 case of donor-derived strongyloidiasis. Donor screening was not performed prior to recovery. Six of the 7 donors had epidemiological risk factors for strongyloidiasis (born in an endemic country). Eleven of the 20 recipients (55%) developed donor-derived disease, and 2 (18%) died of transmission complications.[64] In contrast, an OPO performed targeted screening using *Strongyloides* antibodies; procurement occurred without delay pending test results. Once available, positive results were promptly conveyed to the transplant programs and recipients treated. Using this approach, the OPO did not have *Strongyloides* donor-derived events during the study period.[64] Collectively, these studies describe that the risk of donor-derived *Strongyloides* can be mitigated by donor testing.[65,66] Unfortunately, a survey in 2022 revealed that only 24% of OPOs are currently testing for this parasite.[67]

Toxoplasmosis is caused by infection with the parasite *Toxoplasma gondii*.[68] Seroprevalence varies geographically, with higher prevalence in South America, the Middle East, Eastern and Central Europe, Southeast Asia, and Africa.[69] In the United States, the seroprevalence of toxoplasma is 13.2%.[70] Donor-derived toxoplasmosis can occur when organs from seropositive donors are transplanted into seronegative recipients; the risk can be mitigated with prophylaxis. Although heart transplant recipients are at the highest risk in this scenario, transmission can also occur to non-heart recipients.[71,72] Donor-derived toxoplasmosis presents at a median of 87 (12–7907) days posttransplant. Syndromes include pneumonitis, myocarditis, chorioretinitis, meningitis, brain abscess, and disseminated disease.[71] An analysis of the Toxoplasma PDDTE reported to the OPTN identified the lack of universal toxoplasma donor testing as a contributing factor.[73] This analysis guided the development of a policy to test all deceased donors for toxoplasmosis by IgG. The overarching goal of the policy was to allow transplant programs to stratify the need for toxoplasma prophylaxis based on toxoplasma IgG donor and recipient testing.[74]

T cruzi is the third most common parasite transmitted via transplantation.[5] The epidemiology of *T cruzi* infection has changed, in part, because of the migration of individuals outside of endemic regions.[75] In the United States, more than 300,000 immigrants are infected.[76,77] From 2001 to 2011, the CDC investigated unintentional *T cruzi* PDDTE from seropositive donors. The transmission was confirmed in 9 of the 19 recipients from 6 organ donors. In these events, the donor or the donor's mother was born in Latin America. Five recipients had symptomatic disease, and 4 were detected by PCR monitoring; all received therapy. One of the recipients with symptomatic disease died of *T cruzi* myocarditis, whereas none of the recipients detected by PCR died of Chagas-related complications.[78] To prevent donor-derived *T cruzi* infection, organ donors with epidemiological risk factors should be screened by serology.[68] Unfortunately, a survey in 2019 revealed that only 37% of OPOs are currently testing for this parasite.[67] The ideal screening test would be accessible to OPOs, have adequate diagnostic performance, and a short turn-around time. These characteristics will minimize the risk of donor-derived infection and organ discard. The Food and Drug Administration has cleared the Ortho ELISA and Abbott's Alinity for donor screening. The potential drawback of screening with these tests is the possibility of false positives in a low pretest probability setting, given the performance of the available assays. Non-heart donors with a positive screening test can be used for transplantation with adequate informed consent. The recipient must be aware of the need to confirm donor infection with a second assay and serial monitoring by PCR.[75,79–82] A single positive *T cruzi* PCR in a recipient of infected organs will warrant treatment with benznidazole or nifurtimox. Current recommendations advocate against recovering hearts for transplantation from donors with a positive *T cruzi* screening test, albeit there is a single case report describing good outcomes despite transmission.[68,78]

Donor-Derived Tuberculosis

Tuberculosis (TB) is responsible for 4% of donor-derived infections.[5] The DTAC analyzed 51 TB of PDDTE from 2008 to 2018.[83] Nine donors transmitted disease to at least one recipient and exposed 35 recipients. Eleven (31% penetrance) of them developed evidence of infection at a median time of 104 days (0–165) and 9 (88%) had allograft involvement. TB risk factors in the donors included: birth in a TB-endemic country (6/9, 67%) and a known diagnosis of LTBI (3/9, 33%). Abnormal radiographic findings concerning TB were present in a third of the donors. Four had AFB smears and cultures performed; the smears were negative, and the cultures were positive in 2 (1 from a BAL and 1 splenocytes). The donor with a positive culture from splenocytes also had a positive TB PCR. Four donors had histopathology performed without findings suggestive of TB. Although some have advocated for TB donor screening for latent TB by IGRA, it does not perform adequately in this population because of the high proportion of indeterminate results.[84] Screening with culture and PCR is limited by the low pretest probability of active TB, the turn-around time, and the availability of these assays to OPOs. Collectively, these studies suggest that we need to identify TB risk factors in deceased donors, monitor their recipients clinically, and identify donors with active TB.[85]

Although disease transmission via transplantation is rare, analyzing aggregate data has identified avenues to minimize the risk and improve transplantation safety in the United States.[5] In addition, PDDTE should be taken seriously, because 1 in 6 events reviewed by the OPTN DTAC transmits to at least one recipient. Reporting PDDTE is required by policy. It may allow for the implementation of measures that mitigate the risk of transmission, morbidity, and mortality, as well as organ loss in other recipients from the same donor.

DECEASED DONOR EVALUATION—CURRENT POLICIES AND AREAS FOR IMPROVEMENT

The host OPO is responsible for evaluating the deceased organ donor (Policy 2.2). The evaluation includes the donor's medical and behavioral history. Transplant hospitals will use this information to identify risk factors or the presence of transmissible diseases. The host OPO is also responsible (Policy 2.9) for completing a series of infectious disease tests (**Box 1**) in Clinical Laboratory Improvement Amendments certified laboratories or laboratories meeting equivalent requirements as determined by the Centers for Medicare and Medicaid Services. Notably, the US transplant system has a low incidence of donor-derived diseases. The low risk of donor-derived disease is partly the result of the above policies and donor selection. With the goal of

---

Box 1
Required deceased donor infectious disease testing[a]

1. Blood and urine cultures

2. Sputum Gram stain, with description of sputum, for deceased lung donors only

3. Infectious disease testing for all potential deceased organ donors using FDA licensed, approved, or cleared tests, as listed below:
   a. HIV antibody donor screening test or HIV antigen/antibody combination test
   b. HIV ribonucleic acid by donor screening or diagnostic nucleic acid test
   c. Hepatitis B surface antigen donor screening test
   d. Hepatitis B core antibody donor screening test
   e. Hepatitis B deoxyribonucleic acid by donor screening or diagnostic nucleic acid test
   f. Hepatitis C antibody donor screening test
   g. Hepatitis C ribonucleic acid by donor screening or diagnostic nucleic acid test
   h. Cytomegalovirus antibody donor screening or diagnostic test
   i. Epstein-Barr virus antibody donor screening or diagnostic test
   j. Syphilis donor screening or diagnostic test
   k. Toxoplasma IgG test

4. Infectious diseases testing for all potential deceased lung donors using an FDA licensed, approved, cleared, or emergency use authorized, lower respiratory specimen test for SARS-CoV-2 by NAT[b]

[a] Donor samples for all required HIV, HBV, and HCV testing must be obtained within 96 h prior to organ procurement. [b] Lower respiratory specimen test results for SARS-CoV-2 by NAT must be available pretransplant of lungs.

Adapted from OPTN, Policy 5.4.A: Nondiscrimination in Organ Allocation, effective April 1, 2021. (Accessed 12/06/22).

---

minimizing organ discard and the risk of donor-derived disease, OPOs could consider consulting with a transplant infectious diseases specialist.

The OPTN needs to provide additional details to Policy 2.9. The policy does not specify donor blood and urine cultures' timing, the technique used to collect them, or the need for susceptibility testing of organisms identified. OPOs should collect blood and urine cultures within a certain number of days of organ recovery. With regards to the technique for collection, in the case of blood cultures, they should be obtained by venipuncture, using adequate skin antisepsis, and collecting at least 2 sets of blood cultures (usually consisting of 1 aerobic bottle and 1 anaerobic bottle) with the correct volume to maximize the yield.[86] In the case of the urine culture, ideally, the sample should be obtained after replacing the bladder catheter to avoid culturing bacteria present in the biofilm of the catheter but not in the bladder.[87] In addition to blood and urine cultures, the policy should also include the need for lower respiratory tract cultures for lung donors. The OPO should also ensure adequate susceptibility testing for clinically relevant microbial isolates, regardless of the culture source. The current policy should also specify the Cytomegalovirus (CMV) and Epstein-Barr Virus (EBV) tests to be performed. The American Society of Transplantation Guidelines recommend screening donors with CMV IgG and EBV VCA IgG, respectively.[88,89] In addition, as discussed in a previous section, the currently available evidence supports donor testing for *Strongyloides*, *T cruzi*, and Mollicutes.

The OPTN members, committees, and board, as well as the donation and transplant communities, play a role in policy development. Those involved in transplantation in the United States are encouraged to participate in policy development. The diversity of ideas will ensure a safer transplant system.

FACTORS TO CONSIDER AT ORGAN ACCEPTANCE AND CONCLUSIONS

At the time of the organ offer, transplant teams and the intended recipient must consider multiple concepts, variables, and factors (**Box 2**). The first concept is perhaps the most important one. Transplantation has inherent risks, and donor-derived disease is one of them. In contrast with living donation, the evaluation of the deceased donor occurs in a compressed time frame. The epidemiological risk factors are obtained indirectly from the next of kin, who may not be aware of all the activities of the deceased donor; thus, misclassification may occur. In addition, screening tests have diagnostic performance, and there is a residual risk. The second concept to remember is the mortality of the waitlist; 20 people die daily in the United States waiting for a transplant. We also need to account for additional variables that may increase the risk of mortality on the waitlist beyond what may be estimated by the listing MELD, LAS, or heart transplant listing status, for example, recipient size and panel reactivity antibodies.

Third, organ decline is associated with increased mortality risk on the waitlist.[90,91] On average, patients who died waiting for a kidney had 16 offers that were declined and ultimately transplanted into other patients.[92] The fourth variable is allograft quality; the next offer may have lower quality in specific scenarios.[90] Fifth, during organ acceptance, we need to balance the real risk of mortality on the waitlist with the potential risk of donor-derived disease. During the process, we need to avoid overestimating the risks of disease transmission and underestimating the risk of mortality on the waitlist. Sixth, transplant teams assessing the risk of disease transmission should include the following: risk factors in the donor, biology of the disease, including infectivity period,

---

Box 2
Concepts, variables, and factors to consider at the time of an organ offer

1. Transplantation carries an inherent risk of donor-derived disease. A program with a zero tolerance for donor-derived disease may face higher pretransplant mortality rates.

2. Pretransplant mortality rate of the intended recipient.
   a. As the risk of mortality on the waitlist increases, so should the tolerance to accept the risk of donor-derived disease
   b. Account for additional variables (eg, patient size and panel reactivity antibodies) that may increase the risk of mortality on the waitlist beyond what may be estimated by the listing MELD or LAS score or heart transplant listing status.

3. Organ decline is associated with a risk of pretransplant mortality.

4. Allograft quality. The next offer may have lower quality.

5. Donor–recipient match. For example, the degree of human leukocyte antigen matching may require additional immunosuppression or provide a lower risk of rejection, or any other peculiarities that make this the ideal donor for the recipient.

6. Assess the risk of donor-derived disease. Consider the following:
   a. Donor risk factors
   b. Biology of the disease, including the infectivity period
   c. Risk of transmission depends on the penetrance of the disease and allograft type
   d. Clinical presentation of the donor and diagnostic certainty
   e. Donor mechanism of death
   f. Posttest probability if the donor was screened
   g. Prior therapies received by the deceased organ donor
   h. Availability of prophylactic and treatment strategies to mitigate risk
   i. Morbidity and mortality associated with the specific potential donor-derived disease, including impact on long-term outcomes

risk of transmission depending on the penetrance of the disease and allograft type, clinical presentation of the donor and diagnostic certainty, donor mechanism of death (donors with an unknown central nervous system disorder may carry a high risk),[41] the posttest probability if the donor was screened, morbidity and mortality associated with the specific donor-derived disease, including impact on long-term outcomes, and available prophylactic and treatment strategies for the recipient, as well as prior therapies in the deceased donor.

For example, on one end of the spectrum, we could have a donor with proven pan-susceptible *Streptococcus pneumoniae* meningitis who is now afebrile and hemodynamically stable and has received days of antimicrobials. In this case, the risk of disease transmission is low and further mitigated by using antimicrobials. On the opposite end of the spectrum, we could have a deceased donor with a proven West Nile virus neuroinvasive disease. In this situation, the penetrance of disease and morbidity of donor-derived disease are high, and there are no effective prophylactic or treatment strategies. Finally, somewhere along that spectrum, we have the donor with HCV viremia, where the risk of disease transmission is high but the disease has a high rate of cure with effective therapy without apparent long-term allograft or patient survival. Also along the spectrum is the SARS-CoV-2 NAT + donor, where the biology of the disease and current knowledge suggest a low risk for non-lung recipients with good short-term outcomes.[93–98]

The result of the analysis contrasts the risk of disease transmission with the mortality on the waitlist. If the mortality on the waitlist is many fold higher, accepting the organ will likely benefit the recipient. As the mortality on the waitlist increases, so should the tolerance to accept a risk of donor-derived disease. A program or system with zero tolerance for disease transmission will likely face a higher risk of mortality on the waitlist.

SUMMARY

Once listed for transplantation, the optimal care of the transplant candidate balances access to transplantation in a timely manner with good long-term outcomes. The waitlist mortality metric depends on various factors, including effective organ donation and utilization.[99] In the United States, despite the advances in transplantation, pretransplant mortality remains high.[100–103] Reducing pretransplant mortality rates requires synergy between OPOs, transplant centers, education, guidance documents, and policy development to optimize the use of potentially available deceased donors.

We all must contribute to reducing pretransplant mortality rates, including transplant infectious disease specialists. Regarding emerging and reemerging infections, Anthony Fauci said, "It ain't over till it's over… but it's never over".[104] Therefore, in the future, a challenge that transplant infectious disease specialists will face is to remain objective and avoid organ discard from emerging donor populations that, based on the available information, pose minor risks to transplant candidates.[105–107]

DISCLOSURE

The author of this manuscript has no conflicts of interest to disclose.

REFERENCES

1. National Organ Transplant Act, 42 U.S.C.§274e (1984). Act from Congress - https://www.congress.gov/bill/98th-congress/senate-bill/2048.

2. The Organ Procurement and Transplantation Network Final Rule of 2000, 42 U.S.C. § 12 (2000). https://www.ecfr.gov/current/title-42/chapter-I/subchapter-K/part-121.
3. OPTN Policies. Available at: https://optn.transplant.hrsa.gov/media/eavh5bf3/optn_policies.pdf. Accessed July 12 2022.
4. Green M. Introduction: Infections in solid organ transplantation. Am J Transplant 2013;13(Suppl 4):3–8.
5. Kaul DR, Vece G, Blumberg E, et al. Ten years of donor-derived disease: A report of the disease transmission advisory committee. Am J Transplant 2021; 21(2):689–702.
6. Jones JM, Kracalik I, Levi ME, et al. Assessing Solid Organ Donors and Monitoring Transplant Recipients for Human Immunodeficiency Virus, Hepatitis B Virus, and Hepatitis C Virus Infection - U.S. Public Health Service Guideline, 2020. MMWR Recomm Rep (Morb Mortal Wkly Rep) 2020;69(4):1–16.
7. Vece G, La Hoz RM, Wolfe CR, et al. 88. Public Health Service (PHS) Increased-Risk Factors in Organ Donors: A Review of the OPTN Ad hoc Disease Transmission Advisory Committee (DTAC). Open Forum Infect Dis 2019; 6(Supplement_2):S5–6.
8. Bixler D, Annambhotla P, Montgomery MP, et al. Unexpected Hepatitis B Virus Infection After Liver Transplantation - United States, 2014-2019. MMWR Morb Mortal Wkly Rep 2021;70(27):961–6.
9. Theodoropoulos NM, La Hoz RM, Wolfe C, et al. Donor derived hepatitis B virus infection: Analysis of the Organ Procurement & Transplantation Network/United Network for Organ Sharing Ad Hoc Disease Transmission Advisory Committee. Transpl Infect Dis 2021;23(1):e13458.
10. Contributors to the Ca. C4 article: Implications of COVID-19 in transplantation. Am J Transplant 2021;21(5):1801–15.
11. Booker SE, Jett C, Fox C, et al. OPTN required SARS-CoV-2 lower respiratory testing for lung donors: Striking the balance. Transpl Infect Dis 2023;e14048.
12. Anesi JA, Blumberg EA, Han JH, et al. Risk factors for multidrug-resistant organisms among deceased organ donors. Am J Transplant 2019;19(9):2468–78.
13. Anesi JA, Blumberg EA, Han JH, et al. Impact of donor multidrug-resistant organisms on solid organ transplant recipient outcomes. Transpl Infect Dis 2022;24(1):e13783.
14. Anesi JA, Han JH, Lautenbach E, et al. Impact of deceased donor multidrug-resistant bacterial organisms on organ utilization. Am J Transplant 2020;20(9): 2559–66.
15. Anesi JA, Lautenbach E, Han J, et al. Antibiotic Utilization in Deceased Organ Donors. Clin Infect Dis 2021;73(7):1284–7.
16. Ashraf N, Kubat RC, Poplin V, et al. Re-drawing the Maps for Endemic Mycoses. Mycopathologia 2020;185(5):843–65.
17. McCormack WM, Almeida PC, Bailey PE, et al. Sexual activity and vaginal colonization with genital mycoplasmas. JAMA 1972;221(12):1375–7.
18. McCormack WM, Rosner B, Alpert S, et al. Vaginal colonization with mycoplasma hominis and ureaplasma urealyticum. Sex Transm Dis 1986;13(2): 67–70.
19. Klein JO, Buckland D, Finland M. Colonization of newborn infants by mycoplasmas. N Engl J Med 1969;280(19):1025–30.
20. Taylor-Robinson D, Furr PM, Liberman MM. The occurrence of genital mycoplasmas in babies with and without respiratory distress. Acta Paediatr Scand 1984;73(3):383–6.

21. Mufson MA. Mycoplasma hominis: a review of its role as a respiratory tract pathogen of humans. Sex Transm Dis 1983;10(4 Suppl):335–40.

22. Roberts SC, Malik W, Ison MG. Hyperammonemia syndrome in immunosuppressed individuals. Curr Opin Infect Dis 2022;35(3):262–8.

23. Wang X, Karau MJ, Greenwood-Quaintance KE, et al. Ureaplasma urealyticum Causes Hyperammonemia in an Experimental Immunocompromised Murine Model. PLoS One 2016;11(8):e0161214.

24. Wang X, Greenwood-Quaintance KE, Karau MJ, et al. Ureaplasma parvum causes hyperammonemia in a pharmacologically immunocompromised murine model. Eur J Clin Microbiol Infect Dis 2017;36(3):517–22.

25. Roberts SC, Bharat A, Kurihara C, et al. Impact of Screening and Treatment of Ureaplasma species on Hyperammonemia Syndrome in Lung Transplant Recipients: A Single Center Experience. Clin Infect Dis 2021;73(9):e2531–7.

26. Vijayvargiya P, Esquer Garrigos Z, Kennedy CC, et al. Routine Donor and Recipient Screening for Mycoplasma hominis and Ureaplasma Species in Lung Transplant Recipients. Open Forum Infect Dis 2022;9(11):ofac607.

27. Tam PC, Alexander BD, Lee MJ, et al. 632. Donor-Derived Mollicute Infections in Lung Transplant Recipients: a Prospective Study of Donor Respiratory Tract Screening and Recipient Outcomes. Open Forum Infect Dis 2022; 9(Supplement_2).

28. La Hoz RM, Loyd JE, Wheat LJ, et al. How I treat histoplasmosis. Current Fungal Infection Reports 2013;7(1):36–43.

29. Freeman Weiss Z, Leon A, Koo S. The Evolving Landscape of Fungal Diagnostics, Current and Emerging Microbiological Approaches. J Fungi (Basel). 2021;7(2).

30. Thompson GR 3rd, Boulware DR, Bahr NC, et al. Noninvasive Testing and Surrogate Markers in Invasive Fungal Diseases. Open Forum Infect Dis 2022;9(6): ofac112.

31. Wisplinghoff H, Bischoff T, Tallent SM, et al. Nosocomial bloodstream infections in US hospitals: analysis of 24,179 cases from a prospective nationwide surveillance study. Clin Infect Dis 2004;39(3):309–17.

32. Pappas PG, Lionakis MS, Arendrup MC, et al. Invasive candidiasis. Nat Rev Dis Primers 2018;4:18026.

33. Kullberg BJ, Arendrup MC. Invasive Candidiasis. N Engl J Med 2015;373(15): 1445–56.

34. Clancy CJ, Nguyen MH. Finding the "missing 50%" of invasive candidiasis: how nonculture diagnostics will improve understanding of disease spectrum and transform patient care. Clin Infect Dis 2013;56(9):1284–92.

35. Singh N, Huprikar S, Burdette SD, et al. Donor-derived fungal infections in organ transplant recipients: guidelines of the American Society of Transplantation, infectious diseases community of practice. Am J Transplant 2012;12(9):2414–28.

36. Pappas PG, Perfect JR, Cloud GA, et al. Cryptococcosis in human immunodeficiency virus-negative patients in the era of effective azole therapy. Clin Infect Dis 2001;33(5):690–9.

37. La Hoz RM, Pappas PG. Cryptococcal infections: changing epidemiology and implications for therapy. Drugs 2013;73(6):495–504.

38. Hevey MA, George IA, Rauseo AM, et al. Performance of the Lateral Flow Assay and the Latex Agglutination Serum Cryptococcal Antigen Test in Cryptococcal Disease in Patients with and without HIV. J Clin Microbiol 2020;58(11).

39. Pappas PG, Alexander BD, Andes DR, et al. Invasive fungal infections among organ transplant recipients: results of the Transplant-Associated Infection Surveillance Network (TRANSNET). Clin Infect Dis 2010;50(8):1101–11.
40. Penumarthi LR, La Hoz RM, Wolfe CR, et al. Cryptococcus transmission through solid organ transplantation in the United States: A report from the Ad Hoc Disease Transmission Advisory Committee. Am J Transplant 2021;21(5):1911–23.
41. Kaul DR, Covington S, Taranto S, et al. Solid organ transplant donors with central nervous system infection. Transplantation 2014;98(6):666–70.
42. Camargo JF, Simkins J, Schain DC, et al. A cluster of donor-derived Cryptococcus neoformans infection affecting lung, liver, and kidney transplant recipients: Case report and review of literature. Transpl Infect Dis 2018;20(2):e12836.
43. Miller R, Assi M, Practice ASTIDCo. Endemic fungal infections in solid organ transplant recipients-Guidelines from the American Society of Transplantation Infectious Diseases Community of Practice. Clin Transplant 2019;33(9):e13553.
44. Vikram HR, Blair JE. Coccidioidomycosis in transplant recipients: a primer for clinicians in nonendemic areas. Curr Opin Organ Transplant 2009;14(6):606–12.
45. Blair JE, Logan JL. Coccidioidomycosis in solid organ transplantation. Clin Infect Dis 2001;33(9):1536–44.
46. Blair JE, Douglas DD, Mulligan DC. Early results of targeted prophylaxis for coccidioidomycosis in patients undergoing orthotopic liver transplantation within an endemic area. Transpl Infect Dis 2003;5(1):3–8.
47. Kusne S, Taranto S, Covington S, et al. Coccidioidomycosis Transmission Through Organ Transplantation: A Report of the OPTN Ad Hoc Disease Transmission Advisory Committee. Am J Transplant 2016;16(12):3562–7.
48. Tripathy U, Yung GL, Kriett JM, et al. Donor transfer of pulmonary coccidioidomycosis in lung transplantation. Ann Thorac Surg 2002;73(1):306–8.
49. Wright PW, Pappagianis D, Wilson M, et al. Donor-related coccidioidomycosis in organ transplant recipients. Clin Infect Dis 2003;37(9):1265–9.
50. Miller MB, Hendren R, Gilligan PH. Posttransplantation disseminated coccidioidomycosis acquired from donor lungs. J Clin Microbiol 2004;42(5):2347–9.
51. Brugiere O, Forget E, Biondi G, et al. Coccidioidomycosis in a lung transplant recipient acquired from the donor graft in France. Transplantation 2009;88(11):1319–20.
52. Engelthaler DM, Chiller T, Schupp JA, et al. Next-generation sequencing of Coccidioides immitis isolated during cluster investigation. Emerg Infect Dis 2011;17(2):227–32.
53. Blodget E, Geiseler PJ, Larsen RA, et al. Donor-derived Coccidioides immitis fungemia in solid organ transplant recipients. Transpl Infect Dis 2012;14(3):305–10.
54. Dierberg KL, Marr KA, Subramanian A, et al. Donor-derived organ transplant transmission of coccidioidomycosis. Transpl Infect Dis 2012;14(3):300–4.
55. Nelson JK, Giraldeau G, Montoya JG, et al. Donor-Derived Coccidioides immitis Endocarditis and Disseminated Infection in the Setting of Solid Organ Transplantation. Open Forum Infect Dis 2016;3(3):ofw086.
56. Mazi PB, Sahrmann JM, Olsen MA, et al. The Geographic Distribution of Dimorphic Mycoses in the United States for the Modern Era. Clin Infect Dis 2023;76(7):1295–301.
57. Bisoffi Z, Buonfrate D, Montresor A, et al. Strongyloides stercoralis: a plea for action. PLoS Neglected Trop Dis 2013;7(5):e2214.
58. Siddiqui AA, Berk SL. Diagnosis of Strongyloides stercoralis infection. Clin Infect Dis 2001;33(7):1040–7.

59. Russell ES, Gray EB, Marshall RE, et al. Prevalence of Strongyloides stercoralis antibodies among a rural Appalachian population–Kentucky, 2013. Am J Trop Med Hyg 2014;91(5):1000–1.

60. McKenna ML, McAtee S, Bryan PE, et al. Human Intestinal Parasite Burden and Poor Sanitation in Rural Alabama. Am J Trop Med Hyg 2017;97(5):1623–8.

61. Singer R, Sarkar S. Modeling strongyloidiasis risk in the United States. Int J Infect Dis 2020;100:366–72.

62. Singer R, Xu TH, Herrera LNS, et al. Prevalence of Intestinal Parasites in a Low-Income Texas Community. Am J Trop Med Hyg 2020;102(6):1386–95.

63. Pelletier LL Jr, Gabre-Kidan T. Chronic strongyloidiasis in Vietnam veterans. Am J Med 1985;78(1):139–40.

64. Abanyie FA, Gray EB, Delli Carpini KW, et al. Donor-derived Strongyloides stercoralis infection in solid organ transplant recipients in the United States, 2009-2013. Am J Transplant 2015;15(5):1369–75.

65. La Hoz RM, Morris MI, Practice ASTIDCo. Intestinal Parasites including Cryptosporidium, Cyclospora, Giardia, & Microsporidia, Entamoeba histolytica, Strongyloides, Schistosomiasis, & Echinococcus: Guidelines from the American Society of Transplantation Infectious Diseases Community of Practice. Clin Transplant 2019;e13618.

66. La Hoz RM, Vece G, Danziger-Isakov L, et al. Donor Derived Strongyloidiasis, a Preventable Event. Paper presented at: American Transplant Congress2019.

67. Theodoropoulos NM, Greenwald MA, Chin-Hong P, et al. Testing deceased organ donors for infections: An organ procurement organization survey. Am J Transplant 2021;21(5):1924–30.

68. La Hoz RM, Morris MI. Infectious Diseases Community of Practice of the American Society of T. Tissue and blood protozoa including toxoplasmosis, Chagas disease, leishmaniasis, Babesia, Acanthamoeba, Balamuthia, and Naegleria in solid organ transplant recipients- Guidelines from the American Society of Transplantation Infectious Diseases Community of Practice. Clin Transplant 2019;33(9):e13546.

69. Pappas G, Roussos N, Falagas ME. Toxoplasmosis snapshots: global status of Toxoplasma gondii seroprevalence and implications for pregnancy and congenital toxoplasmosis. Int J Parasitol 2009;39(12):1385–94.

70. Jones JL, Kruszon-Moran D, Rivera HN, et al. Toxoplasma gondii seroprevalence in the United States 2009-2010 and comparison with the past two decades. Am J Trop Med Hyg 2014;90(6):1135–9.

71. Fernandez-Sabe N, Cervera C, Farinas MC, et al. Risk factors, clinical features, and outcomes of toxoplasmosis in solid-organ transplant recipients: a matched case-control study. Clin Infect Dis 2012;54(3):355–61.

72. Dhakal R, Gajurel K, Montoya JG. Toxoplasmosis in the non-orthotopic heart transplant recipient population, how common is it? Any indication for prophylaxis? Curr Opin Organ Transplant 2018;23(4):407–16.

73. Wolfe C, Wilk A, Tlusty S, et al. Donor-Derived Toxoplasmosis in Solid Organ Transplant 2008-2015: Opportunities for Improvement. Am J Transplant 2016; 16(Suppl 3).

74. United Network of Organ Sharing, 2017, Toxoplasmosis testing of all donors is now required. https://unos.org/news/coming-soon-opos-should-plan-for-required-toxoplasmosis-testing-of-all-donors/.

75. La Hoz RM. Transplantation for chagas' disease: closing the knowledge gap. Curr Opin Infect Dis 2022;35(5):397–403.

76. Bern C, Montgomery SP. An estimate of the burden of Chagas disease in the United States. Clin Infect Dis 2009;49(5):e52–4.

77. Manne-Goehler J, Umeh CA, Montgomery SP, et al. Estimating the Burden of Chagas Disease in the United States. PLoS Neglected Trop Dis 2016;10(11): e0005033.

78. Huprikar S, Bosserman E, Patel G, et al. Donor-Derived Trypanosoma cruzi Infection in Solid Organ Recipients in the United States, 2001-2011. Am J Transplant 2013;13(9):2418–25.

79. Riarte A, Luna C, Sabatiello R, et al. Chagas' disease in patients with kidney transplants: 7 years of experience 1989-1996. Clin Infect Dis 1999;29(3):561–7.

80. Cura CI, Lattes R, Nagel C, et al. Early Molecular Diagnosis of Acute Chagas Disease After Transplantation With Organs From Trypanosoma cruzi-Infected Donors. Am J Transplant 2013;13(12):3253–61.

81. Salvador F, Sanchez-Montalva A, Sulleiro E, et al. Case Report: Successful Lung Transplantation from a Donor Seropositive for Trypanosoma cruzi Infection (Chagas Disease) to a Seronegative Recipient. Am J Trop Med Hyg 2017;97(4): 1147–50.

82. Gray AEB, La Hoz RM, Green JS, et al. Reactivation of Chagas disease among heart transplant recipients in the United States, 2012-2016. Transpl Infect Dis 2018;e12996.

83. Malinis M, La Hoz RM, Vece G, et al. Donor-derived tuberculosis among solid organ transplant recipients in the United States-2008 to 2018. Transpl Infect Dis 2022;24(2):e13800.

84. Schmidt T, Schub D, Wolf M, et al. Comparative analysis of assays for detection of cell-mediated immunity toward cytomegalovirus and M. tuberculosis in samples from deceased organ donors. Am J Transplant 2014;14(9):2159–67.

85. Morris MI, Daly JS, Blumberg E, et al. Diagnosis and management of tuberculosis in transplant donors: a donor-derived infections consensus conference report. Am J Transplant 2012;12(9):2288–300.

86. Doern GV, Carroll KC, Diekema DJ, et al. Practical Guidance for Clinical Microbiology Laboratories: A Comprehensive Update on the Problem of Blood Culture Contamination and a Discussion of Methods for Addressing the Problem. Clin Microbiol Rev 2019;33(1).

87. Hooton TM, Bradley SF, Cardenas DD, et al. Diagnosis, prevention, and treatment of catheter-associated urinary tract infection in adults: 2009 International Clinical Practice Guidelines from the Infectious Diseases Society of America. Clin Infect Dis 2010;50(5):625–63.

88. Allen UD, Preiksaitis JK, Practice ASTIDCo. Post-transplant lymphoproliferative disorders, Epstein-Barr virus infection, and disease in solid organ transplantation: Guidelines from the American Society of Transplantation Infectious Diseases Community of Practice. Clin Transplant 2019;33(9):e13652.

89. Razonable RR, Humar A. Cytomegalovirus in solid organ transplant recipients-Guidelines of the American Society of Transplantation Infectious Diseases Community of Practice. Clin Transplant 2019;33(9):e13512.

90. Bowring MG, Holscher CM, Zhou S, et al. Turn down for what? Patient outcomes associated with declining increased infectious risk kidneys. Am J Transplant 2018;18(3):617–24.

91. Haugen CE, Bowring MG, Holscher CM, et al. Survival benefit of accepting livers from deceased donors over 70 years old. Am J Transplant 2019;19(7): 2020–8.

92. Husain SA, King KL, Pastan S, et al. Association Between Declined Offers of Deceased Donor Kidney Allograft and Outcomes in Kidney Transplant Candidates. JAMA Netw Open 2019;2(8):e1910312.
93. Jones JM, Kracalik I, Rana MM, et al. SARS-CoV-2 Infections among Recent Organ Recipients, March-May 2020, United States. Emerg Infect Dis 2021;27(2): 552–5.
94. La Hoz RM, Danziger-Isakov LA, Klassen DK, et al. Risk and reward: Balancing safety and maximizing lung donors during the COVID-19 pandemic. Am J Transplant 2021;21(8):2635–6.
95. Free RJ, Annambhotla P, La Hoz RM, et al. Risk of Severe Acute Respiratory Syndrome Coronavirus 2 Transmission Through Solid Organ Transplantation and Outcomes of Coronavirus Disease 2019 Among Recent Transplant Recipients. Open Forum Infect Dis 2022;9(7):ofac221.
96. La Hoz RM, Mufti AR, Vagefi PA. Short-term liver transplant outcomes from SARS-CoV-2 lower respiratory tract NAT positive donors. Transpl Infect Dis 2022;24(1):e13757.
97. Sanchez-Vivaldi JA, Patel MS, Shah JA, et al. Short-term kidney transplant outcomes from severe acute respiratory syndrome coronavirus 2 lower respiratory tract positive donors. Transpl Infect Dis 2022;24(4):e13890.
98. Goldman JD, Pouch SM, Woolley AE, et al. Transplant of organs from donors with positive SARS-CoV-2 nucleic acid testing: A report from the organ procurement and transplantation network ad hoc disease transmission advisory committee. Transpl Infect Dis 2023;25(1):e14013.
99. La Hoz RM, Green M. SARS-CoV-2 NAT+ donors for pediatric solid organ transplant recipients-Are they safe and provide good outcomes? Pediatr Transplant 2022;26(8):e14406.
100. Lentine KL, Smith JM, Hart A, et al. OPTN/SRTR 2020 Annual Data Report: Kidney. Am J Transplant 2022;22(Suppl 2):21–136.
101. Kwong AJ, Ebel NH, Kim WR, et al. OPTN/SRTR 2020 Annual Data Report: Liver. Am J Transplant 2022;22(Suppl 2):204–309.
102. Colvin M, Smith JM, Ahn Y, et al. OPTN/SRTR 2020 Annual Data Report: Heart. Am J Transplant 2022;22(Suppl 2):350–437.
103. Valapour M, Lehr CJ, Skeans MA, et al. OPTN/SRTR 2020 Annual Data Report: Lung. Am J Transplant 2022;22(Suppl 2):438–518.
104. Fauci AS. It Ain't Over Till It's Over … but It's Never Over - Emerging and Reemerging Infectious Diseases. N Engl J Med 2022;387(22):2009–11.
105. Michaels MG, La Hoz RM, Danziger-Isakov L, et al. Coronavirus disease 2019: Implications of emerging infections for transplantation. Am J Transplant 2020; 20(7):1768–72.
106. Dollard SC, Annambhotla P, Wong P, et al. Donor-derived human herpesvirus 8 and development of Kaposi sarcoma among 6 recipients of organs from donors with high-risk sexual and substance use behavior. Am J Transplant 2021;21(2): 681–8.
107. Durand CM, Florman S, Motter JD, et al. HOPE in action: A prospective multicenter pilot study of liver transplantation from donors with HIV to recipients with HIV. Am J Transplant 2022;22(3):853–64.

COVID-19 Prevention in Solid Organ Transplant Recipients: Current State of the Evidence

Maria Tsikala Vafea, MD[a], Ghady Haidar, MD[b],*

KEYWORDS

- COVID-19 • SARS-CoV-2 • Solid organ transplant • mRNA vaccine • Antibody
- T-cell

KEY POINTS

- COVID-19 vaccine responses in solid organ transplant (SOT) are poor.
- Three or greater vaccine doses result in superior antibody responses compared to two doses, but some people do not respond, especially those who are older, who have been vaccinated within a year of SOT, who are receiving mycophenolate, or who have received BNT162b2.
- Vaccine effectiveness in SOT is suboptimal but improved by boosters.
- Safety and efficacy of immunosuppression reduction around vaccination warrant further study.
- Monoclonal antibody pre-exposure prophylaxis with tixagevimab–cilgavimab may be protective but is no longer authorized for use in the United States as of January 26, 2023, due to the increased prevalence of variants with reduced in vitro susceptibility to tixagevimab–cilgavimab.

INTRODUCTION

Solid organ transplant (SOT) recipients are at risk for poor COVID-19-related outcomes due to the use of immunosuppressive medications and the presence of comorbidities.[1] Although the advent of direct-acting antivirals such as monoclonal antibodies (none of which are currently authorized in the United States due to the dominance of resistant variants), remdesivir, nirmatrelvir-ritonavir, and molnupiravir

[a] Divison of Internal Medicine, University of Pittsburgh School of Medicine, UPMC, 200 Lothrop Street, Pittsburgh, PA 15213, USA; [b] Division of Infectious Diseases, University of Pittsburgh School of Medicine, 3601 Fifth Avenue, Falk Medical Building, Suite 5B, Pittsburgh, PA 15213, USA
* Corresponding author.
E-mail address: haidarg@upmc.edu

Infect Dis Clin N Am 37 (2023) 459–473
https://doi.org/10.1016/j.idc.2023.03.002
0891-5520/23/© 2023 Elsevier Inc. All rights reserved.

appears to have ameliorated COVID-19 outcomes after transplantation,[2–5] it remains critical to optimize preventing Severe Acute Respiratory Syndrome Coronavirus 2 (SARS-CoV-2) infection, particularly in vulnerable populations. Unfortunately, although COVID-19 vaccines after SOT are safe, SOT recipients have generally not reaped the benefits of COVID-19 vaccination, with multiple studies establishing that they exhibit extremely attenuated humoral and cellular immune responses compared to their non-immunocompromised counterparts. Exacerbating this problem is the remarkable plasticity of SARS-CoV-2, whereby novel variants—particularly Omicron—are capable of escaping antibody-inducted neutralization.[6] Although novel variants do not appear to evade T-cell-mediated responses elicited by ancestral variants,[7] all these variables have contributed to the high rates of COVID-19 hospitalizations experienced by immunocompromised patients, including SOT recipients.[8] Here, we review the evidence regarding COVID-19 prevention in SOT recipients to date. We discuss humoral and T-cell responses to existing COVID-19 vaccines, as well as clinical effectiveness. We also review the preliminary data on the safety and efficacy of immunosuppression modulation around the time of vaccination, as well as monoclonal antibody pre-exposure prophylaxis and current US Centers for Disease Control and Prevention (CDC) and Food and Drug Administration (FDA) recommendations for COVID-19 prevention. Although we briefly discuss adenovirus vector vaccines, we focus our review on homologous vaccination with monovalent messenger RNA (mRNA) vaccines, as most studies thus far have evaluated these vaccination modalities. We do not discuss bivalent or protein subunit vaccines, as there are currently no data on SOT recipients.

HUMORAL IMMUNE RESPONSES
First mRNA Vaccine Dose

In the first published study of humoral immune responses to COVID-19 vaccines among SOT recipients, Boyarsky and colleagues[9] demonstrated that only 17% of patients had a detectable anti-Spike IgG antibody level after a single dose of either the BNT162b2 or mRNA-1273 vaccine. The extremely low seropositivity starkly contrasted with the results of early mRNA vaccine trials among healthy individuals, which showed 100% seroconversion after a single mRNA-1273 or BNT162b2 dose.[10,11] Other studies evaluating antibody responses after a single mRNA vaccine dose demonstrated similarly poor responses, with only 4% to 10% of SOT developing anti-Spike IgG antibodies, and with almost negligible in vitro neutralization of SARS-CoV-2.[12,13] Importantly, these early studies also identified certain risk factors associated with poor antibody responses, such as the use of anti-metabolites, advanced age, vaccination within 1 year of SOT, and the use of BNT162b2 as opposed to mRNA-1273.[9,12]

Second mRNA Vaccine Dose

Humoral responses after a second mRNA vaccine dose, which for a limited time constituted the primary vaccination series in SOT recipients, are also blunted compared to those of non-immunocompromised individuals, with 0% to 64% of SOT recipients becoming seropositive.[14–21] Several longitudinal studies have followed patients after one then two mRNA vaccine doses. Two small studies showed an increase in the seropositive proportion of transplant patients from approximately 5% to only around 35% after the first and then second mRNA vaccine dose, with comparable increases in neutralization titers.[22,23] By contrast, in a study of 50 heart transplant recipients, 90% of patients had no humoral response after both the first and second mRNA vaccine dose; the second dose also failed to meaningfully increase neutralizing anti-SARS-

CoV2 antibody titers.[13] In a prospective cohort study of 658 solid SOT recipients that longitudinally tracked antibody responses after mRNA vaccination, 15% had a detectable antibody response after dose 1 and dose 2, 46% had no antibody response after dose 1 or dose 2, and 39% had no antibody response after dose 1 but subsequently developed an antibody response after dose 2. Use of anti-metabolites, vaccination with BNT162b2, advanced age, and vaccination within 1 year of SOT were among the variables associated with poor responses.[24] In another prospective observational study which compared humoral responses to two doses of BNT162b2 or mRNA-1273 among over 1200 immunocompromised versus non-immunocompromised individuals, SOT recipients exhibited the lowest seropositivity, with only 30.7% of participants developing a positive anti-Spike IgG response, compared to 92.4% of non-immunocompromised individuals, 50% of patients with hematologic malignancies, and approximately 80% of patients with autoimmune conditions, HIV infection, or solid tumors.[21] In this study, age > 45 years, vaccination with BNT162b2 versus mRNA-1273, vaccination within 1 year of SOT, administration of ≥ 2 immunosuppressive medications, and non-liver transplant status were among the variables associated with lower odds of seropositivity.[21] Lung transplant recipients had particularly poor vaccine responses.[21] Similar predictors of an attenuated humoral response to vaccines have also been reported in other studies, with anti-metabolites such as mycophenolate emerging as a potentially modifiable risk factor.[25] Of note, the underlying etiologies for the superior antibody responses observed with mRNA-1273 compared to BNT162b2 are thought to be related to the higher mRNA dose in the mRNA-1273 vaccine, the longer interval between doses, or other unknown reasons.

Data regarding the durability of antibody responses after two mRNA vaccine doses in transplant patients are more mixed. For instance, 3 months after administration of the second mRNA vaccine, antibody titers decreased in 35% of patients, increased in 43%, and remained stable in 21%.[26] However, 4% of patients with detectable antibodies at 1 month became seronegative by 3 months, while 19% of patients with high-positive titers at 1 month had low-positive titers at 3 months.[26] Another study found that at 6 months after the second mRNA vaccine dose, anti-Spike IgG antibody titers increased in 27% of patients, decrease in 12%, and remained stable in 61%.[27]

Third mRNA Vaccine Dose

As of the writing of this manuscript, three monovalent mRNA vaccine doses are considered to be part of the primary vaccine series for all immunocompromised individuals, including SOT recipients (see the section on CDC and FDA recommendations).[28] In general, metrics of humoral immune responses improve with a third dose, with similar findings for both the mRNA-1273 and BNT162b2 vaccines. In a randomized, placebo-controlled trial of 120 SOT recipients who received either a third mRNA-1273 vaccine dose or placebo, there was a significantly greater proportion of patients with detectable anti-receptor binding domain (RBD) antibodies in the mRNA-1273 vaccine group compared to the placebo group (55% vs 18%, respectively).[29] Similarly, viral neutralization ability was significantly higher in the mRNA-1273 group versus the placebo group (median 71% vs 13%, respectively).[29] The antibody level after the second dose also appears to predict humoral responses after the third dose. For instance, in an observational study of two versus three mRNA-1273 doses, SOT recipients who had a low-positive response after the second dose were more likely to develop an antibody response after the third dose compared with those without an antibody response.[30]

Multiple observational studies have sought to evaluate risk factors for poor humoral responses. In a prospective study of 101 SOT recipients (most of whom were kidney transplant recipients), seropositivity increased from 40% after the second dose to 68% after the third dose, with advanced age, higher degree of immunosuppression, and lower glomerular filtration rate (GFR) being associated with an inability to mount an antibody response.[31] A study of 96 heart transplant recipients, which demonstrated that a third BNT162b2 dose resulted in a nine-fold increase in SARS-CoV-2 neutralization antibody titers, also identified that the use of mycophenolate and lower GFR predicted a reduced likelihood of developing a humoral immune response.[32]

Unfortunately, waning antibody responses and the emergence of novel viral variants capable of immune escape can limit the protection conferred by a third mRNA vaccine dose. For instance, in a prospective study of 103 heart transplant recipients, a third BNT162b2 vaccine dose resulted in significantly greater neutralization titers against wild-type SARS-CoV-2 compared to Delta, with minimal neutralization against Omicron.[33] Neutralizing activity substantially declined at 6 months but was still high versus the wild-type virus and the Delta variant. By contrast, neutralization activity was essentially negligible against the Omicron variant.[33] These observations provided the rationale for additional vaccine doses ("boosters") in immunocompromised patients, as discussed further in the next section. By comparison, among the general population, neutralizing antibodies against Omicron continue to be detected at 6 months, although they are up to six-fold lower than those of other variants and appear to decline more quickly.[34]

Fourth and Fifth mRNA Vaccine Doses

Before the bivalent mRNA vaccine recommendations that were released in the fall of 2022, the US CDC had recommended that all immunocompromised patients, including SOT recipients, receive two additional or booster monovalent mRNA vaccine doses after their three-dose primary mRNA vaccination series.[28] However, practical experience with these boosters remains limited, with less robust adherence to these booster recommendations than was seen with the primary two- then three-dose mRNA vaccine series[28] Nonetheless, a few studies have evaluated metrics of humoral immunity after four or five mRNA vaccine doses. In a study of kidney transplant recipients 19.1%, 29.4%, 55.6%, and 57.5% of patients became seropositive after a second, third, fourth, and fifth mRNA vaccine dose, respectively.[35] Factors associated with an improved response after the fourth dose were baseline low-positive anti-SARS-Cov2-S-protein IgG titers, younger age, and greater time elapsed since transplant, while factors associated with a reduced response were treatment with belatacept or higher mycophenolate doses.[35]

In another study with 25 SOTs, a fourth dose of mRNA-1273 resulted in higher antibody titers and improved neutralizing activity against all variants except Omicron.[36] Indeed, median neutralization activity after the fourth dose increased for the Alpha, Beta, Gamma, and Delta variants, but paradoxically decreased for the Omicron variant.[36] In one small study assessing a fifth vaccine dose, all 17 SOT recipients who were seropositive before the fifth dose exhibited an increase in antibody titers following the fifth dose (some to antibody levels mirroring those of the general population). However, one patient who was receiving high-dose mycophenolate and was seronegative at baseline remained seronegative after the fifth dose.[37] Thus, it is evident that even after up to 4 or 5 mRNA vaccine doses, some SOT recipients will fail to mount any humoral responses to vaccination.

Adenovirus Vaccines

Limited studies have been published evaluating humoral responses after administration of adenovirus vaccines in SOT recipients. However, the results overall appear to mirror those of mRNA vaccines. In a study of 25 kidney transplant recipients without humoral responses after two doses of BNT162b2, administration of a third dose of either heterologous ChAdOx1 (adenovirus vector vaccine) or homologous BNT162b2 resulted in 36% of patients seroconverting at day 27 after vaccination.[38] In a study with 99 heart transplant recipients who received ChAdOx1, 24% of patients had detectable antibody levels after the first dose, which increased to 34.8% after the second dose.[39] As has been demonstrated with mRNA vaccines, risk factors associated with a lack of response included the use of mycophenolate and chronic kidney disease.[39]

Clinical Utility of Antibody Level Measurements

Anti-SARS-CoV-2 Spike IgG levels appear to positively correlate with viral neutralization,[21] with high antibody levels being associated with more potent in vitro neutralization. Thus, there has been interest in the use of anti-SARS-CoV-2 antibody levels to determine the level of protection against COVID-19; indeed, the availability of such a biomarker would have drastic implications on clinical care and would allow clinicians to provide individualized counseling to their patients about how well-protected they are against SARS-CoV-2 infection. However, as indicated above, the neutralizing activity of SARS-CoV-2 antibodies is a "moving target" that is influenced by the dominant variant of concern, making it difficult if not impossible to identify a fixed and accurate immune correlate of protection. For instance, a given anti-SARS-CoV-2 Spike IgG assay result may be associated with robust neutralization against an ancestral variant such as D614G but negligible neutralization against emerging variants such as the Omicron subvariants. As a result, a simple antibody-based biomarker that accurately and consistently estimates the degree of protection does not currently exist. Furthermore, existing anti-Spike or anti-RBD IgG assays cannot distinguish between antibodies elicited by vaccines or circulating antibody levels detected as a result of prior monoclonal antibody administration (as all monoclonal antibodies to date target the Spike protein),[40,41] including tixagevimab–cilgavimab, which may continue to be detected for over 6 months after injection. Any antibody-based correlates of protection should be focused on neutralizing antibody titers and should be updated as new variants come along.[42] At this stage, both the FDA and the American Society of Transplantation recommend against routine measurements of anti-SARS-CoV-2 antibody levels for clinical care,[43,44] because currently authorized SARS-CoV-2 antibody tests are not validated to evaluate specific immunity or protection from SARS-CoV-2 infection.

T-CELL RESPONSES

The proportion of SOT recipients with a detectable T-cell response after COVID-19 vaccination has varied from approximately 50% to 79% after two mRNA vaccine doses,[20,45] and approximately 47.9% to 78% after three doses.[29,32] Not surprisingly, SOT recipients also have diminished T-cell responses compared to the general population. For instance, T-cell reactivity (measured by an interferon-γ release assay) was diminished in cardiothoracic transplant recipients compared to non-immunocompromised individuals after two BNT162b2 vaccine doses.[13] Similarly, kidney transplant recipients were found to have reduced T helper cell responses compared to immunocompetent individuals after BNT162b2 vaccination, as well as impairments in effector cytokine production, memory differentiation, and activation-related signatures.[16] Variables associated with the absence of cellular immunity included advanced age, diabetes, receiving lymphocyte depletion with anti-thymocyte globulin within the past year, lymphopenia, vaccination within 1 year of transplant, and lower eGFR.[45]

Interestingly, in certain SOT recipients, T-cell responses are present even in the absence of a humoral response,[13,46] suggesting that some SOT recipients may potentially remain protected against severe COVID-19 despite mounting no meaningful antibody response. In one study, 10% of SOT recipients who did not develop a humoral response developed a T-cell response after two doses of the BNT162b2 vaccine.[25] None of the clinical risk factors associated with absence of humoral responses were associated with the absence of T-cell responses; however, the presence of lower anti-RBD antibody titers was associated with a lack of T-cell responses.[25] Furthermore, in a randomized trial comparing a third mRNA-1273 vaccine dose to a placebo, 46.2% of SOT recipients with a negative anti-RBD IgG titer still had a positive CD4+ T-cell response.[23] A study of heart transplant recipients showed that a T-cell response was present in a small subset of individuals with absent serum neutralization; there was no correlation between the SARS-CoV-2-specific T-cell response and neutralization.[32] However, the correlation between T-cell responses and vaccine clinical effectiveness is not currently known.

Cellular immune responses appear to persist longer than humoral responses.[46] A third dose of BNT162b2 administered to heart transplant recipients induced a T-cell response which persisted through 6 months, in contrast with the levels of neutralizing antibodies, which rapidly declined.[33] Finally, although immune evasion of T-cell immunity with novel variants has not emerged as a major phenomenon in the general population, it remains unknown whether this holds true for SOT recipients. Thus, although the FDA has authorized the use of certain SARS-CoV-2 T-cell reactivity assays,[47] the utility of these assays and how they correlate with protection against SARS-CoV-2 infection is unknown. Therefore, the routine use of these T-cell assays to guide clinical care cannot be recommended at this time.

CLINICAL EFFECTIVENESS

The low immunogenicity of COVID-19 vaccines in SOT recipients has expectedly resulted in poor clinical effectiveness. In a cohort of transplant patients who received either one or two doses of BNT162b2 or mRNA-1273, 0.6% of patients developed a breakthrough infection, which is over ten-fold higher than the rate of 0.05% reported in the general population.[48,49] SOT recipients with breakthrough infection also had undetectable or low-positive anti-Spike antibodies, and their clinical course was similar to that of unvaccinated SOT recipients with COVID-19.[48] In a follow-up multicenter study of SOT recipients who were vaccinated during the two-mRNA vaccine dose era, 0.83% of patients developed breakthrough infection, a rate that was 82-fold higher than that of healthy adults.[50] Furthermore, 0.48% of patients were hospitalized and 0.077% died after breakthrough COVID-19, representing a 485-fold higher risk of breakthrough infection with associated hospitalization and death compared to the general population. However, the authors noted that the incidence of both infection and death was lower than that reported in unvaccinated SOTs in the literature (approximately 5% and 20.5% at the time, respectively).[51,52] By contrast, another study found that SOT recipients who developed medically attended COVID-19 following one- or two-dose mRNA vaccination experienced similar disease severity to unvaccinated SOT recipients with COVID-19, supporting recommendations for additional vaccine doses in these patients.[53] However, it is encouraging that vaccine effectiveness against infection in SOT recipients appears to increase with additional vaccine doses. In a population-based study from Canada which included data for the BNT162b2, mRNA-1273, and ChAdOx1 vaccines, vaccine effectiveness against any SARS-CoV-2 infection was 31%, 46%, and 72% after one, two, and three doses, respectively.[54] Importantly, vaccine effectiveness against hospitalization or death also incrementally increased with one, two, and then three vaccine doses (38%, 54% and 67%, respectively).[54]

IMMUNOSUPPRESSION MODULATION TO IMPROVE VACCINE RESPONSES

Antimetabolite immunosuppression has been associated with a reduced likelihood of developing a humoral response to COVID-19 vaccines.[9,24,32,35] Additionally, studies in patients with autoimmune and rheumatologic conditions have shown that temporary discontinuation of mycophenolate is safe and is associated with improved vaccine responses.[55] These observations have led to the hypothesis that temporary antimetabolite cessation around the time of vaccination might augment humoral response to vaccines in SOT recipients. However, in transplant patients, there is a concern that temporary discontinuation of anti-rejection therapy may precipitate allograft rejection.

Nonetheless, a few observational studies have begun to shed light on the safety and effectiveness of this approach. In a study of kidney transplant recipients who failed to mount a humoral immune response after three mRNA vaccine doses, stopping mycophenolate or azathioprine for 5 weeks led to seroconversion with neutralizing activity in over 70% of patients, accompanied by robust increases in other metrics of SARS-CoV-2 immunity, including T-cell responses.[56] Reassuringly, no de novo human keukocyte antigen (HLA) antibodies developed, and biomarkers for subclinical allograft rejection did not increase.[56] In another study of kidney transplant recipients, stopping mycophenolate and adding 5 mg of prednisone before the fourth vaccine dose and maintaining this low net-state of immunosuppression for 4 to 8 weeks resulted in an increase in serological response rates of 75% compared to no dose adjustment (52% response) or mycophenolate dose reduction without cessation (46% response).[35] Among patients in whom mycophenolate was held, only 1% each developed de novo donor-specific antibodies or T-cell mediated rejection; these patients required additional immunosuppressive therapy.[35] Although these results are reassuring, they require validation in randomized trials. Furthermore, whether these findings are generalizable to other SOT recipients, particularly lung transplant recipients who are at a greater risk for acute rejection, requires further evaluation. An ongoing, multicenter randomized trial is being conducted to determine the safety and efficacy of immunosuppression reduction around the time of COVID-19 vaccination in kidney transplant and liver transplant recipients (NCT05077254).

MONOCLONAL ANTIBODIES

Passive administration of monoclonal antibodies with neutralizing activity against SARS-CoV-2 may confer rapid protection against COVID-19 among high-risk individuals who do not respond to or cannot tolerate vaccines.[57] The monoclonal antibody combination tixagevimab–cilgavimab, has been shown to prevent COVID-19.[57] In a randomized trial that did not include SOT recipients, tixagevimab–cilgavimab was associated with a 76.7% relative risk reduction of developing COVID-19.[57] Several "real world" studies have since shown clinical effectiveness of tixagevimab–cilgavimab in immunocompromised patients. In a preprint of a retrospective study of over 1800 patients from the Veterans Affairs database (over 92% of whom were immunocompromised), patients receiving tixagevimab–cilgavimab had a lower incidence of COVID-19, hospitalization, and all-cause mortality.[58] In another retrospective cohort study evaluating 444 SOT recipients, tixagevimab–cilgavimab was associated with a lower incidence of breakthrough infection, especially in kidney transplant and lung transplant recipients.[59] Tixagevimab–cilgavimab conferred protection regardless of vaccination history and number of vaccine doses, but was not associated with a reduced incidence of COVID-19 among previously infected SOT recipients.[59]

Despite these promising findings, new SARS-CoV-2 variants with reduced susceptibility to tixagevimab–cilgavimab have emerged, as was the case for therapeutic monoclonal antibodies. Tixagevimab–cilgavimab seems to maintain its neutralizing activity against Omicron BA.2,[60] while partially neutralizing BA.1.[61] However, new emerging Omicron subvariants, including BQ.1, BQ.1.1, BA.4.6, BF.7, and BA.2.75.2 exhibit reduced susceptibility and even resistance to tixagevimab–cilgavimab in vitro.[62] Thus, as of January 26, 2023, the US FDA has paused its authorization of tixagevimab–cilgavimab because the national prevalence of SARS-CoV-2 variants with reduced susceptibility to this drug is now greater than 90%.[63] As a result, tixagevimab–cilgavimab is no longer available in the United States, as it was only authorized for use when the combined frequency of non-susceptible variants is less than or equal to 90%.[62] A clinical trial evaluating the safety and efficacy of a new next-generation long-acting monoclonal antibody (AZD3153) as pre-exposure prophylaxis of COVID-19 among immunocompromised individuals is currently underway.[64] This monoclonal antibody is thought to have broad neutralizing activity against multiple SARS-CoV-2 variants, including those that are resistant to neutralization by tixagevimab–cilgavimab.

POST-EXPOSURE PROPHYLAXIS

Post-exposure prophylaxis of COVID-19 was shown to be effective with the monoclonal antibody casirivimab-imdevimab.[65] However, this strategy was only briefly implemented in the United States because the authorization of this monoclonal antibody was revoked due to the rapid emergence of variants with reduced susceptibility to casirivimab-imdevimab.[66] In contrast, post-exposure prophylaxis using nirmatrelvir-ritonavir[67] was not effective. Given the poor immune responses of SOT recipients to COVID-19 vaccines and the pause of the authorization of tixagevimab–cilgavimab for pre-exposure prophylaxis, post-exposure prophylaxis is a potential option to protect these vulnerable individuals from COVID-19. As no agent is currently authorized for this indication, future trials should re-evaluate the efficacy of novel monoclonal antibodies or antivirals for post-exposure prophylaxis of COVID-19, with a focus on SOT recipients and other immunocompromised individuals.

CENTERS FOR DISEASE CONTROL AND PREVENTION AND FOOD AND DRUG ADMINISTRATION RECOMMENDATIONS (AS OF JANUARY 31, 2023)

CDC recommendations (current as of January 31, 2023) for COVID-19 vaccination in immunocompromised patients, including SOT recipients, are found in **Table 1**.[68] Prior to the withdrawal of tixagevimab–cilgavimab's authorization, the CDC had recommended that it be administered every 6 months for pre-exposure prophylaxis, and at least 2 weeks after a COVID-19 vaccine.[69] However, as outlined in **Table 1**, tixagevimab–cilgavimab is no longer authorized in the United States at this time. Because of the rapidly evolving landscape of COVID-19 prevention recommendations, the reader is encouraged to review the CDC website for the most up to date vaccine and prophylaxis guidelines.

FUTURE DIRECTIONS

In the coming years, ongoing data collection is needed to define humoral and cellular immune responses to vaccines targeting novel variants, such as the bivalent mRNA

Table 1
Fall 2022 US Centers for Disease Control COVID-19 vaccine/prophylaxis recommendations in immunocompromised patients

Strategy	Dose 1	Interval	Dose 2	Interval	Dose 3	Interval	Booster	Tixagevimab–Cilgavimab
			Primary Vaccine Series					
Option 1	mRNA: BNT162b2 (Pfizer, ages 5 or greater) or mRNA-1273 (Moderna, ages 6 or greater)	3 weeks if BNT162b2; 4 weeks if mRNA-1273	mRNA (preferably the same)	At least 4 weeks	mRNA (preferably the same)	At least 2 months	Any age-appropriate bivalent mRNA vaccine[a], irrespective of prior number of boosters	Not currently authorized (as of January 26, 2023). Prior to January 26, 2023, the recommendation was: "at least 2 weeks after any COVID-19 vaccine dose; once tixagevimab–cilgavimab given, no minimum interval for next vaccine."
Option 2 (12 years and older)	Protein subunit (NVX-CoV2373, Novavax)	3 weeks	Protein subunit (NVX-CoV2373, Novavax)	NA	NA			
Option 3 (18 years and older)	Ad26.COV2.S (Janssen, only brand available in the United States)	At least 4 weeks	Additional mRNA vaccine (any brand)	NA	NA			

Abbreviation: NA, not applicable.
[a] Pfizer bivalent booster authorized for ages 5 and greater; Moderna bivalent booster authorized for ages 6 and greater. Table up to date as of January 31, 2023.
Data from Refs.[62,63,68,69]

vaccines, as well as the clinical effectiveness of these vaccines. Determining whether temporary discontinuation of immunosuppressive drugs will bolster immune responses without precipitating allograft rejection is an unmet need; randomized clinical trial data across the different SOT types are needed to truly determine the safety and efficacy of this approach. Newer generation prophylactic monoclonal antibodies will also be expected to add an extra layer of protection to SOT recipients.[64] Finally, post-exposure prophylaxis should continue to be evaluated in trials.

CLINICS CARE POINTS

- COVID-19 vaccines in SOT recipients are safe
- SOT recipients exhibit poor humoral and cellular immune responses to COVID-19 vaccines
- A three-dose primary mRNA vaccine series results in better immune responses than one or two-dose mRNA vaccination, but a substantial proportion of SOT recipients remains seronegative even after three doses
- mRNA vaccine boosters improve antibody responses, though some patients, especially those who are highly immunosuppressed, remain seronegative
- Risk factors for poor humoral immune responses include advanced age, degree of immunosuppression, mycophenolate use, chronic kidney disease, vaccination within 1 year of transplant, and use of BNT162b2 instead of mRNA-1273
- Although T-cell responses in SOT recipients are worse than those of immunocompetent individuals, some SOT recipients exhibit T-cell responses without humoral responses
- Immune correlates of protection after vaccination are not defined; routine measurement of antibody levels of T-cell reactivity is therefore not currently recommended
- Clinical effectiveness of mRNA vaccines in SOT recipients is significantly worse than the general population (for infection, hospitalization, and death). However, clinical effectiveness is improved by booster vaccine doses
- Immunosuppression reduction around the time of vaccination may improve immune responses, but additional studies of efficacy and safety (particularly as it relates to rejection) are needed
- The monoclonal antibody combination tixagevimab–cilgavimab appears to protect SOT recipients from COVID-19, but it is no longer available for use in the United States (as of January 26, 2023) due to the increased prevalence (>90%) of variants with reduced susceptibility to this agent
- No drugs are currently authorized for post-exposure prophylaxis of COVID-19
- CDC COVID-19 vaccine recommendations (current as of January 31, 2023) for SOT recipients include a three-dose primary mRNA vaccine series, or a two-dose primary protein subunit, or a one-dose adenovirus vector vaccine followed by one mRNA vaccine dose, all followed at least 2 months later by a bivalent mRNA vaccine booster. These recommendations are updated periodically.

FUNDING SOURCE

None.

CONFLICT OF INTEREST/DISCLOSURES

G. Haidar is a recipient of research grants from Allovir, Karius, and AstraZeneca. G. Haidar also serves on the scientific advisory boards of Karius and AstraZeneca and has received honoraria from the International AIDS Society and MDOutlook. The rest of the author has no disclosures.

REFERENCES

1. Cochran W, Shah P, Barker L, et al. COVID-19 clinical outcomes in solid organ transplant recipients during the omicron surge. Transplantation 2022;106(7): e346–7.
2. Hedvat J, Lange NW, Salerno DM, et al. COVID-19 therapeutics and outcomes among solid organ transplant recipients during the Omicron BA.1 era. Am J Transplant 2022;22(11):2682–8.
3. Solera JT, Arbol BG, Bahinskaya I, et al. Short-course early outpatient remdesivir prevents severe disease due to COVID-19 in organ transplant recipients during the omicron BA.2 wave. Am J Transplant 2022. https://doi.org/10.1111/ajt.17199.
4. Villamarin M, Marquez-Algaba E, Esperalba J, et al. Preliminary clinical experience of molnupiravir to prevent progression of COVID-19 in kidney transplant recipients. Transplantation 2022;106(11):2200–4.
5. Yetmar ZA, Beam E, O'Horo JC, et al. Outcomes of bebtelovimab and sotrovimab treatment of solid organ transplant recipients with mild-to-moderate coronavirus disease 2019 during the Omicron epoch. Transpl Infect Dis 2022;24(4):e13901.
6. Jacobs JL, Haidar G, Mellors JW. COVID-19: challenges of viral variants. Annu Rev Med 2022. https://doi.org/10.1146/annurev-med-042921-020956.
7. Geers D, Shamier MC, Bogers S, et al. SARS-CoV-2 variants of concern partially escape humoral but not T-cell responses in COVID-19 convalescent donors and vaccinees. Sci Immunol 2021;6(59). https://doi.org/10.1126/sciimmunol.abj1750.
8. Singson JRC, Kirley PD, Pham H, et al. Factors associated with severe outcomes among immunocompromised adults hospitalized for COVID-19 - COVID-NET, 10 States, March 2020-February 2022. MMWR Morb Mortal Wkly Rep 2022;71(27): 878–84.
9. Boyarsky BJ, Werbel WA, Avery RK, et al. Immunogenicity of a single dose of SARS-CoV-2 Messenger RNA vaccine in solid organ transplant recipients. JAMA 2021;325(17):1784–6.
10. Jackson LA, Anderson EJ, Rouphael NG, et al. An mRNA vaccine against SARS-CoV-2 - preliminary report. N Engl J Med 2020;383(20):1920–31.
11. Walsh EE, Frenck RW Jr, Falsey AR, et al. Safety and immunogenicity of Two RNA-Based Covid-19 vaccine candidates. N Engl J Med 2020;383(25):2439–50.
12. Benotmane I, Gautier-Vargas G, Cognard N, et al. Weak anti-SARS-CoV-2 antibody response after the first injection of an mRNA COVID-19 vaccine in kidney transplant recipients. Kidney Int 2021;99(6):1487–9.
13. Schramm R, Costard-Jackle A, Rivinius R, et al. Poor humoral and T-cell response to two-dose SARS-CoV-2 messenger RNA vaccine BNT162b2 in cardiothoracic transplant recipients. Clin Res Cardiol 2021;110(8):1142–9.
14. Aslam S, Danziger-Isakov L, Mehra MR. COVID-19 vaccination immune paresis in heart and lung transplantation. J Heart Lung Transplant 2021;40(8):763–6.
15. Peled Y, Ram E, Lavee J, et al. BNT162b2 vaccination in heart transplant recipients: clinical experience and antibody response. J Heart Lung Transplant 2021; 40(8):759–62.
16. Sattler A, Schrezenmeier E, Weber UA, et al. Impaired humoral and cellular immunity after SARS-CoV-2 BNT162b2 (tozinameran) prime-boost vaccination in kidney transplant recipients. J Clin Invest 2021;131(14). https://doi.org/10.1172/JCI150175.

17. Rincon-Arevalo H, Choi M, Stefanski AL, et al. Impaired humoral immunity to SARS-CoV-2 BNT162b2 vaccine in kidney transplant recipients and dialysis patients. Sci Immunol 2021;6(60). https://doi.org/10.1126/sciimmunol.abj1031.
18. Havlin J, Svorcova M, Dvorackova E, et al. Immunogenicity of BNT162b2 mRNA COVID-19 vaccine and SARS-CoV-2 infection in lung transplant recipients. J Heart Lung Transplant 2021;40(8):754–8.
19. Grupper A, Rabinowich L, Schwartz D, et al. Reduced humoral response to mRNA SARS-CoV-2 BNT162b2 vaccine in kidney transplant recipients without prior exposure to the virus. Am J Transplant 2021;21(8):2719–26.
20. Herrera S, Colmenero J, Pascal M, et al. Cellular and humoral immune response after mRNA-1273 SARS-CoV-2 vaccine in liver and heart transplant recipients. Am J Transplant 2021;21(12):3971–9.
21. Haidar G, Agha M, Bilderback A, et al. Prospective Evaluation Of Coronavirus Disease 2019 (COVID-19) vaccine responses across a broad spectrum of immunocompromising conditions: the COVID-19 vaccination in the immunocompromised study (COVICS). Clin Infect Dis 2022;75(1):e630–44.
22. Schmidt T, Klemis V, Schub D, et al. Cellular immunity predominates over humoral immunity after homologous and heterologous mRNA and vector-based COVID-19 vaccine regimens in solid organ transplant recipients. Am J Transplant 2021; 21(12):3990–4002.
23. Hall VG, Ferreira VH, Ierullo M, et al. Humoral and cellular immune response and safety of two-dose SARS-CoV-2 mRNA-1273 vaccine in solid organ transplant recipients. Am J Transplant 2021;21(12):3980–9.
24. Boyarsky BJ, Werbel WA, Avery RK, et al. Antibody response to 2-Dose SARS-CoV-2 mRNA vaccine series in solid organ transplant recipients. JAMA 2021; 325(21):2204–6.
25. Hamm SR, Moller DL, Perez-Alos L, et al. Decline in antibody concentration 6 months after two doses of SARS-CoV-2 BNT162b2 vaccine in solid organ transplant recipients and healthy controls. Front Immunol 2022;13:832501.
26. Boyarsky BJ, Chiang TP, Teles AT, et al. Antibody kinetics and durability in SARS-CoV-2 mRNA vaccinated solid organ transplant recipients. Transplantation 2021; 105(10):e137–8.
27. Alejo JL, Mitchell J, Chiang TP, et al. Six-month Antibody Kinetics and Durability in SARS-CoV-2 mRNA vaccinated solid organ transplant recipients. Transplantation 2022;106(1):e109–10.
28. Boosters Work. Available at: https://www.cdc.gov/coronavirus/2019-ncov/covid-data/covidview/past-reports/02112022.html. Accessed 31 January, 2023.
29. Hall VG, Ferreira VH, Ku T, et al. Randomized trial of a third dose of mRNA-1273 vaccine in transplant recipients. N Engl J Med 2021;385(13):1244–6.
30. Benotmane I, Gautier G, Perrin P, et al. Antibody response after a third dose of the mRNA-1273 SARS-CoV-2 vaccine in kidney transplant recipients with minimal serologic response to 2 doses. JAMA 2021. https://doi.org/10.1001/jama.2021. 12339.
31. Kamar N, Abravanel F, Marion O, et al. Three doses of an mRNA Covid-19 vaccine in solid-organ transplant recipients. N Engl J Med 2021;385(7):661–2.
32. Peled Y, Ram E, Lavee J, et al. Third dose of the BNT162b2 vaccine in heart transplant recipients: immunogenicity and clinical experience. J Heart Lung Transplant 2022;41(2):148–57.
33. Peled Y, Patel JK, Afek A, et al. Kinetics of cellular and humoral responses to third BNT162B2 COVID-19 vaccine over six months in heart transplant recipients -

Implications for the omicron variant: correspondence. J Heart Lung Transplant 2022. https://doi.org/10.1016/j.healun.2022.07.012.

34. Pajon R, Doria-Rose NA, Shen X, et al. SARS-CoV-2 omicron variant neutralization after mRNA-1273 booster vaccination. N Engl J Med 2022;386(11):1088–91.

35. Osmanodja B, Ronicke S, Budde K, et al. Serological response to three, four and five doses of SARS-CoV-2 vaccine in kidney transplant recipients. J Clin Med 2022;11(9). https://doi.org/10.3390/jcm11092565.

36. Karaba AH, Johnston TS, Aytenfisu TY, et al. A fourth dose of COVID-19 Vaccine does not induce neutralization of the omicron variant among solid organ transplant recipients with suboptimal vaccine response. Transplantation 2022; 106(7):1440–4.

37. Abedon AT, Teles MS, Alejo JL, et al. Improved antibody response after a fifth dose of a SARS-CoV-2 vaccine in solid organ transplant recipients: a case series. Transplantation 2022;106(5):e262–3.

38. Schrezenmeier E, Rincon-Arevalo H, Stefanski AL, et al. B and T Cell responses after a third dose of SARS-CoV-2 vaccine in kidney transplant recipients. J Am Soc Nephrol 2021. https://doi.org/10.1681/ASN.2021070966.

39. Tanner R, Starr N, Chan G, et al. Humoral response to SARS-CoV-2 adenovirus vector vaccination (ChAdOx1 nCoV-19 [AZD1222]) in heart transplant recipients aged 18 to 70 years of age. J Heart Lung Transplant 2022;41(4):492–500.

40. Benotmane I, Velay A, Vargas GG, et al. A rapid decline in the anti-receptor-binding domain of the SARS-CoV-2 spike protein IgG titer in kidney transplant recipients after tixagevimab-cilgavimab administration. Kidney Int 2022;102(5): 1188–90.

41. Sasaki H, Miyata N, Yoshimura Y, et al. High titer of antibody against the SARS-CoV-2 spike protein among patients receiving neutralizing antibody cocktail therapy with REGN-COV. Infection 2022;50(3):771–4.

42. Gilbert PB, Donis RO, Koup RA, et al. A Covid-19 milestone attained - a correlate of protection for vaccines. N Engl J Med 2022;387(24):2203–6.

43. COVID-19 Vaccine FAQ Sheet updated 1/12/2023. Available at: https://www.myast. org/sites/default/files/01012023%20AST%20Vaccine%20Prof%20FAQ%20FINAL. pdf. Accessed 31 January, 2023.

44. Antibody Testing Is Not Currently Recommended to Assess Immunity After COVID-19 Vaccination: FDA Safety Communication. Available at: https://www.fda.gov/medical-devices/safety-communications/antibody-testing-not-currently-recommended-assess-immunity-after-covid-19-vaccination-fda-safety. Accessed 31 January, 2023.

45. Cucchiari D, Egri N, Bodro M, et al. Cellular and humoral response after MRNA-1273 SARS-CoV-2 vaccine in kidney transplant recipients. Am J Transplant 2021; 21(8):2727–39.

46. Haidar G. Immunity to a third BNT162B2 COVID-19 vaccine after heart transplantation: bridging the knowledge gap to end the pandemic for organ transplant recipients. J Heart Lung Transplant 2022;41(10):1426–8.

47. Emergency use authorization (EUA) summary T-detect COVID test. adaptive biotechnologies corporation. Updated: September 2, 2021. Available at: https://www.fda.gov/media/146481/download. Accessed 31 January, 2023.

48. Wadei HM, Gonwa TA, Leoni JC, et al. COVID-19 infection in solid organ transplant recipients after SARS-CoV-2 vaccination. Am J Transplant 2021;21(10): 3496–9.

49. Keehner J, Horton LE, Pfeffer MA, et al. SARS-CoV-2 infection after vaccination in health care workers in california. N Engl J Med 2021;384(18):1774–5.

50. Qin CX, Moore LW, Anjan S, et al. Risk of breakthrough SARS-CoV-2 infections in adult transplant recipients. Transplantation 2021;105(11):e265–6.
51. Elias M, Pievani D, Randoux C, et al. COVID-19 infection in kidney transplant recipients: disease incidence and clinical outcomes. J Am Soc Nephrol 2020; 31(10):2413–23.
52. Kates OS, Haydel BM, Florman SS, et al. Coronavirus disease 2019 in solid organ transplant: a multicenter cohort study. Clin Infect Dis 2021;73(11):e4090–9.
53. Hall VG, Al-Alahmadi G, Solera JT, et al. Outcomes of SARS-CoV-2 infection in unvaccinated compared with vaccinated solid organ transplant recipients: a propensity matched cohort study. Transplantation 2022;106(8):1622–8.
54. Naylor KL, Kim SJ, Smith G, et al. Effectiveness of first, second, and third COVID-19 vaccine doses in solid organ transplant recipients: a population-based cohort study from Canada. Am J Transplant 2022;22(9):2228–36.
55. Connolly CM, Chiang TP, Boyarsky BJ, et al. Temporary hold of mycophenolate augments humoral response to SARS-CoV-2 vaccination in patients with rheumatic and musculoskeletal diseases: a case series. Ann Rheum Dis 2022; 81(2):293–5.
56. Schrezenmeier E, Rincon-Arevalo H, Jens A, et al. Temporary antimetabolite treatment hold boosts SARS-CoV-2 vaccination-specific humoral and cellular immunity in kidney transplant recipients. JCI Insight 2022;7(9). https://doi.org/10.1172/jci.insight.157836.
57. Levin MJ, Ustianowski A, De Wit S, et al. Intramuscular AZD7442 (Tixagevimab-Cilgavimab) for prevention of Covid-19. N Engl J Med 2022;386(23):2188–200.
58. Young-Xu Y, Epstein L, Marconi VC, et al. Tixagevimab/Cilgavimab for Prevention of COVID-19 during the omicron surge: retrospective analysis of national VA electronic data. medRxiv 2022. https://doi.org/10.1101/2022.05.28.22275716. 2022.05.28.22275716.
59. Al Jurdi A, Morena L, Cote M, et al. Tixagevimab/cilgavimab pre-exposure prophylaxis is associated with lower breakthrough infection risk in vaccinated solid organ transplant recipients during the omicron wave. Am J Transplant 2022. https://doi.org/10.1111/ajt.17128.
60. Takashita E, Kinoshita N, Yamayoshi S, et al. Efficacy of antiviral agents against the SARS-CoV-2 omicron subvariant BA.2. N Engl J Med 2022;386(15):1475–7.
61. Planas D, Saunders N, Maes P, et al. Considerable escape of SARS-CoV-2 Omicron to antibody neutralization. Nature 2022;602(7898):671–5.
62. Fact sheet for healthcare providers: emergency use authorization for evusheldtm (tixagevimab co-packaged with cilgavimab). Available at: https://www.fda.gov/media/154701/download. Accessed 31 January, 2023.
63. FDA announces Evusheld is not currently authorized for emergency use in the U.S. Available at: https://www.fda.gov/drugs/drug-safety-and-availability/fda-announces-evusheld-not-currently-authorized-emergency-use-us. Accessed 31 January, 2023.
64. First participant dosed in SUPERNOVA Phase I/III trial evaluating AZD5156, a next-generation long-acting antibody combination, for prevention of COVID-19. Available at: https://www.astrazeneca-us.com/media/statements/2022/first-participant-dosed-in-supernova-phase-I-III-trial-evaluating-azd5156-a-next-generation-long-acting-antibody-combination-for-prevention-of-covid-19.html. Accessed 31 January, 2023.
65. O'Brien MP, Forleo-Neto E, Musser BJ, et al. Subcutaneous REGEN-COV Antibody Combination to Prevent Covid-19. N Engl J Med 2021;385(13):1184–95.

66. Fact sheet for health care providers emergency use authorization (EUA) OF RE-GEN-COV® (casirivimab and imdevimab). Available at: https://www.fda.gov/media/145611/download. Accessed 31 January, 2023.
67. Pfizer Shares Top-Line Results from Phase 2/3 EPIC-PEP Study of PAXLOVID™ for Post-Exposure Prophylactic Use. Available at: https://www.pfizer.com/news/press-release/press-release-detail/pfizer-shares-top-line-results-phase-23-epic-pep-study/. Accessed 13 December, 2022.
68. COVID-19 Vaccines for People Who Are Moderately or Severely Immunocompromised. Available at: https://www.cdc.gov/coronavirus/2019-ncov/vaccines/recommendations/immuno.html. Accessed 31 January, 2023.
69. Pre-exposure Prophylaxis with EVUSHELD™. Available at: https://www.cdc.gov/coronavirus/2019-ncov/hcp/clinical-care/pre-exposure-prophylaxis.html. Accessed 31 January, 2023.

Coronavirus Disease 2019 Management Strategies in Solid Organ Transplant Recipients

Maria Alejandra Mendoza, MD[a,b],
Raymund R. Razonable, MD[a,b],*

KEYWORDS

- Anti-spike monoclonal antibodies • Coronavirus disease-2019 • COVID-19
- Molnupiravir • Nirmatrelvir • Remdesivir • Transplantation

KEY POINTS

- Solid organ transplant recipients are at high risk of severe coronavirus disease-2019 (COVID-19). If left untreated, COVID-19 in transplant patients results in high rates of hospitalization, need for intensive care unit level of care, and death.
- When diagnosed early at the mild-to-moderate COVID-19 state, treatment with remdesivir, ritonavir-boosted nirmatrelvir, or an anti-spike neutralizing monoclonal antibody may prevent its progression to severe and critical COVID-19. However, the effectivity of the anti-spike monoclonal antibodies is highly variable depending on specific variants and subvariants.
- Among solid organ transplant patients with severe and critical COVID-19, treatment with intravenous remdesivir with or without immunomodulation with dexamethasone, tocilizumab, or baricitinib is recommended.

INTRODUCTION

Severe acute respiratory syndrome coronavirus-2 (SARS-CoV-2), the RNA virus that is responsible for coronavirus disease 2019 (COVID-19), was initially recognized to cause a cluster of atypical pneumonia cases in Wuhan, China, in December 2019.[1] Since then, the virus had spread rapidly across regions to cause a novel human disease that was declared a pandemic on March 11, 2020. As of December 2022, there have been over 640 million confirmed cases of COVID-19 globally with 6.6 million cumulative deaths; these numbers are likely underestimates of the magnitude of the pandemic as many cases are not reported to authorities.[2]

[a] Division of Public Health, Infectious Diseases and Occupational Medicine, Department of Medicine, Mayo Clinic, Rochester, MN, USA; [b] William J von Liebig Clinic Center for Transplantation and Clinical Regeneration, Mayo Clinic, Rochester, MN, USA
* Corresponding author. 200 First Street Southwest, Rochester, MN 55905.
E-mail address: razonable.raymund@mayo.edu

Infect Dis Clin N Am 37 (2023) 475–493
https://doi.org/10.1016/j.idc.2023.03.003
0891-5520/23/© 2023 Elsevier Inc. All rights reserved.

SARS-CoV-2 causes infection in any person, but the severe and unfavorable outcomes have been most notable among the high-risk immunosuppressed population. At the beginning of the COVID-19 pandemic in 2020, the reported mortality among hospitalized solid organ transplant (SOT) recipients was around 20%, which was generally higher when compared to the general population.[3] However, this reported mortality rate did not account for SOT recipients with mild-to-moderate COVID-19 who did not require hospitalization. Nonetheless, there are multiple factors that could account for the worse outcome of COVID-19 in SOT recipients, including the impaired T-cell-mediated immunity that hampers the host response to the infection,[4] and many other risk factors that co-exist in the SOT recipient, such as having an older age and medical comorbidities.[3]

As the COVID-19 pandemic continually evolved for the last 3 years, the mortality rates in the general and immunocompromised population have fortunately declined. The improvement in outcomes could be substantially attributed to the remarkable and rapid advances in its prevention (such as vaccination and prophylaxis) and effective treatment. In addition, the evolution of SARS-CoV-2 resulted in less virulent variants of concern (VOC). The widespread use of vaccination, for example, has led to more people having underlying immunity that prevents progression to severe clinical disease and death (discussed in a separate article in this issue). The rapid development of antiviral therapeutics such as intravenous remdesivir has also resulted in improved clinical outcomes among outpatients and hospitalized persons. Oral antiviral drugs such as ritonavir-booster nirmatrelvir were developed to reduce the risk of hospitalization and death among high-risk outpatients. Early administration of passive immunotherapy with anti-spike neutralizing monoclonal antibodies has also resulted in a marked reduction in severe disease and hospitalization. Among hospitalized patients with severe and critical COVID-19, the use of remdesivir with or without an immunomodulator such as dexamethasone, baricitinib, and tocilizumab, has resulted in reduced mortality rate.[5] On the other hand, SARS-CoV-2 has evolved into VOC, currently predominated by the Omicron variant, which has been described to cause clinical disease with lower severity and lower associated mortality.[6] This observation has also been observed in the SOT population. One study reported that while the SARS-CoV-2 Omicron variant had higher transmissibility, it was associated with lower disease severity and associated mortality. In this study of 347 infected patients, the hospitalization rate was 26% but the mortality rate was only 2%.[7]

At the time of this writing, on December 15, 2022, the United States National Institutes of Health (NIH) provided updated comprehensive treatment recommendations for patients with SARS-CoV-2. In general, the treatment during the early phase of the disease is focused on antiviral drugs, while the later stages of the disease are mostly focused on treating a dysregulated immunomodulatory response to the virus.[8] In this article, we discuss the available therapies for COVID-19, with specific focus on the use of these drugs in SOT patients, both in the outpatient and inpatient setting (**Figs. 1** and **2**). Notably, there are no randomized clinical trials (RCT) of COVID-19 treatments that are focused on the SOT population, so the data supporting their use in this specific high-risk population are extrapolated from clinical trials in the general non-transplant patients and from real-world experiences described in the multitude of retrospective studies in SOT recipients that have been published to date. Aggressive treatment of the SOT patient is highly recommended since immunosuppressed patients have a well-described blunted antibody response to infection and remain at high-risk of severe outcomes.[9,10]

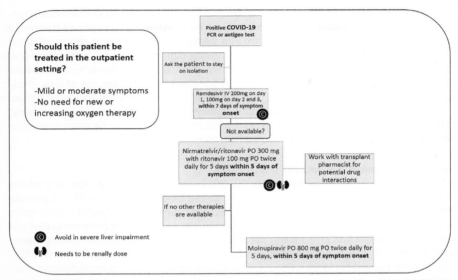

Fig. 1. Outpatient management of solid organ transplant recipients with mild-to-moderate COVID-19. IV, intravenous; PCR, polymerase chain reaction; PO, oral. Anti-spike monoclonal antibodies are no longer available as an option as of December 2022.

Treatment of Solid Organ Transplant Recipients with Early Coronavirus Disease 2019 of Mild-to-Moderate Severity

Supportive care
Among immunocompetent persons without risk factors, the recommended management of mild-to-moderate COVID-19 is supportive care using antipyretics, analgesics,

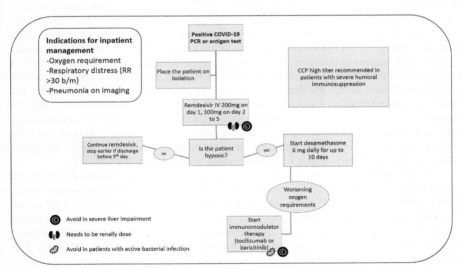

Fig. 2. Recommended management of solid organ transplant recipients with severe COVID-19.

fluids, and rest. However, this approach alone is not sufficient in high-risk individuals, including the SOT population. In one study of SOT patients with mild-to-moderate COVID-19 during the SARS-CoV-2 Omicron period, the cohort of patients who did not receive any COVID-19-directed therapy had a higher rate of hospitalization and death (27.1% and 6.3%, respectively), when compared to those who received virus-directed treatment (13.5% and 0%, respectively).[11] The results of this study have been replicated in many others, as discussed with the different therapies below, and highlights the need for all symptomatic patients to be tested and diagnosed early, so that SOT patients, even those with mild–moderate disease, can be treated early as they will benefit from the available outpatient therapies.

Anti-spike neutralizing monoclonal antibodies

From November 9, 2020, to November 30, 3022, monoclonal antibodies against the SARS-CoV-2 spike protein were a backbone for the treatment of high-risk outpatients with mild-to-moderate COVID-19, including SOT recipients.[12] The SARS-CoV-2 spike protein is an essential component used by the virus to enter human cells through virus-host cell membrane fusion.[13] Initially identified in the blood of a patient who recovered from COVID-19, these immunoglobulin-G molecules were subsequently manufactured in pharmaceutical laboratories as immunotherapies aimed to impede virus entry and improve clinical outcomes.

The first two anti-spike monoclonal antibody preparations, bamlanivimab and casirivimab-imdevimab, were investigated in randomized, placebo-controlled clinical trials of high-risk outpatients with mild-to-moderate COVID-19. These monoclonal antibody products reduced hospitalization and emergency department (ED) visits (bamlanivimab, 1.6% vs 6.3%) or medically attended visits (casirivimab-imdevimab, 3% vs 6%) when compared to placebo.[14,15] As a result of these seminal studies, these products were granted emergency use authorizations (EUA) by the US FDA in November 2020 for the treatment of high-risk outpatients with mild-to-moderate COVID-19, including SOT recipients. Since November 2020, there have been a total of five anti-spike monoclonal antibodies authorized for emergency use as treatment of high-risk patients with mild-to-moderate COVID-19. These include bamlanivimab, bamlanivimab-etesevimab, casirivimab-etesevimab, sotrovimab, and bebtelovimab—the clinical effectivity of each of these monoclonal antibody products was highly variable depending on the circulating VOC in the communities, as discussed below.

These anti-spike monoclonal antibodies are recommended for early treatment of laboratory-confirmed mild-to-moderate COVID-19, including SOT patients. Patients should be treated within the first 7 to 10 days of symptom onset, emphasizing the need for early diagnosis. Patients who present with severe disease, as indicated by hypoxia and respiratory distress, and those hospitalized for COVID-19 indications or requiring oxygen supplementation, are excluded from treatment based on EUA criteria; the use of anti-spike monoclonal antibodies in these later-stage situations characterized by severe illness have not proven to be beneficial.

There are no RCTs that specifically assessed the efficacy and safety of anti-spike monoclonal antibodies in SOT patients. The evidence for the use of anti-spike monoclonal antibodies in SOT recipients is extrapolated from the original RCTs that included standard-risk and high-risk patients.[16,17] However, subsequent observational retrospective studies of anti-spike monoclonal antibodies in high-risk patients, including SOT recipients, have shown reductions in hospitalizations, ED visits, ICU admission, and mortality.[18–20]

Based on these observational retrospective studies, SOT patients who received anti-spike monoclonal antibodies have rates of hospitalization ranging from 0% to

16.7%, ICU admission rates of 0% to 8.3%, and mortality rates of 0% to 4.2%.[21–23] These rates are comparably lower than previous historical cohorts. From studies with a defined comparator group, there were lower rates of progression to severe disease,[24] ED visits,[23] hospitalization,[23,25,26] and mortality[24,26] among those who received anti-spike monoclonal antibodies. A higher burden of comorbid medical conditions and immunocompromised status has been associated with a higher chance of hospitalization despite treatment with anti-spike monoclonal antibodies.[27] Nonetheless, treatment with an anti-spike monoclonal antibody was protective from hospitalization or ED visit after adjustment for age, chronic kidney disease, race, and ethnicity.[23]

Anti-spike monoclonal antibodies have greater efficacy among seronegative patients.[28] However, serology to assess the presence of anti-SARS-CoV-2 antibodies is not a routine or standard of care. Nonetheless, this observation suggests that these passive immunotherapies appear to confer most benefit when given earlier in the disease course, before the development of endogenous antibodies.[21,29] SOT recipients, especially those who have received B-cell-depleting agents, are a group of persons who may not mount a sufficient humoral immune response,[30] and may benefit from passive immunotherapy with these anti-spike monoclonal antibody treatments.

Anti-spike monoclonal antibody therapy appears beneficial even among vaccinated high-risk patients, including SOT patients, who develop breakthrough COVID-19.[31] One study of high-risk vaccinated patients, including SOT recipients, found casirivimab-imdevimab treatment was associated with lower risk of hospitalization.[32] Another large cohort of fully vaccinated high-risk patients, including SOT recipients, found anti-spike monoclonal antibody therapy to reduce hospitalization. This beneficial effect was greater among patients with more comorbid conditions.[33] An observational study of fully vaccinated SOT recipients with breakthrough COVID-19 reported that 14.3% developed severe disease.[34] However, among those who presented with mild-to-moderate disease and were treated early with anti-spike monoclonal antibody therapy, only 3.4% progressed to a severe disease requiring hospitalization. Smaller cohort studies have also reported similar outcomes.[35]

Despite the limitations of real-world retrospective studies, the collective data suggest a beneficial role of anti-spike monoclonal antibody therapy in the treatment of SOT recipients with mild-to-moderate COVID-19. However, SARS-CoV-2 continually evolved, and VOC have rapidly developed that affected the clinical utility and effectivity of anti-spike monoclonal antibodies. The emergence of SARS-COV-2 B.1351 (Beta) and P.1 (Gamma) in early 2021 led to the revocation of EUA of bamlanivimab monotherapy, while the emergence of B.1.1.529 (Omicron) in December 2021 made bamlanivimab-etesevimab and casirivimab-imdevimab ineffective. Sotrovimab was useful during SARS-COV-2 Omicron B.1.1.529 period, but its clinical utility dissipated with the emergence of Omicron BA.2 and BA.5 subvariants in March 2022.[11] Bebtelovimab maintained activity against Omicron BA.2 and BA.5 subvariants[36] but its authorization for treatment was revoked on November 30, 2022, when Omicron BQ.1 and BQ.1.1 became the dominant VOC. As of this writing, there is no longer any anti-spike monoclonal antibody that is currently authorized for the treatment of mild-to-moderate COVID-19. Nonetheless, there are ongoing efforts to develop novel monoclonal antibody products for the prevention and treatment of COVID-19.

Intravenous remdesivir

As a nucleotide prodrug of an adenosine analog, remdesivir binds to the SARS-CoV-2 RNA-dependent RNA polymerase and inhibits viral replication by prematurely terminating RNA transcription. Remdesivir was initially approved for the treatment of hospitalized patients with severe disease, including those requiring oxygen supplementation by nasal cannula.[37]

Remdesivir was later evaluated in high-risk outpatients with mild-to-moderate COVID-19. In the landmark PINETREE trial, high-risk outpatients within 7 days of onset of mild-to-moderate COVID-19 were randomized to either receive remdesivir 200 mg on day 1 and 100 mg on days 2 and 3, versus placebo. The primary endpoints, which were COVID-19-related visits or death at day 28, occurred in only two patients (0.7%) in the remdesivir group and in 15 (5.3%) in the placebo group (HR, 0.13; 95% confidence interval [CI], 0.03–0.59; $P =$ .008). In addition, COVID-19-related visit was higher in the placebo group (HR, 0.19; 95% CI, 0.07–0.56). This trial highlighted the benefits of early administration of an antiviral drug in the outpatient setting. In this study, only 4.1% of the patients were labeled as immunocompromised.[38] Nonetheless, the reassuring results allowed for the use of intravenous remdesivir in SOT recipients with mild-to-moderate COVID-19 in real-world settings (especially now that there is no longer an option for anti-spike monoclonal antibodies, as discussed above). The logistics of administering IV remdesivir once daily in the outpatient setting can be challenging in certain places.

There have been studies that evaluated intravenous remdesivir in SOT patients. In one prospective cohort study conducted during the Omicron BA.2 wave, the effectiveness of the 3-day remdesivir treatment course was evaluated in a cohort of 192 SOT patients. The early administration of remdesivir decreased the hospitalization rate of treated patients, with an adjusted HR of 0.12 (95%CI: 0.03–0.057); the adjusted number needed to treat with intravenous remdesivir to prevent one hospitalization was 15.2.[39] Another study compared remdesivir or sotrovimab to no treatment in a retrospective cohort study, and found that patients treated with remdesivir were significantly less likely to be hospitalized or visit the ED within 29 days from symptom onset (11% vs 23.3%; odds ratio (OR) = 0.41, 95% CI = 0.17–0.95).[40]

There is clear evidence that early administration of intravenous remdesivir in SOT patients with mild-to-moderate COVID-19 appears safe and beneficial. Intravenous remdesivir is active against all SARS-CoV-2 variants to date, and there are only very rare reports of drug resistance. As the anti-spike monoclonal antibodies are no longer an option, intravenous remdesivir offers the potential for good outcomes. However, the logistics of administering this intravenous medication once daily for 3 consecutive days can be very challenging, especially among patients who reside in remote areas with limited access to an infusion center. Remdesivir is a minor inhibitor of CYP3A1 enzymes, but the clinical significance of this is minimal; so far, there are no reported complications of remdesivir interactions, which is very important in the SOT population who receive drugs with a high likelihood of potentially relevant drug interactions.[8]

Ritonavir-boosted nirmatrelvir

Nirmatrelvir is an oral SARS-CoV-2 main protease inhibitor that is active against M[pro], a viral protease that is essential in viral replication by cleaving two viral polyproteins. The systemic level of nirmatrelvir is pharmacologically boosted by its co-administration with ritonavir, a well-known HIV-1 protease inhibitor whose cytochrome P450-3A inhibitor activity increases the levels of many drugs including nirmatrelvir.[41,42] On its own, however, ritonavir does not have any activity against SARS-CoV-2. Nirmatrelvir plus ritonavir combination was evaluated in a randomized controlled trial of symptomatic, unvaccinated, non-hospitalized patients with COVID-19. In this trial, the incidence of COVID-19-related hospitalization or death by day 28 was reduced by 87% in the nirmatrelvir–ritonavir group when compared to the placebo group. However, this clinical study did not include transplant patients.[43]

Several small studies have reported on the real-world use of ritonavir-boosted nirmatrelvir in SOT patients with mild-to-moderate COVID-19. In one of the first studies reporting on the use of nirmatrelvir–ritonavir in 25 SOT patients with mild COVID-19, three patients subsequently required hospitalization, but no deaths were reported; however, the authors highlight that the lack of control group and the small study size hinders the interpretation on its efficacy.[44] In a larger retrospective study of 154 SOT patients who were infected during the Omicron period, patients who received nirmatrelvir–ritonavir (or sotrovimab) experienced a lower rate of 30-day hospitalization or mortality when compared to patients who did not receive treatment ($P =.009$). When adjusted for organ transplant type, nirmatrelvir–ritonavir treatment (adjusted risk ratio [aRR] 0.21, 95% CI: 0.06–0.71) was associated with lower risk for 30-day hospitalization or death.[45]

Nirmatrelvir–ritonavir is a remarkable therapeutic advance in COVID-19 therapeutics because it is given orally, allowing for its convenient use in the outpatient setting (see **Fig. 1**). However, the major concern with using nirmatrelvir–ritonavir is its potential for drug interactions that could have mild to life-threatening clinical implications. Its pharmacologic booster, ritonavir, inhibits CYP 450, and consequently leads to the accumulation of certain drugs. This effect is very concerning particularly in SOT population as ritonavir will result in a markedly increased concentration of specific immunosuppressants such as calcineurin inhibitors (tacrolimus, cyclosporine) or mammalian target of rapamycin inhibitors (sirolimus, everolimus). There have been anecdotal reports of supratherapeutic tacrolimus levels among patients who were treated with nirmatrelvir–ritonavir. To ensure that it is administered safely, there are published recommendations on the management of medications such as tacrolimus,[46,47] and our protocol for mitigating this drug interaction is depicted in **Fig. 3**, as an example. These protocols and recommendations may not be fully applicable everywhere as patients may not have close access to therapeutic drug monitoring.

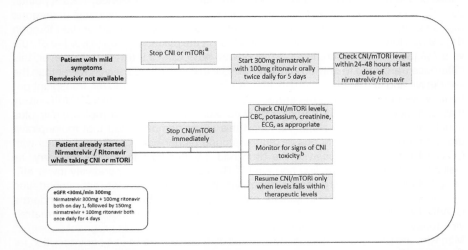

Fig. 3. Proposed management of solid organ transplant patients receiving ritonavir-boosted nirmatrelvir for COVID-19. [a]If a patient is on belatacept, recommend using nirmatrelvir–ritonavir as first line over remdesivir. [b]Severe headaches, tremors, confusion, visual disturbances, palpitations, changes in blood pressure, diarrhea, and oral ulcers. CBC, complete blood count; CNI, calcineurin inhibitors (tacrolimus, cyclosporine); ECG, electrocardiogram; IS, immunosuppression; mTORi, inhibition of mTORi (everolimus, sirolimus); NR, nirmatrelvir/ritonavir.

Indeed, it is recommended that alternative treatment of COVID-19 should be considered if strategies that ensure safe administration of nirmatrelvir–ritonavir is not available.

In addition to the impact of nirmatrelvir–ritonavir on tacrolimus and sirolimus levels, it is important to point out that SOT patients may be receiving other medications for their comorbid medical conditions, and these medications will also need to be adjusted, such as antifungals (voriconazole, posaconazole), anticoagulants (clopidogrel, warfarin), antihypertensives (amlodipine), cholesterol-lowering drugs (rosuvastatin), among others. Accordingly, nirmatrelvir–ritonavir use in SOT requires a detailed assessment and a more individualized, and often difficult, treatment approach.

Another concern with the use of nirmatrelvir–ritonavir is the recurrence of symptoms in a subset of patients after completion of treatment—a condition initially termed as rebound syndrome.[48] Studies have shown that rebound is uncommon[49,50] and has occurred even in untreated patients and those who received other therapies. Accordingly, rebound may be a feature of the natural history of COVID-19.[51] Among the SOT population, a retrospective study reported that two of 14 kidney transplant recipients who received nirmatrelvir-ritonavir developed early relapse with associated increased viral loads; however, it is difficult to extrapolate from this small study.[52] Nonetheless, these observations suggest the need to maintain continuous clinical monitoring of SOT patients during the treatment of COVID-19.

Molnupiravir. Molnupiravir is an oral prodrug that is metabolized to cytidine nucleoside analog N-hydroxycytidine, which when phosphorylated will cause mutations in the viral genome, thereby inhibiting the production of viable virus.[41] Molnupiravir was investigated in the MOVE-OUT trial, a double-blind randomized placebo-controlled trial where patients were randomized to receive the medication or matching placebo within 5 days of the onset of symptoms. The risk of hospitalization for any cause or death through day 29 was lower with molnupiravir (difference, -6.8% points; 95% CI, -11.3 to -2.4; $P =.001$). In the analysis of all participants who had undergone randomization, the percentage of participants who were hospitalized or died through day 29 was lower in the molnupiravir group than in the placebo group (6.8% [48 of 709] vs 9.7% [68 of 699]; difference, -3.0% points; 95% CI, -5.9 to -0.1). However, this difference translated to only 36% risk reduction; this was comparatively lower than the remdesivir and nirmatrelvir–ritonavir trials (discussed above). Moreover, transplant patients were not included in the study.[53] Subsequent to this, the PANORAMIC study was conducted in 25,783 participants who were randomized to molnupiravir plus usual care or usual care alone. Although this study demonstrated that molnupiravir did not reduce hospitalizations or deaths among higher-risk, vaccinated adults with COVID-19, those who received the drug had a faster time to clinical recovery, as well as reduced viral detection and load.[54] Because of the comparatively lower efficacy (relative to remdesivir and nirmatrelvir–ritonavir), the current recommendation by the NIH is to use molnupiravir only among patients with mild-to-moderate COVID-19 disease who do not have access to intravenous remdesivir or nirmatrelvir–ritonavir. In addition, molnupiravir is contraindicated for use in pregnant patients.[8] Men who are prescribed molnupiravir should also be advised to use contraception for 3 months after use of the drug. Among women of childbearing age, barrier contraception should be used and in patients taking hormonal contraception, the current guidance is to use an alternative method during the treatment period until one complete menstrual cycle after stopping the antiviral treatment.[55]

Because of the lower efficacy reported in clinical trials, the clinical use of molnupiravir has been lagging behind other therapies. Accordingly, there have only been a few small-scale studies regarding the use of molnupiravir in transplant patients. In a report of a small prospective study of nine kidney transplant patients, only one of the patients experienced clinical deterioration despite molnupiravir treatment and developed pneumonia requiring hospital admission. None of the patients suffered adverse effects attributed to molnupiravir and no adjustment of tacrolimus dose was needed.[56] Another retrospective cohort study of 16 kidney transplant patients showed that molnupiravir resulted in improvement of clinical symptoms and no serious side effects were reported, but then, this was not compared to any control.[57] Therefore, given the NIH recommendation as well as the lack of data to support its use in the transplant population, molnupiravir should be used only when the first-line options of remdesivir or nirmatrelvir–ritonavir are not available. Molnupiravir offers the advantage of oral administration and the lack of drug-to-drug interactions.

Treatment of Solid Organ Transplant Patients with Severe to Critical Coronavirus Disease 2019

Severe COVID-19 is indicated by the need for oxygen supplementation (or increasing oxygen requirement among those with long-term oxygen supplementation) and the need for hospitalization. SOT patients with severe COVID-19 may no longer benefit from the use of anti-spike monoclonal antibodies, nirmatrelvir–ritonavir, or molnupiravir, as these therapies have not been proven to be effective for the treatment of severe to critical COVID-19. Remdesivir is the only backbone antiviral drug for the treatment of severe COVID-19 (see **Fig. 2**).

Intravenous Remdesivir

Remdesivir was first approved for use in hospitalized patients with severe COVID-19.[58] It was first evaluated in the ACTT-1 trial in 2020, which enrolled 1062 hospitalized patients. It was associated with shortened time of recovery as well as decreased progression to lower respiratory infection. Moreover, Kaplan–Meier estimates of mortality were 6.7% with remdesivir and 11.9% with placebo by day 15, and 11.4% with remdesivir and 15.2% with placebo by day 29.[37] As a result of this seminal study, the NIH recommends remdesivir as a first line of therapy among patients hospitalized for COVID-19 and among high-risk patients with mild disease but are hospitalized for other non-COVID-19 reasons. However, among patients who are already requiring higher amount of oxygen supplementation, such as the use of high-flow nasal cannula or mechanical ventilation, the benefit of remdesivir is not as proven, hence there is no recommendation to use remdesivir in this setting.[8] Recently, there was a retrospective multicenter comparative effectiveness study of more than 96,000 patients who were hospitalized for the first episode of COVID-19 at one of the Hospital Corporation of America hospitals in the United States between February 2020 and February 2021. Among patients with their first COVID-19-related hospitalization, 43.9% received remdesivir, and these remdesivir-treated patients were significantly more likely to show clinical improvement by 28 days (aHR, 1.19). In this study, 6.2% of patients were transplant recipients, although no transplant-specific analysis was performed.[59]

Remdesivir is not approved for use in patients with eGFR of less than 30 mL/min because of the potential for accumulation of the excipients of the drug. This is an important issue to highlight among transplant patients, since it is not uncommon for these patients to have a low eGFR. However, a secondary analysis study from the CATCO randomized trial evaluated the safety of remdesivir in patients with kidney dysfunction (ie, those patients with eGFR <30 mL/min at baseline). There was no increased risk of transaminitis or toxic kidney effects at day 5 among patients with renal dysfunction and who received remdesivir.[60]

There have been only a few studies, and mostly in kidney transplant patients, that assessed the use of remdesivir for COVID-19. A multicenter cohort study from Spain with 51 hospitalized kidney transplant patients, reported that the remdesivir was well tolerated and safe in terms of renal and hepatic toxicity.[61] Another case-control study of 15 SOT patients from Hungary reported that remdesivir was safe, although there was a high mortality in the remdesivir group driven by the lung transplant patients.[62] In another retrospective study of 245 transplants, including mostly kidney and liver recipients, remdesivir was associated with a reduction in the hospitalization period in the hospital and the intensive care unit, as well as the mortality rates.[63]

Dexamethasone

The clinical benefit of the anti-inflammatory dexamethasone was conclusively shown in the landmark trial RECOVERY, where the reported mortality benefits were evident among patients receiving invasive mechanical ventilation or oxygen supplementation alone, but not among those who did not require any respiratory support. As in most studies, the study was not specific for transplant patients, which were generally not included in these studies.[64] This clinical benefit of dexamethasone was later supported by the CODEX trial from Brazil, which showed that the mean number of alive days and free from ventilation were greater than the control group.[65] In the REMAP Trial, ICU patients given hydrocortisone had higher odds of improvement in organ support-free days compared to patients who received placebo.[66] Based on these studies, dexamethasone is recommended for use in hospitalized patients with COVID-19 and who are requiring conventional oxygen supplementation to mechanical ventilation or ECMO. These patients may receive dexamethasone 6 mg once daily for up to 10 days.[8]

There are no good clinical trials available to evaluate the efficacy of dexamethasone for severe COVID-19 in the SOT population. However, the mortality benefit of dexamethasone has been so well-described in other clinical trials that there probably is not going to be a future trial that will further evaluate this intervention. However, there is concern about the safety of adding dexamethasone among SOT recipients who are already immunosuppressed at baseline. The question arises if adding dexamethasone is still needed among immunosuppressed patients, or will it further enhance the immunosuppression state and increase the risk of infections including reactivation of latent pathogens such as viral hepatitis B, cytomegalovirus, tuberculosis, or even strongyloidiasis, among others. Larger clinical trials, including the RECOVERY trial, did not provide data regarding the risk of secondary infections with the use of dexamethasone. Other studies have reported that steroid therapy may have been associated with higher rates of fungal infections such as coronavirus-associated pulmonary aspergillosis or mucormycosis. However, some of these patients also received other immunomodulators, so it is difficult to solely attribute this risk to steroids alone.[67] One retrospective multicenter study from Norway found that the risk of superinfections is higher among those who received steroids, however, the occurrence of a superinfection did not alter mortality. Indeed, higher mortality was associated with not using steroids.[68]

Based on these studies, clinicians should have heightened clinical suspicion for the occurrence of secondary infections in SOT recipients who received dexamethasone for severe COVID-19. Until more studies indicate otherwise, transplant status is not a contraindication per se for the use of dexamethasone, considering that the benefit is higher than the potential risk.

Immunomodulators

Tocilizumab acts by inhibiting the IL-6 signaling thereby dampening the cytokine release responsible for the pro-inflammatory phase of COVID-19.[69] Baricitinib, on the other hand, decreases cytokine signaling and release by inhibiting the JAK pathway.[70] The NIH treatment guidelines recommend the use of these immunomodulators, tocilizumab or baricitinib, among patients with severe to critical COVID-19 who have increasing oxygen requirements as well as patients in non-invasive and invasive ventilation. The rationale behind this recommendation is the observation that later in the clinical course of SARS-CoV-2 infection, the clinical severity of the disease is primarily driven by a dysregulated inflammatory response to the virus infection.[8]

The RECOVERY trial, which included 4116 patients who received tocilizumab, which was combined with steroids in the majority (82%), found reduced mortality at 28 days (rate ratio $0·85$; 95% CI $0·76–0·94$; $P = 0·0028$).[71] The REMAP-CAP trial also demonstrated similar findings with the use of IL-6 antagonists with a 90-day survival risk of 1.61 (95% CI, 1.25–2.08).[72]

Another cohort in the RECOVERY trial, which included 8156 patients who received baricitinib, demonstrated a decreased mortality in the baricitinib group (age-adjusted rate ratio 0.87; 95% CI 0.77–0.99; $P = 0·028$) when compared to usual care,[73] however, this reduction in mortality is reportedly smaller compared to other studies. In a metanalysis of the nine trials, there was a reduction of mortality of 20% (rate ratio 0.80; 95% CI 0.72–0.89; $P < .0001$). In the ACTT-2 Trial, over 1000 hospitalized patients were randomized to receive remdesivir plus either baricitinib or placebo. The time to recovery was significantly reduced with remdesivir–baricitinib combination treatment, with the most pronounced effect observed among patients who required high-flow oxygenation or non-invasive ventilation.[70] On the safety side, the COV-BARRIER study showed that even though there was no significant reduction in disease progression, the frequency of serious adverse effects, infections, and thromboembolic events were similar among groups.[74]

Although the benefit of survival from use of baricitinib and tocilizumab has been shown in the general population, the data on their use in transplant recipients are limited. So far, there are two small-scale studies highlighting the clinical experience of these immunomodulators in the SOT population. In one small retrospective matched cohort study of 29 patients receiving tocilizumab, there was no statistically significant mortality difference among the groups, even after adjusting for age and steroids. Reassuringly, there was no increase in secondary infections.[75] Another cohort study of 21 patients that received tocilizumab matched to standard-of-care patients also found no clear difference in mortality or mechanical ventilation requirement, but they did find that the hospital stay was shorter in the tocilizumab group.[76] These studies are limited by their retrospective study design and small cohort of SOT populations.

The main concern about the use of tocilizumab and baricitinib, similar to dexamethasone, has been the potential increased risk of superinfections. Small-scale studies have not demonstrated these potential risks. More studies involving larger cohort of patients are needed to assess the risk of opportunistic and secondary infections in SOT recipients with severe to critical COVID-19 treated with tocilizumab or baricitinib. Specifically, it will be important to document the rates and types of specific infections so their use can be further guided in the future.

Convalescent Plasma

Convalescent plasma is recovered plasma from donors who have recovered from COVID-19.[77] It contains polyclonal antibody components that could bind to SARS-CoV-2 and prevent virus entry into human cells. The use of convalescent plasma in the general population with COVID-19 has had conflicting clinical outcomes since the product was first authorized for use under the expanded access program. Several clinical trials have been conducted since then, with inconsistent results. In 2021, a national registry of 3082 patients who received convalescent plasma showed that patients who received high-titer convalescent plasma had a lower risk of death within 30 days compared to the low-titer group. However, this beneficial effect was not observed in patients who required mechanical ventilation.[78] Another study showed a reduction in mortality within 28 days in patients who received a transfusion with convalescent plasma with an anti-spike protein receptor binding domain titer of greater than 1:1350, within 72 hours of admission. This suggests the possible benefits of high-titer convalescent plasma when given earlier in the course of infection.[79] Indeed, a randomized clinical trial in older adults showed that early administration of high-titer convalescent plasma in elderly patients with mild COVID-19 can reduce the progression of COVID-19 disease.[80] However, other studies, including RCT and meta-analyses, did not consistently find a benefit of this intervention. In one such study, the administration of COVID-19 convalescent plasma to high-risk outpatients within 1 week after the onset of symptoms of COVID-19 did not prevent disease progression.[81] The RECOVERY trial analyzed the effect of convalescent plasma in 5795 hospitalized patients, and failed to find any clinical benefits on survival or progression to mechanical ventilation.[82]

Currently, high-titer convalescent plasma is not included as first-line treatment option since there is insufficient evidence to recommend its use. However, it is considered an option among immunosuppressed patients, especially when the preferred antiviral drugs are not available. Most of the data that showed the potential benefit of high-titer convalescent plasma involved immunosuppressed patients with underlying B cell hematologic malignancies.[83,84] However, in SOT populations, there are not enough controlled studies that support its use in this population.[85]

SUMMARY AND FUTURE DIRECTIONS

SOT recipients are at high risk of severe COVID-19. Before the availability of vaccination, passive immunotherapies, and effective antiviral therapeutics, the outcomes of COVID-19 in transplant recipients were devastating, with high morbidity and mortality. Primary vaccination and booster programs have reduced disease severity in most populations, including SOT patients, but their immune response to vaccines is notably suboptimal. Breakthrough COVID-19 may occur among vaccinated patients, and those with immunosuppression and high-risk comorbidities remain at increased risk of severe disease progression and death.

The administration of therapeutics, as early in the course of infection as possible, has led to a reduction in severe disease progression and death among high-risk patients, including SOT recipients. Anti-spike neutralizing monoclonal antibodies have been demonstrated to be highly effective and safe, but their therapeutic lifespan was dependent on the emerging VOC. After the successful clinical use of anti-spike monoclonal antibodies during the past 2 years, there is no longer an effective product in the clinical setting. Since they are safe and effective, we encourage efforts for further discovery and clinical development of these products for passive immunotherapy. Their niche is especially for the immunosuppressed patients who have impaired or are unable to mount an immune response to vaccination and natural infection. Accordingly, these patients are particularly prone to develop prolonged and protracted infections, and antibody-based therapies may improve their outcomes. In addition, the safety profile of monoclonal antibodies would allow for their use among high-risk patients who may not be safely given any of the available antiviral drugs, due to the adverse risk of drug interactions.

Three different antiviral drugs have been proven effective for treatment of COVID-19, and the clinical evidence for their use in SOT is extrapolated from clinical trials in general high-risk persons. Intravenous remdesivir is an effective option for the treatment of COVID-19 from mild-to-moderate and for those with severe infection. Its main disadvantage is the need for intravenous administration for 3 or 5 consecutive days, depending on clinical disease severity. Oral nirmatrelvir boosted by ritonavir is also highly effective in reducing severe disease progression, if given to patients early during the mild-to-moderate phase. It is convenient for patients as it is given orally, but the potential for drug interactions has been a major hurdle for use among some patient groups, including SOT patients who are on calcineurin inhibitors. Such drug interactions can be mitigated by a systematic approach to ensure patient safety. Oral molnupiravir is also an alternative oral option for early treatment of mild-to-moderate COVID-19 when remdesivir and nirmatrelvir–ritonavir are not available as first-line options. There are only minimal data in the medical literature on the use of nirmatrelvir–ritonavir and molnupiravir, and we encourage larger-scale studies to assess real-world outcomes of SOT recipients treated with these oral antiviral drugs. In addition, since the three antiviral drugs act on different aspects of the life cycle of SARS-CoV-2, it is also possible to consider clinical trials to assess the clinical outcomes of combination therapy. In this context, it will be important to consider trials to assess antiviral drug combination or a combination of an antiviral drug with a monoclonal antibody. These combination regimens are particularly attractive to examine in the highest risk immunosuppressed patients, such as SOT recipients, to assess their efficacy, safety, and potential to reduce the risk of resistance development.

The use of immunomodulators remains debated in SOT patients. Although data to support their use has been demonstrated in the general population, survival benefit from these immunomodulators in SOT recipients has not yet been demonstrated. No large-scale studies have been conducted, even retrospective study design, to assess the benefit of these strategies. We, therefore, encourage multicenter collaboration to conduct clinical trials. This is especially important in SOT and immunosuppressed populations because of the potential safety concern of opportunistic and superinfections.

In conclusion, there has been rapid development of life-saving antiviral therapeutics and passive antibody immunotherapies for the treatment of COVID-19. The use of these products has benefited SOT populations, where remarkable improvements in clinical outcomes have been observed. However, there remains the need to address unmet needs, especially among immunosuppressed patients, where the current therapeutic options have characteristics that limit their widespread use in SOT patients.

CLINICS CARE POINTS

- Early diagnosis of COVID-19 in solid organ transplant recipients allows for early treatment with antivirals and anti-spike monoclonal anitbodies.

- Treatment of mild to moderate COVID-19 in solid organ transplant recipients consists of a 3 day IV remdesivir course or a 5 day course of ritonavir-boosted nirmatrelvir. If available, anti-spike monoclonal antibodies are also highly effective.

- Treatment of severe COVID-19 among hospitalized solid organ transplant patients consists of a 5-day course of IV remdesivir. Dexamethasone is given to patients needing oxygen supplementation. The role of tocilizumab and baricitinib in solid organ transplant patients is not clear.

DISCLOSURE

R. Razonable: research grants (funds to the institution) from Gilead, United States, Regeneron, United States and Roche, United States; member of Data Safety Monitoring Board for Allovir and Novartis; member of the Board of Director of American Society of Transplantation. M.A. Mendoza: no conflicts.

REFERENCES

1. Huang C, Wang Y, Li X, et al. Clinical features of patients infected with 2019 novel coronavirus in Wuhan, China. Lancet 2020;395(10223):497–506.
2. WHO coronavirus (COVID-19) dashboard. World Health Organization; 2022. Available at: https://covid19.who.int/. Accessed 12 August, 2022.
3. Kates OS, Haydel BM, Florman SS, et al. Coronavirus Disease 2019 in Solid Organ Transplant: A Multicenter Cohort Study. Clin Infect Dis 2021;73(11):e4090–9.
4. L'Huillier AG, Ferreira VH, Hirzel C, et al. T-cell responses following Natural Influenza Infection or Vaccination in Solid Organ Transplant Recipients. Sci Rep 2020; 10(1):10104.
5. Heldman MR, Kates OS, Safa K, et al. Changing trends in mortality among solid organ transplant recipients hospitalized for COVID-19 during the course of the pandemic. Am J Transplant 2022;22(1):279–88.
6. Prevention CfDCa. Trends in Disease Severity and Health Care Utilization During the Early Omicron Variant Period Compared with Previous SARS-CoV-2 High Transmission Periods — United States, December 2020–January 2022, 2022. Available at: https://www.cdc.gov/mmwr/volumes/71/wr/mm7104e4.htm?s_cid=mm7104e4_w. Accessed 12 August, 2022.
7. Cochran W, Shah P, Barker L, et al. COVID-19 Clinical Outcomes in Solid Organ Transplant Recipients During the Omicron Surge. Transplantation 2022;106(7): e346–7.
8. Health NIo. COVID-19 Treatment Guidelines. Available at: https://www.covid19treatmentguidelines.nih.gov/management/. Accessed 12 August, 2022.
9. Stock PG, Henrich TJ, Segev DL, et al. Interpreting and addressing suboptimal immune responses after COVID-19 vaccination in solid-organ transplant recipients. J Clin Invest 2021;15(14):131. https://doi.org/10.1172/JCI151178.
10. Koff A, Malinis M. Suboptimal Antispike Antibody Levels Following Vaccination in Recipients of Solid Organ Transplant-Variance of Concern. JAMA Netw Open 2022;5(4):e226880.
11. Radcliffe C, Palacios CF, Azar MM, et al. Real-world experience with available, outpatient COVID-19 therapies in solid organ transplant recipients during the omicron surge. Am J Transplant 2022;22(10):2458–63.
12. Administration FaD. FDA Announces Bebtelovimab is Not Currently Authorized in Any US Region. 2022. Available at: https://www.fda.gov/drugs/drug-safety-and-availability/fda-announces-bebtelovimab-not-currently-authorized-any-us-region#:~:text=FDA%20Announces%20Bebtelovimab%20is%20Not%20Currently%20Authorized%20in%20Any%20US%20Region,-Share&text=%5B11%2F30%2F2022%5D,to%20neutralize%20Omicron%20subvariants%20BQ.
13. Jiang S, Hillyer C, Du L. Neutralizing Antibodies against SARS-CoV-2 and Other Human Coronaviruses. Trends Immunol 2020;41(5):355–9.
14. Chen P, Nirula A, Heller B, et al. SARS-CoV-2 Neutralizing Antibody LY-CoV555 in Outpatients with Covid-19. N Engl J Med 2021;384(3):229–37.

15. Weinreich DM, Sivapalasingam S, Norton T, et al. REGN-COV2, a Neutralizing Antibody Cocktail, in Outpatients with Covid-19. N Engl J Med 2021;384(3): 238–51.
16. Gottlieb RL, Nirula A, Chen P, et al. Effect of Bamlanivimab as Monotherapy or in Combination With Etesevimab on Viral Load in Patients With Mild to Moderate COVID-19: A Randomized Clinical Trial. JAMA 2021;325(7):632–44.
17. Dougan M, Nirula A, Azizad M, et al. Bamlanivimab plus Etesevimab in Mild or Moderate Covid-19. N Engl J Med 2021;385(15):1382–92.
18. Ganesh R, Pawlowski CF, O'Horo JC, et al. Intravenous bamlanivimab use associates with reduced hospitalization in high-risk patients with mild to moderate COVID-19. J Clin Invest 2021;(19):131. https://doi.org/10.1172/JCI151697.
19. Webb BJ, Buckel W, Vento T, et al. Real-world Effectiveness and Tolerability of Monoclonal Antibody Therapy for Ambulatory Patients With Early COVID-19. Open Forum Infect Dis 2021;8(7):ofab331.
20. Razonable RR, Pawlowski C, O'Horo JC, et al. Casirivimab-Imdevimab treatment is associated with reduced rates of hospitalization among high-risk patients with mild to moderate coronavirus disease-19. EClinicalMedicine 2021;40:101102.
21. Yetmar ZA, Beam E, O'Horo JC, et al. Monoclonal Antibody Therapy for COVID-19 in Solid Organ Transplant Recipients. Open Forum Infect Dis 2021;8(6): ofab255.
22. Dhand A, Lobo SA, Wolfe K, et al. Casirivimab-imdevimab for Treatment of COVID-19 in Solid Organ Transplant Recipients: An Early Experience. Transplantation 2021;105(7):e68–9.
23. Klein EJ, Hardesty A, Vieira K, et al. Use of anti-spike monoclonal antibodies in kidney transplant recipients with COVID-19: Efficacy, ethnic and racial disparities. Am J Transplant 2022;22(2):640–5.
24. Del Bello A, Marion O, Vellas C, et al. Anti-SARS-CoV-2 Monoclonal Antibodies in Solid-organ Transplant Patients. Transplantation 2021;105(10):e146–7.
25. Sarrell BA, Bloch K, El Chediak A, et al. Monoclonal antibody treatment for COVID-19 in solid organ transplant recipients. Transpl Infect Dis 2022;24(1): e13759.
26. Ahearn AJ, Thin Maw T, Mehta R, et al. A Programmatic Response, Including Bamlanivimab or Casirivimab-imdevimab Administration, Reduces Hospitalization and Death in COVID-19 Positive Abdominal Transplant Recipients. Transplantation 2022;106(2):e153–7.
27. Ganesh R, Philpot LM, Bierle DM, et al. Real-World Clinical Outcomes of Bamlanivimab and Casirivimab-Imdevimab Among High-Risk Patients With Mild to Moderate Coronavirus Disease 2019. J Infect Dis 2021;224(8):1278–86.
28. Group RC. Casirivimab and imdevimab in patients admitted to hospital with COVID-19 (RECOVERY): a randomised, controlled, open-label, platform trial. Lancet 2022;399(10325):665–76.
29. Verderese JP, Stepanova M, Lam B, et al. Neutralizing Monoclonal Antibody Treatment Reduces Hospitalization for Mild and Moderate Coronavirus Disease 2019 (COVID-19): A Real-World Experience. Clin Infect Dis 2022;74(6):1063–9.
30. Boyarsky BJ, Werbel WA, Avery RK, et al. Antibody Response to 2-Dose SARS-CoV-2 mRNA Vaccine Series in Solid Organ Transplant Recipients. JAMA 2021; 325(21):2204–6.
31. Yetmar ZA, O'Horo JC, Seville MT, et al. Outcomes of Solid Organ Transplant Recipients Treated With Antispike Monoclonal Antibodies for Coronavirus Disease 2019 Across Variant Epochs: Impact of Comorbidities and Vaccination. Transplantation 2022;106(11):e507–9.

32. Bierle DM, Ganesh R, Razonable RR. Breakthrough COVID-19 and casirivimab-imdevimab treatment during a SARS-CoV-2 B1.617.2 (Delta) surge. J Clin Virol 2021;145:105026.

33. Bierle DM, Ganesh R, Tulledge-Scheitel S, et al. Monoclonal Antibody Treatment of Breakthrough COVID-19 in Fully Vaccinated Individuals with High-Risk Comorbidities. J Infect Dis 2022;225(4):598–602.

34. Yetmar ZA, Bhaimia E, Bierle DM, et al. Breakthrough COVID-19 after SARS-CoV-2 vaccination in solid organ transplant recipients: An analysis of symptomatic cases and monoclonal antibody therapy. Transpl Infect Dis 2022;24(2):e13779.

35. Anjan S, Natori Y, Fernandez Betances AA, et al. Breakthrough COVID-19 Infections After mRNA Vaccination in Solid Organ Transplant Recipients in Miami, Florida. Transplantation 2021;105(10):e139–41.

36. Yetmar ZA, Beam E, O'Horo JC, et al. Outcomes of bebtelovimab and sotrovimab treatment of solid organ transplant recipients with mild-to-moderate coronavirus disease 2019 during the Omicron epoch. Transpl Infect Dis 2022;24(4):e13901.

37. Beigel JH, Tomashek KM, Dodd LE, et al. Remdesivir for the Treatment of Covid-19 - Final Report. N Engl J Med 2020;383(19):1813–26.

38. Gottlieb RL, Vaca CE, Paredes R, et al. Early Remdesivir to Prevent Progression to Severe Covid-19 in Outpatients. N Engl J Med 27 2022;386(4):305–15.

39. Solera JT, Arbol BG, Bahinskaya I, et al. Short-course Early Outpatient Remdesivir Prevents Severe Disease due to COVID-19 in Organ Transplant Recipients During the Omicron BA.2 Wave. Am J Transplant 2022. https://doi.org/10.1111/ajt.17199.

40. Piccicacco N, Zeitler K, Ing A, et al. Real-world effectiveness of early remdesivir and sotrovimab in the highest-risk COVID-19 outpatients during the Omicron surge. J Antimicrob Chemother 2022;77(10):2693–700.

41. Saravolatz LD, Depcinski S, Sharma M. Molnupiravir and Nirmatrelvir-Ritonavir: Oral COVID Antiviral Drugs. Clin Infect Dis 2022. https://doi.org/10.1093/cid/ciac180.

42. Owen DR, Allerton CMN, Anderson AS, et al. An oral SARS-CoV-2 M(pro) inhibitor clinical candidate for the treatment of COVID-19. Science 2021;374(6575):1586–93.

43. Hammond J, Leister-Tebbe H, Gardner A, et al. Oral Nirmatrelvir for High-Risk, Nonhospitalized Adults with Covid-19. N Engl J Med 2022;386(15):1397–408.

44. Salerno DM, Jennings DL, Lange NW, et al. Early clinical experience with nirmatrelvir/ritonavir for the treatment of COVID-19 in solid organ transplant recipients. Am J Transplant 2022;22(8):2083–8.

45. Hedvat J, Lange NW, Salerno DM, et al. COVID-19 therapeutics and outcomes among solid organ transplant recipients during the Omicron BA.1 era. Am J Transplant 2022;22(11):2682–8.

46. Lemaitre F. Yes We Can (Use Nirmatrelvir/Ritonavir Even in High Immunological Risk Patients Treated with Immunosuppressive Drugs). Clin Pharmacokinet 2022;61(8):1071–3.

47. Lange NW, Salerno DM, Jennings DL, et al. Nirmatrelvir/ritonavir use: Managing clinically significant drug-drug interactions with transplant immunosuppressants. Am J Transplant 2022;22(7):1925–6.

48. Charness ME, Gupta K, Stack G, et al. Rebound of SARS-CoV-2 Infection after Nirmatrelvir-Ritonavir Treatment. N Engl J Med 2022;387(11):1045–7.

49. Wong GL, Yip TC, Lai MS, et al. Incidence of Viral Rebound After Treatment With Nirmatrelvir-Ritonavir and Molnupiravir. JAMA Netw Open 2022;5(12):e2245086.

50. Ranganath N, O'Horo JC, Challener DW, et al. Rebound Phenomenon after Nirmatrelvir/Ritonavir Treatment of Coronavirus Disease-2019 in High-Risk Persons. Clin Infect Dis 2022. https://doi.org/10.1093/cid/ciac481.

51. Anderson AS, Caubel P, Rusnak JM, et al. Nirmatrelvir-Ritonavir and Viral Load Rebound in Covid-19. N Engl J Med 2022;387(11):1047–9.

52. Devresse A, Sebastien B, De Greef J, et al. Safety, Efficacy, and Relapse of Nirmatrelvir-Ritonavir in Kidney Transplant Recipients Infected With SARS-CoV-2. Kidney Int Rep 2022;7(11):2356–63.

53. Jayk Bernal A, Gomes da Silva MM, Musungaie DB, et al. Molnupiravir for Oral Treatment of Covid-19 in Nonhospitalized Patients. N Engl J Med 2022;386(6): 509–20.

54. Butler C. Molnupiravir plus usual care versus usual care alone as early treatment for adults with COVID-19 at increased risk of adverse outcomes (PANORAMIC): preliminary analysis from the United Kingdom randomised, controlled open-label, platform adaptive trial. 17 2022.

55. Organization WH. Administration of nirmatrelvir-ritonavir for COVID-19. Accessed 2022, Available at: https://apps.who.int/iris/bitstream/handle/10665/359758/WHO-2019-nCoV-Therapeutics-Nirmatrelvir-ritonavir-Poster-B-2022.1-eng.pdf.

56. Villamarin M, Marquez-Algaba E, Esperalba J, et al. Preliminary Clinical Experience of Molnupiravir to Prevent Progression of COVID-19 in Kidney Transplant Recipients. Transplantation 2022;106(11):2200–4.

57. Poznanski P, Augustyniak-Bartosik H, Magiera-Zak A, et al. Molnupiravir When Used Alone Seems to Be Safe and Effective as Outpatient COVID-19 Therapy for Hemodialyzed Patients and Kidney Transplant Recipients. Viruses 2022; 14(10). https://doi.org/10.3390/v14102224.

58. Kokic G, Hillen HS, Tegunov D, et al. Mechanism of SARS-CoV-2 polymerase stalling by remdesivir. Nat Commun 2021;12(1):279.

59. Garibaldi BT, Wang K, Robinson ML, et al. Real-World Effectiveness of Remdesivir in Adults Hospitalized With Coronavirus Disease 2019 (COVID-19): A Retrospective, Multicenter Comparative Effectiveness Study. Clin Infect Dis 2022; 75(1):e516–24.

60. Cheng M, Fowler R, Murthy S, et al. Remdesivir in Patients With Severe Kidney Dysfunction: A Secondary Analysis of the CATCO Randomized Trial. JAMA Netw Open 2022;5(8):e2229236.

61. Buxeda A, Arias-Cabrales C, Perez-Saez MJ, et al. Use and Safety of Remdesivir in Kidney Transplant Recipients With COVID-19. Kidney Int Rep 2021;6(9): 2305–15.

62. Fesu D, Bohacs A, Hidvegi E, et al. Remdesivir in Solid Organ Recipients for COVID-19 Pneumonia. Transplant Proc 2022. https://doi.org/10.1016/j.transproceed.2022.10.043.

63. Shafiekhani M, Shahabinezhad F, Niknam T, et al. Evaluation of the therapeutic regimen in COVID-19 in transplant patients: where do immunomodulatory and antivirals stand? Virol J 2021;18(1):228.

64. Group RC, Horby P, Lim WS, et al. Dexamethasone in Hospitalized Patients with Covid-19. N Engl J Med 2021;384(8):693–704.

65. Tomazini BM, Maia IS, Cavalcanti AB, et al. Effect of Dexamethasone on Days Alive and Ventilator-Free in Patients With Moderate or Severe Acute Respiratory Distress Syndrome and COVID-19: The CoDEX Randomized Clinical Trial. JAMA 2020;324(13):1307–16.

66. Angus DC, Derde L, Al-Beidh F, et al. Effect of Hydrocortisone on Mortality and Organ Support in Patients With Severe COVID-19: The REMAP-CAP COVID-19 Corticosteroid Domain Randomized Clinical Trial. JAMA 2020;324(13):1317–29.

67. Bartoletti M, Pascale R, Cricca M, et al. Epidemiology of Invasive Pulmonary Aspergillosis Among Intubated Patients With COVID-19: A Prospective Study. Clin Infect Dis 2021;73(11):e3606–14.

68. Sovik S, Barrat-Due A, Kasine T, et al. Corticosteroids and superinfections in COVID-19 patients on invasive mechanical ventilation. J Infect 2022;85(1):57–63.

69. Sebba A. Tocilizumab: the first interleukin-6-receptor inhibitor. Am J Health Syst Pharm 2008;65(15):1413–8.

70. Kalil AC, Patterson TF, Mehta AK, et al. Baricitinib plus Remdesivir for Hospitalized Adults with Covid-19. N Engl J Med 2021;384(9):795–807.

71. Group RC. Tocilizumab in patients admitted to hospital with COVID-19 (RECOVERY): a randomised, controlled, open-label, platform trial. Lancet 2021; 397(10285):1637–45.

72. Investigators R-C, Gordon AC, Mouncey PR, et al. Interleukin-6 Receptor Antagonists in Critically Ill Patients with Covid-19. N Engl J Med 2021;384(16): 1491–502.

73. Group RC. Baricitinib in patients admitted to hospital with COVID-19 (RECOVERY): a randomised, controlled, open-label, platform trial and updated meta-analysis. Lancet 2022;400(10349):359–68.

74. Marconi VC, Ramanan AV, de Bono S, et al. Efficacy and safety of baricitinib for the treatment of hospitalised adults with COVID-19 (COV-BARRIER): a randomised, double-blind, parallel-group, placebo-controlled phase 3 trial. Lancet Respir Med 2021;9(12):1407–18.

75. Pereira MR, Aversa MM, Farr MA, et al. Tocilizumab for severe COVID-19 in solid organ transplant recipients: a matched cohort study. Am J Transplant 2020; 20(11):3198–205.

76. Yamani AH, Alraddadi BM, Almaghrabi RS, et al. Early use of tocilizumab in solid organ transplant recipients with COVID-19: A retrospective cohort study in Saudi Arabia. Immun Inflamm Dis 2022;10(3):e587.

77. Wang X, Guo X, Xin Q, et al. Neutralizing Antibody Responses to Severe Acute Respiratory Syndrome Coronavirus 2 in Coronavirus Disease 2019 Inpatients and Convalescent Patients. Clin Infect Dis 2020;71(10):2688–94.

78. Joyner MJ, Carter RE, Senefeld JW, et al. Convalescent Plasma Antibody Levels and the Risk of Death from Covid-19. N Engl J Med 2021;384(11):1015–27.

79. Salazar E, Christensen PA, Graviss EA, et al. Treatment of Coronavirus Disease 2019 Patients with Convalescent Plasma Reveals a Signal of Significantly Decreased Mortality. Am J Pathol 2020;190(11):2290–303.

80. Libster R, Perez Marc G, Wappner D, et al. Early High-Titer Plasma Therapy to Prevent Severe Covid-19 in Older Adults. N Engl J Med 2021;384(7):610–8.

81. Korley FK, Durkalski-Mauldin V, Yeatts SD, et al. Early Convalescent Plasma for High-Risk Outpatients with Covid-19. N Engl J Med 2021;385(21):1951–60.

82. Group RC. Convalescent plasma in patients admitted to hospital with COVID-19 (RECOVERY): a randomised controlled, open-label, platform trial. Lancet 2021; 397(10289):2049–59.

83. Lanza F, Monaco F, Ciceri F, et al. Lack of efficacy of convalescent plasma in COVID-19 patients with concomitant hematological malignancies: An Italian retrospective study. Hematol Oncol 2022;40(5):857–63.

84. Thompson MA, Henderson JP, Shah PK, et al. Association of Convalescent Plasma Therapy With Survival in Patients With Hematologic Cancers and COVID-19. JAMA Oncol 2021;7(8):1167–75.
85. Cristelli MP, Langhi Junior DM, Viana LA, et al. Efficacy of Convalescent Plasma to Treat Mild to Moderate COVID-19 in Kidney Transplant Patients: A Propensity Score Matching Analysis. Transplantation 2022;106(1):e92–4.

Updates in Molecular Diagnostics in Solid Organ Transplantation Recipients

James Everhart, DO[a],*, Nancy G. Henshaw, MPH, PhD[b]

KEYWORDS

- Solid organ transplantation • Metagenomic next-generation sequencing
- Broad-range PCR • Multiplex PCR • Advances in molecular diagnostics

KEY POINTS

- Advanced molecular diagnostics have both advantages and disadvantages. Advantages include high sensitivity and culture-independent methods. The disadvantages are potential false positive results, cost, time, and questionable clinical impact.
- Clinical scenario, previous test results, anatomic location, and the assays performance for different specimen types should all be considered when choosing advanced molecular diagnostic assays.
- Unexpected findings should be confirmed (by orthogonal testing) when using highly sensitive molecular assays.

INTRODUCTION

Advances in molecular diagnostics have the potential to improve patient care among solid organ transplant (SOT) recipients by reducing time to pathogen identification and informing directed therapy. Although cultures remain the cornerstone of traditional microbiology, advanced molecular diagnostics, such as Metagenomic Next-Generation Sequencing (mNGS), may increase detection of pathogens. This is particularly true in the settings of prior antibiotic exposure, and when causative organisms are fastidious (ie, *Coxiella* spp, *Bartonella* spp). mNGS also offers a hypothesis-free diagnostic method of testing. This is useful in situations whereby the differential is broad or when the infectious agent is unlikely to be detected by routine methods. Furthermore, mNGS of plasma cell-free DNA (cfDNA) offers a noninvasive diagnostic option when specimen collection is too high risk.

[a] Duke University Medical Center, 2351 Erwin Road, Wadsworth Building, Room 0170, Durham, NC 27705, USA; [b] Duke University Medical Center, 2351 Erwin Road, Wadsworth Building, Room 0170, Durham, NC 27705, USA
* Corresponding author.
E-mail address: James.everhart@duke.edu

Infect Dis Clin N Am 37 (2023) 495–513
https://doi.org/10.1016/j.idc.2023.04.002
0891-5520/23/© 2023 Elsevier Inc. All rights reserved.

id.theclinics.com

Syndromic multiplex polymerase chain reaction (PCR) panels have become widely used adjunct tests and are highly sensitive, have short turnaround times, and offer a diagnostic panel for the most common infectious causes for their corresponding clinical syndromes.

Given the increasing number of available diagnostics assays, it is important for clinicians to familiarize themselves with their various strengths and weaknesses. This article discusses advances in molecular diagnostic assays and their advantages and disadvantages, with an emphasis on their utility for SOT recipients.

OVERVIEW OF SEQUENCING TECHNOLOGY

In order to understand current sequencing technology, it is necessary to understand the difference between traditional Sanger sequencing and next-generation sequencing (NGS; **Fig. 1**). It is also important to recognize the differences between targeted and unbiased (shotgun) NGS. Traditional Sanger sequencing involves sequencing one single DNA strand at a time and requires preamplification of a known target (eg, 16S rDNA) from a sample that is ideally monomicrobial. NGS is massive parallel sequencing that simultaneously sequences hundreds of millions of DNA fragments during a single run. The fragments are read, and contiguous sequences are aligned. The resulting data are compared with a library of known sequences to determine if the sample DNA is from a microorganism included in the library. NGS approaches may be either targeted or unbiased. Targeted NGS uses primers and/or capture probes to interrogate regions of interest (ie, hypervariable regions, 16s/18s) and then uses NGS technology to provide genetic information about microbial sequences in the sample. The potential benefit of targeted NGS is the ability to resolve mixtures of sequences generated from polymicrobial communities as well as differentiate minor variants within a heterogenous population of a single organism. In contrast to targeted approaches, unbiased (also known as metagenomic or shotgun) NGS

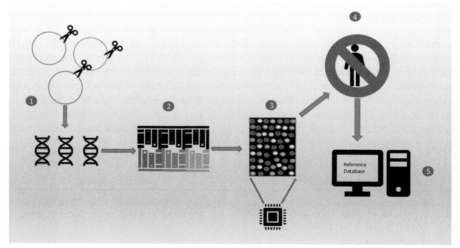

Fig. 1. Overview of mNGS process. (1) DNA is extracted and fragmented. (2) Adaptors are attached with barcoding sequences to prepare a library. (3) Millions of fragments are simultaneously sequenced. (4) Human DNA is removed. (5) Continuous sequences are aligned and compared with a reference library to determine organism identification.

randomly denatures all microbial DNA and then amplifies the fragments and compiles them into larger fragments that are then sorted and compared with sequence libraries.

METAGENOMIC NEXT-GENERATION SEQUENCING

mNGS technology allows pathogens to be detected from clinical specimens by interrogating all nucleic acids within a sample, including both host and microbial sequences. Bioinformatic tools along with depletion methods are used to filter out human DNA and identify remaining pathogen nucleic acid by comparing it with a reference genome library.[1]

In general, the diagnostic yield of NGS-based methods is higher than traditional Sanger sequencing. For example, when used in combination with 16s/18s rDNA PCR, Sanger sequencing has a positivity rate similar to traditional bacterial cultures, whereas targeted NGS increases positivity rates and sensitivity above standard cultures.[2] This is particularly true in patients who have received prior antibiotic therapy.[2,3]

It has also been shown that mNGS outperforms traditional culture methods for detection of fungi, viruses, certain anaerobic bacteria, and possibly *Nocardia* spp.[3]

Although there are many advantages to mNGS, it is not without disadvantages. With such a highly sensitive assay comes the difficulty of distinguishing true pathogens from commensal organisms and contaminants.[4,5] Given that SOT patients are often immunosuppressed, it takes clinical acumen or orthogonal testing (ie, confirmation of the presence of microbial nucleic acid by an alternative methods) to avoid overtreatment and unnecessary diagnostic tests (**Table 1**).

Extensive quality control processes, including internal and external controls, reagent purity, and library and sequencing quality as well as database accuracy, are needed to ensure the quality of this multistep assay. In addition, human DNA has to be filtered out, which can result in a loss of sensitivity. Databases used for analysis must also be updated and validated. There are many organisms from various kingdoms, and detecting these simultaneously makes validation of NGS strategies challenging.[6,7]

NEXT-GENERATION SEQUENCING OF MICROBIAL CELL-FREE DNA FROM PLASMA

The Karius laboratory is certified under the Clinical Laboratory Improvement Amendments of 1988 (CLIA'88) and is accredited by the College of American Pathologists (CAP) to perform high-complexity clinical laboratory testing. The Karius test is an mNGS test that detects circulating degraded microbial DNA; however, it is not Food and Drug Administration (FDA) cleared or approved. It is able to detect the DNA of 1250 bacteria, viruses, fungi, and parasites released into plasma, but does not detect RNA viruses. Results are expressed as molecules of microbial cfDNA per microliter of plasma.[8] The major advantages of the Karius test are detection of culture-negative infections, and ability to sometimes detect deep-seated infections noninvasively.[9] The major disadvantages are cost, varying sensitivity for nonendovascular infections, and the potential for false positive results. In this article, the authors define false positive results from mNGS as the identification of microbial DNA that is either a contaminant or a commensal organism that is not the cause of disease being evaluated.

The performance of cfDNA mNGS has been shown to have similar performance to blood cultures for the diagnoses of endovascular infections and endocarditis.[10,11] One single-center study[10] compared the Karius test with standard blood cultures in 30 patients with suspected bacterial endocarditis of which 23 had proven infective endocarditis. In this study, both blood cultures and the Karius test had a sensitivity of 87% for the microbial cause of endocarditis (gold-standard diagnosis was an adjudication

Table 1
Diagnostic stewardship recommendations

Microbial cfDNA mNGS (Karius test)	We recommend against performing this assay before initial blood cultures are negative
Microbial cfDNA mNGS (Karius test)	For rare pathogens (ie, Brucella and Coxiella) that can be diagnosed with serologic tests, consider sending serology in lieu of Karius test, especially in settings whereby serology assays have good performance
Microbial cfDNA mNGS (Karius test)	For scenarios in which specimen collection is too high risk, Karius test may be appropriate to diagnose deep-seated infections. However, if specimens can safely be acquired, conventional testing (culture, pathology, and so forth), is recommended with BRPCR (16s/18s testing) as an adjunct test when traditional testing does not yield a diagnosis and specimens can be readily obtained
mNGS of CSF	The authors recommend that this assay be reserved for when atypical pathogens are suspected. The most common causes of encephalitis and meningitis can typically be elucidated within 48 h by conventional means (culture and syndromic panels). The authors recommend performing these assays first
mNGS of CSF	Consider collecting an extra tube of CSF during lumbar puncture (LP) or communicating with the microbiology laboratory about saving CSF if atypical pathogens are suspected initially. If conventional tests are negative, then additional or saved CSF can then be sent for mNGS
mNGS of nonsterile specimens	There is low utility of performing mNGS on stool or urine. The authors recommend against using mNGS on these specimen types The authors do not recommend performing mNGS of respiratory specimens. Future applications of transcriptome analysis may increase the clinical utility of performing mNGS on respiratory specimens, but there are currently no available commercially assays that combine mNGS and transcriptome analysis in the United States
BRPCR (16s/18s)	Do not use as a "rule-out" test when conventional cultures are positive. It is unlikely that BRPCR will yield any additional significant pathogens missed by culture. This is especially true when culture results are consistent with the clinical scenario
BRPCR (16s/18s)	Consider that BRPCR has poor performance when microorganisms cannot be seen in pathology specimens. This assay will have low yield in these scenarios
BRPCR (16s/18s)	This assay has poor performance and low utility when used on specimens from nonsterile sites. The authors do not recommend the routine use of

(continued on next page)

Table 1 *(continued)*	
	this assay for blood, BALF, urine, or stool specimens
Syndromic panels	Multiplex PCR assays have high sensitivity and should only be used when the appropriate clinical scenario is present. The authors recommend using these assays as screening tests in asymptomatic patients. In addition, clinicians should keep in mind that these tests are highly sensitive, and the possibility for false positives exists. When an unexpected or atypical pathogen is identified, results should be verified with orthogonal tests. This is especially true when the clinical picture does not align with the result from a syndromic panel

panel of clinicians) despite the Karius test being collected an average of 11 days later than initial blood cultures. Another single-center study[11] examined 175 patients with either *Staphylococcus aureus* or gram-negative bacteremia. Detection of cfDNA persisted longer (median of 15 days vs 2 days) when compared with blood cultures. The authors suggested that there may be future application for the Karius test to determine antibiotic duration in certain patient populations. However, there are currently no data that there is an advantage to using Karius to determine response to therapy and antibiotic duration over traditional means.

MICROBIAL CELL-FREE DNA FOR INVASIVE FUNGAL INFECTIONS

Invasive fungal infections are associated with significant morbidity and mortality among SOT patients. In 2018, Hong and colleagues[12] reported that in patients with invasive fungal disease, plasma cfDNA sequencing identified the fungal organism in 7 of 9 cases when compared with biopsy tissue isolates. In one case, cfDNA was more accurate to species level than conventional testing, identifying *Aspergillus lentulus* as opposed to conventional testing, which identified this isolate as *Aspergillus fumigatus* species complex. *A lentulus* has similar macroscopic, microscopic, and phenotypic characteristics to *A fumigatus sensu stricto*; however, unlike *A fumigatus*, *A lentulus* commonly has resistance to triazoles and amphotericin B. The correct identification of *A lentulus* resulted in a change of treatment. This illustrates that this diagnostic modality can be used to distinguish cryptic species from more common species of molds. Another important point that this study illustrates is that molds that are difficult to grow in culture can be identified more quickly and noninvasively.

One retrospective single-center study[13] of hematopoietic cell transplant recipients examined 114 patients with proven invasive mold infections (IMIs). In the 75 participants with proven or positive IMIs, the sensitivity was 51%. The sensitivity for non–*Aspergillus* IMI was higher (79%) than the sensitivity for IMI caused by *Aspergillus* species (31%). Overall sensitivity was low, and specificity was high. It is unclear why there was a difference in sensitivity between the *Aspergillus* and non–*Aspergillus* species groups in this study. There may have been several factors that contributed to this difference. First of all, the non–*Aspergillus* group contained highly invasive molds (ie, *Rhizopus*, *Scedosporium* spp). This could have resulted in a higher rate of vascular invasion and circulating microbial DNA. One could also consider timing and choice of antifungal prophylaxis as a contributing factors as well. However, given that this is a culture-independent method of detection, antifungal therapy may not have had a significant effect on sensitivity. Another consideration is that the small number of non–*Aspergillus* species in this study may have skewed sensitivity. More studies are needed to determine if cfDNA mNGS is more sensitive at detecting non–*Aspergillus* species of IMI compared with *Aspergillus* spp.

One particularly challenging area of specimen collection is the central nervous system (CNS). In addition, brain imaging cannot accurately predict the cause of brain lesions.

Several case reports describe fungal brain abscesses that have been diagnosed using the Karius test.[14–16] No comparative studies of this method with the gold standard (brain biopsy and culture) have been performed. The Karius test may be a useful adjunct to routine testing in diagnosing CNS infections, as brain biopsy may be contraindicated, and empiric antimicrobials are often necessary before a biopsy can occur.

In summary, the detection of IMIs using cfDNA at a variety of anatomic locations appears to have relatively low sensitivity with high specificity. Thus, a positive result may be helpful, but negative results do not rule out IMIs. When possible, culture should still be attempted to obtain an isolate for susceptibility testing.

CLINICAL IMPACT OF MICROBIAL CELL-FREE DNA TESTING

Clinical impact study results for the Karius test have been mixed, possibly owing, at least in part, to the use of different definitions to define clinical impact. The definitions used by the studies cited in later discussion are summarized in **Table 2**. One retrospective review of 82 Karius tests, that included a large number of immunosuppressed patients (65%), had a positivity rate of 61% (50 out of 82 tests identified a microorganism). Half of the positive tests were monomicrobial (bacteria, virus, and fungi), and 50% identified more than one microorganism. No parasites were identified in this study. The most common indication for ordering a Karius test was fever of unknown origin (23.2%), followed by suspected respiratory infection (13.4%), sepsis (9.8%), suspected endocarditis (8.5%), and febrile neutropenia (7.3%). The study concluded that there was a 7.3% positive and 3.7% negative clinical impact. For 86.6% of tests performed, there was no clinical impact. The remaining 2.4% of tests were inconclusive. Sixty percent of patients in this study received a microbiologic diagnosis before testing, which may have affected the clinical impact of the Karius test.[17]

Another retrospective study included 59 tests from 54 patients and found that immunocompromised status was the only patient characteristic that trended toward a significant clinical impact.[18] The Karius test led to a change in antimicrobial treatment in 8 (14%) cases, and 7 of these 8 patients were immunocompromised.[9]

An additional retrospective study of 80 patients evaluating the clinical impact of the Karius test concluded a positive impact in 43% and a negative impact in 3%. The positive impact was higher in SOT (71.4%) and in patients with sepsis (71.4%). Positive impact was influenced primarily by de-escalation of antibiotics in the patients.[18]

METAGENOMICS FOR CENTRAL NERVOUS SYSTEM INFECTIONS

The University of California, San Francisco (UCSF) offers an mNGS test to diagnose pathogens causing meningitis and encephalitis. Sequences of both DNA and RNA from cerebrospinal fluid (CSF) are identified that align with pathogens in the GenBank database. The combination of sequencing RNA viruses is useful in that many

Table 2
List of definitions of clinical impact in studies cited in this article

Reference	Definition of Clinical Impact

Lee et al,[9] 2020	Positive clinical impact
	  De-escalation of antibiotics if team used mNGS results
	  New diagnosis or targeted therapy
	  Different diagnosis and additional therapy
	No clinical impact
	  Redundant information; antibiotics and clinical plan were not changed
	  No additional information
	  Not-relevant organism

Hogan et al,[17] 2021	Positive
	  New diagnosis based on Karius result and not confirmed by conventional microbiologic methods
	  Earlier diagnosis based on Karius result and later confirmed but conventional microbiologic methods
	  Karius result enabled avoidance of invasive surgical biopsy
	  Karius result enabled initiation of appropriate therapy
	  Karius result enabled de-escalation of therapy
	  Karius result enabled escalation of therapy
	  Karius result confirmed clinical diagnosis
	Negative
	  Karius result led to unnecessary treatment
	  Karius result led to additional unnecessary diagnostic interventions
	  Karius result led to longer length of stay
	None
	  Karius result showed new organism but result not acted upon
	  Karius result confirmed conventional microbiologic diagnosis and not acted upon
	  Karius result was negative and not acted upon
	  Patient died before Karius test result was available
	Indeterminate
	  Could not determine clinical impact from chart review

Shishido et al,[18] 2022	Positive clinical impact
	  Test result led to a new diagnosis when conventional tests were negative
	  Test result confirmed clinical diagnosis
	  Test result led to an earlier diagnosis
	  Test result negated invasive or costly procedure or tests
	  Test result helped to reduce hospital length of stay
	  Test result led to the initiation of appropriate antimicrobial therapy
	  Test led to de-escalation or discontinuation of antimicrobial therapies
	Negative impact
	  Test led to unnecessary diagnostic intervention or procedures
	  Test result led to unnecessary antimicrobial treatment
	  Test result led to an unnecessarily prolonged hospital stay
	Uncertain or no impact
	  Test result did not change clinical management or unable to determine the clinical impact

arboviruses and uncommon causes of meningitis or encephalitis are caused by RNA viruses. Turnaround time is about 1 week, including shipping.

In a comparison study of UCSF mNGS and conventional testing for meningitis and encephalitis among 204 pediatric and adult patients, the mNGS test detected 58 infections in 57 patients. The hospitals' routine microbiologic testing missed 13 (22%)

infections. Seven of the 13 infections detected only by mNGS resulted in targeted treatment with improved clinical effect.[19]

Although there are case reports of mNGS identifying viruses normally diagnosed by serology, mNGS is less sensitive than serology for arboviral encephalitis. These viruses are transient in the human host and unlikely to be present in the specimen at the time of collection. In the immunocompetent host, these viruses are present early in the asymptomatic phase of illness[20,21] and may persist longer than immunocompetent patients. It is uncertain if this assay performs better in SOT patients compared with immunocompetent patients, and additional studies would be required to make that determination.

Another study noted increased detection of atypical bacteria from tick-borne illnesses,[22] and several other case studies have illustrated the ability of mNGS to detect rare pathogens.[23,24]

Metagenomic NGS of CSF can be a useful adjunct for the diagnosis of meningitis and encephalitis in immunocompromised patients if unusual organisms are suspected, especially when routine testing and syndromic PCR panels are negative. However, it is important to note that PCR-based methods are generally more sensitive than mNGS,[25]with the caveat that a viral variant may decrease the sensitivity of singleplex PCR if there is a mutation at the PCR target site. In addition, both PCR and traditional bacterial cultures typically have a shorter turnaround time than mNGS.

METAGENOMICS FOR MONITORING DNA VIRUSES

The ARC Bio Galileo Pathogen Solution (Arc Bio LLC; EdenRoc Sciences, Cambridge MA, USA and Scotts Valley, CA, USA) is a novel mNGS reagent and bioinformatics pipeline that simultaneously detects and quantitates 10 double-stranded DNA viruses (Adenovirus [ADV], BK virus [BKV], Cytomegalovirus, Epstein-Barr Virus [EBV], Human Herpesvirus 6A [HHV-6A], HHV-6B, Herpes Simplex Virus 1 [HSV-1], HSV-2, JC Virus [JCV], and Varicella-Zoster Virus [VZV]). The 95% limit of quantitation ranged from 14 copies/mL (HHV-6) to 191 copies/mL (BKV). The lower limit of quantitation ranged from 442 IU/mL (EBV) to 661 copies/mL (VZV).[26] An evaluation of 50 plasma samples with at least one DNA virus detected showed total percent agreement of mNGS and quantitative PCR (qPCR) of 89.2% (306/343), with a k statistic of 0.725. The positive agreement was 84.9%, and the negative agreement was 90.7% (233/257). mNGS detected 7 coinfections that were confirmed but not initially requested by qPCR. There was reduced specificity with closely related viruses as seen with high BKV samples showing low levels of JCV signaling. The authors concluded that the mNGS Galileo Pathogen Solution system demonstrated analytical performance comparable to qPCR for DNA viruses. However, the authors noted that this technique will not replace routine monitoring of transplant patients by qPCR, as qPCR is readily available, is less laborious, is less costly, and is calibrated to the international standard. Although Galileo mNGS can simultaneously detect and quantitate viruses important in transplant patients, the assay takes 48 hours; in comparison, qPCR single-target assays require 4 to 6 hours.[27] In addition to the previously reported 10 DNA viruses, a subsequent study by Sam and colleagues[28] detected Parvovirus B19 and Torque Teno Virus (TTV). TTV, a single-stranded DNA virus, could potentially be used to monitor immunosuppression in SOT recipients.

The authors postulate that the Galileo assay system may be deployable to local laboratories, as the Galileo mNGS system pipeline is developed and bioinformatics expertise is not needed. Currently, the Arc Bio Galileo is not commercially available but may be a useful future diagnostic assay in the treatment of SOT recipients.

EVALUATING HOST RESPONSE IN CONJUNCTION WITH UNBIASED METAGENOMIC NEXT-GENERATION SEQUENCING

Some of the disadvantages of using mNGS on nonsterile specimens is detection of commensal organisms and inability to determine if potential pathogenic bacteria are causing illness or merely commensals. One promising potential method of overcoming these disadvantages is evaluating the host transcriptome and response to pathogen. Several studies suggest that measuring host gene expression may be able to differentiate between viral, bacterial, and noninfectious causes of illness and could potentially discriminate between pathogen and commensal organisms.[29–31] Assays that assess host gene expression responses would need to be explicitly validated in an SOT population given their immunosuppressed state and potentially disordered host responses to infection. There are currently no assays commercially available in the United States that use this technology to evaluate host response to infections. Furthermore, there will need to be further studies to evaluate clinical efficacy.

CURRENT CONSENSUS FOR METAGENOMIC NEXT-GENERATION SEQUENCING TESTING

The consensus conference of the American Transplantation Society set forth recommendations for uses of mNGS in its current state of development for SOT recipients.[31] The conference recommended that for all syndromes conventional testing over NGS be prioritized given the limited availability of NGS methods and limited studies defining performance characteristics. In all cases, clinical specimens should be collected and stored early in clinical presentation, ideally before antibiotic therapy, so that in the eventuality that standard testing is negative, NGS has the best chance of producing a result. More specific guidelines are as follows: for focal sites of infection, conventional testing should be prioritized, and if negative, NGS may be applied for infected tissues; plasma-based NGS may be useful when focal infection cannot be accessed for sampling. Second, for sepsis without a localized source/cause, select populations, such as SOT with severe illness, may benefit from plasma NGS in conjunction with conventional testing early in the course of illness. For respiratory infections, NGS of respiratory samples may be useful but with careful interpretation of results to differentiate pathogens from nonpathogens in the respiratory tract. For meningoencephalitis, NGS of CSF is potentially useful in conjunction with standard testing. Although current data show NGS to be of suboptimal sensitivity for invasive fungal infections, in select cases NGS may be useful when standard tests are negative.[31] The negative predictive value of metagenomic sequencing has not been established, and negative results do not exclude invasive infection. Positive results require evaluation within a clinical context. Studies that evaluate the clinical utility of mNGS for specific clinical scenarios in SOT patients could help clinicians better determine when and where to use these assays.

BROAD-RANGE POLYMERASE CHAIN REACTION

Broad-range (16s/18s) polymerase chain reaction (BRPCR) followed by sequencing uses specific primers of conserved 16s/18s ribosomal RNA bacterial gene sequences and/or internal transcribed spacer fungal sequences to detect and identify a wide array of organisms. Sequencing results are compared with validated databases for organism identification. BRPCR pathogen detection is limited to bacteria and fungi. Studies have shown that BRPCR is potentially useful for culture-negative cardiac and joint infections as well as for fungal sinusitis.[32,33] Some limitations of BRPCR are lower sensitivity than targeted, singleplex PCR, inability to distinguish commensals from pathogens, cost, and availability. In addition, Bronchoalveolar Lavage (BAL) specimens have low clinical impact and often identify nonpathogens or oral flora. BRPCR of blood has also been shown to be less sensitive than tissue samples.[34,35]

SYNDROMIC PANELS

Multiplex molecular syndromic panels that detect the most common causes of blood-stream, respiratory, gastrointestinal (GI), and CNS infections are now widely available and generate results within hours. Testing can also be performed directly from patient specimens or positive blood aliquots. In most cases involving the syndromes specific to these panels, multiplex PCR panels should be used before considering mNGS or BRPCR. Similar to other molecular assays, these panels cannot distinguish between infection, colonization, contamination, or prolonged viral shedding.

BLOOD PATHOGEN DETECTION PANELS

There are currently 9 FDA-approved molecular panels to detect bloodstream pathogens (**Table 3**). The Biofire BCID2 panel can detect a total of 33 pathogens and 10 resistance genes. The MEC Right Extremity Junction (MREJ) is also detected and can help differentiate an MEC A gene associated with S aureus or coagulase-negative Staphylococcus species.[36]

One study[37] showed the turnaround time for organism identification from blood collection by the BCID2 was 24.6 hours, whereas traditional methods took 48.1 hours. Of note, sensitivities were decreased (remained >80%) for less common pathogens (Proteus spp, Salmonella spp, Acinetobacter baumannii, Stenotrophomonas malto-philia, Bacteroides fragilis, Staphylococcus lugdunensis).[37]

The ePlex assays (Roche) are notable, as the 3 combined assays (gram-positive, gram-negative, and Candida) detect a large number of pathogens (41 bacteria, 11 yeast, and 11 resistance markers). Among the bacterial targets are 5 common blood culture contaminants, which may differentiate contamination from bacteremia early in the clinical course.

The Accelerate Pheno is a novel system that performs antimicrobial susceptibility testing of 20 different antibiotics within 8 hours using morphokinetic cellular analysis.[38] Performance decreases with polymicrobial bacteremia; the sensitivity significantly drops (98.6%–68.8%). This assay may misidentify coagulase-negative Staphylococci (CONS) as S aureus and Shigella flexneri may be misidentified as Escherichia coli. There have been reports of false positive Candida glabrata results.[39]

The T2Bacteria and T2Candida Biosystems use thermostable PCR, superparamag-netic beads, and T2 Resonance to detect bloodstream infections directly from spec-imens without the need for culture growth. The T2Bacteria detects the ESKAPE (Enterococcus faecium, S aureus, Klebsiella pneumoniae, Pseudomonas aeruginosa, and E coli) bacteria, which are the most common pathogens to cause bacteremia. T2Candida detects Candida albicans/Candida tropicalis, Candida g/Candida krusei, and Candida parapsilosis groups. The major limitations of these assays are the limited number of detectable targets and inability to detect antimicrobial resistance genes. The T2Bacteria shows high sensitivity and specificity (90%–94%/98%–100%),[40] and time to detection was significantly shorter than standard blood cultures.[41] The T2Candida has been shown to have a high sensitivity and specificity in high-risk

Table 3
Syndromic panels to detect bloodstream infections available in the United States

Assay Names	Method	Targets	Resistance Markers/ Susceptibility Testing	Sensitivity/Specificity	Advantages/ Disadvantages
QuickFish (OpGen)	In situ hybridization-based method	S aureus, S epidermidis, E faecalis, E faecium E coli, PsA, K pneumonia, 5 candida species, including Candia galbrata, C albicans, C parapsilosis	None	97%–100%/90%–100%	Quick turnaround time Few targets
AccuProbe (Hologic USA)	In situ hybridization-based method	S pneumoniae, S aureus	None	>97%/81%–100%	5 min assay time Limited targets
Accelerate PhenoTest	In situ hybridization-based method	11 gram-positive bacteria and 8 gram-negative bacteria, 2 Candida spp	20 antimicrobial MICs determined	96%/99%	Antimicrobial susceptibility testing Poor performance for polymicrobial bacteremia
Verigene (Luminex)	DNA-microarray based methods	13 gram-positive bacteria, 9 gram-negative bacteria	mecA, VanA/B, CTX-M, IMP, KPC, NDM, OXA, VIM	81%–100%/>98%	Quick results Resistance genes available Limited targets
FilmArray (bioMerieux) BCID2	Nucleic acid amplification-based methods/film array	15 gram-negative bacteria, 11 gram-positive bacteria, 6 candida species, Cryptococcus neoformans/gattii	mecA/C and MREJ (MRSA) vanA/B bla CTX-M Bla KPC Bla IMP, bla OXA-48, Bla NDM, bla VIM, mcr-1	73.1%–98.1%/98.1%–99.9%	Short assay run time 33 pathogens detected 10 resistance genes Sensitivity of more rare bloodstream pathogens drops but stays above 80%

(continued on next page)

Table 3
(continued)

Assay Names	Method	Targets	Resistance Markers/ Susceptibility Testing	Sensitivity/Specificity	Advantages/ Disadvantages
Xpert MRSA/SA BC (cepheid)	NAAT	MRSA/S aureus	mecA	98%–100%/99%–100%	Assay time 1–2 h Only one pathogen and one resistance gene detected
ePlex BCID	Multiplex PCR and hybridization- based method	3 separate panels. 20 gram-positive bacteria,21 gram-negative, pan gram-positive/gram-negative targets/pan candida targets, 11 candida species, *C neoformans/gattii*, *fusarium*, *Rhodotorula*	mecA/C, VanA/B, CTX-M, IMP, KPC, NDM OXA23, OXA-48, VIM	97%–99%/94%–99%	1-h assay time Combined all 3 assays Covers 52 targets Can identify bacteria that are common contaminants
T2Bacteria	T2 Resonance	*E faecium, S aureus, K pneumoniae, P aeruginosa, and E coli*	None	90%–94%/98%–100%	Can detect blood pathogens before growth Limited number of pathogens
T2Candida	T2 Resonance	*C albicans/C tropicalis, C glabrata/C krusei, and C parapsilosis*	None		Can detect yeast 73 h before standard blood cultures Strong NPV It would be difficult to detect mixed candidemia LOD is 1–3 CFU, which is higher than standard cultures (1 CFU/mL)

Data from Refs.[36–41,54]

populations. The limit of detection (LOD) is 1 to 3 CFU/mL, which is slightly higher than standard blood cultures (1 CFU/mL).[40] Giannella and colleagues[42] conducted a meta-analysis that showed a shorter time to species identification by 72 hours, shorter length of stay for intensive care unit and hospital, but did not show a decrease in mortality.

MENINGITIS/ENCEPHALITIS SYNDROMIC PANEL

The FilmArray Meningitis/Encephalitis (ME) Panel (BioFire; BioMerieux, Salt Lake City, UT, USA) is the only commercial FDA-approved ME panel available. This assay has decreased sensitivity for *Cryptococcus* spp, HSV-1, *Listeria monocytogenes*, *Haemophilus influenzae*, and *E coli*.[31] Detection of *Cryptococcus* spp may be particularly problematic in transplant patients owing to the antifungal properties of calcineurin inhibitors.[43] Currently, the manufacturer of the Biofire ME panel states that cryptococcal antigen (CrAg) and fungal culture are the tests of choice in early cryptococcal meningitis.[44] However, CrAg persists in CSF and is less useful in diagnosing relapse or recurrent infection. Although CrAG titers are poor predictors of recurrent or relapsing infection, significant increases in titers can support recurrent infection. Although multiplex and targeted PCR assays typically have lower sensitivities compared with CrAG, they may have increased clinical utility in these particular situations. Clinicians should also be aware that this assay excludes EBV, JCV, *Mycobacterium tuberculosis*, and *Toxoplasma gondii*.[45] Furthermore, this assay cannot differentiate between an acute or latent viral infection. This is especially true for HHV-6.[45,46] This assay does not generate any information about antimicrobial susceptibility, and the number of pathogens detected is limited. For these reasons, this assay is an important adjunct test in SOT patients but should not be used exclusively for diagnosing meningitis or encephalitis.

UPPER RESPIRATORY PANELS

Currently, there are 4 FDA-approved upper respiratory multiplex panels (Luminex NxTAG RPP, Verigene Nanosphere RP Flex, GenMark eSensor XT-8, ePlex RP2, and the Biofire Film Array RP2.1). Characteristics of these assays are listed in **Table 4**. All of these assays report high sensitivity and specificity. However, these panels lack targets for most common causes of bacterial CAP and do not provide any information about resistance genes. These assays are most useful for detection of viral pathogens.

LOWER RESPIRATORY PANELS

The FilmArray pneumonia panel (FilmArray PP; BioFire Diagnostics, Salt Lake City, UT, USA) is an FDA-approved multiplex panel for sputum, endotracheal, and BAL specimens. One study evaluated the performance in 59 specimens from patients with lower respiratory tract infections compared with standard diagnostic methods.[47] Overall agreement of the FilmArray with standard methods was 79%. FilmArray detected *Legionella pneumophilia* in 2 specimens that were not detected by culture and serology. In addition, it should be noted that there were substantial discrepancies in detection of antimicrobial resistance genes.

The Unyvero LRT panel (OpGen) is the only FDA-cleared molecular diagnostic for *Pneumocystis jirovecii*. It also detects 19 bacterial species and 10 resistance markers. A large multicenter study[48] comparing concordance with bacterial cultures from 1408 specimens reported overall positive and negative percent agreement was 93.4% and

Table 4
Respiratory syndromic panels available in the United States

Assay Name	Upper/Lower Respiratory	Targets
BioFire RP 2.1 Panela and RP 2.1 EZ (BioFire Diagnostics)[55]	Upper	Adenovirus, Coronavirus (229E, HKU1, NL63, OC43), SARS-CoV-2, Human Metapneumovirus, Human Rhinovirus/Enterovirus, Influenza A (A/H1, A/H3, A/H1-2009), Influenza B, Parainfluenza 1, 2, 3, 4, RSV, Bordetella parapertussis, Bordetella pertussis, Chlamydia pneumoniae, Mycoplasma pneumoniae
NxTAG Respiratory Pathogen Panel (Luminex)[57]	Upper	RSV type A and B, influenza A variants, influenza A H1 and H3, influenza B, parainfluenza 1, 2, 3, and 4, metapneumovirus, adenovirus, rhinovirus/enterovirus, coronavirus type HKU1, NL63, 229E, OC43, human bocavirus, C pneumoniae, and M pneumoniae
ePlex RP panel and RP2 Panel (GenMark Diagnostics)[56]	Upper	Adenovirus, Coronavirus (229E, HKU1, NL63, OC43), SARS-CoV-2, Metapneumovirus, Rhinovirus/Enterovirus, Influenza A, Influenza A H1, Influenza A H1-2009, Influenza A H3, RSV A, RSV B, C pneumoniae, M pneumoniae, Influenza B, Parainfluenza 1, 2, 3, 4
Verigene nanosphere RP Flex (Luminex)[58]	Upper	Adenovirus, Human metapneumovirus, Influenza A, Influenza A (subtypes H1, H3), Influenza B, Parainfluenza 1, 2, 3, 4, Rhinovirus, RSVA/B, B pertussis, B parapertussis, Bordetella bronchiseptica, Bordetella holmesii
BioFire Pneumonia Panel (BioFire Diagnostics)[56]	Lower	Acinetobacter calcoaceticus–baumannii complex, Enterobacter cloacae complex, E coli, H influenzae, Klebsiella aerogenes, Klebsiella oxytoca, K pneumoniae group, Pseudomonas aeruginosa, Serratia marcescens, S aureus, Streptococcus agalactiae, Streptococcus pneumoniae, Streptococcus pyogenes, C pneumoniae, L pneumophila, Mycoplasma pneumoniae, Adenovirus, coronavirus, Human metapneumovirus, Human rhinovirus/enterovirus, Influenza A, Influenza B, Parainfluenza virus, RSV, IMP, KPC, NDM, OXA-48-like, VIM, CTX-M, MecA/C, MREJ
Unyvero Lower Respiratory tract panel (OpGen)	Lower	Acinetobacter spp, C pneumoniae, Citrobacter freundii, E cloacae complex, E coli, H influenzae, Klebsiella oxytoca, Klebsiella varicola, Klebsiella pneumophila, Moraxella catarrhalis, Morganella morganii, Mycoplasma pneumoniae, P jirovecii, Proteus spp, P aeruginosa, S marcescens, S aureus, S maltophilia, S pneumoniae, KPC, NDM, Oxa-23, Oxa-24, Oxa-48, Oxa-58, VIM, CTX-M, mecA, TEM

Data from Refs.[55–58]

98.3%, respectively. There were 25 specimens that were positive for *P jirovecii*, and the positive predictive agreement (PPA) compared with standard of care methods (indirect flourescent assay [IFA], direct flourescent assay [DFA], PCR) was 87.5%. Concordance with standard-of-care antimicrobial susceptibility testing was relatively high at 85% (86/101). Another smaller study[49] (175 BALF specimens) showed a phenotypic concordance of antimicrobial susceptibility of 79%.

GASTROINTESTINAL MULTIPLEX PANELS

Currently there are 8 FDA-approved syndromic GI panels. These panels are useful for initial workup of gastroenteritis. However, some infections that are relevant in SOT (ADV other than ADV40/42, and so forth) are not available targets. In addition, the panels have a high rate of false positives in immunocompromised patients without GI symptoms. There have been several pseudo-outbreaks of Salmonella, *Entamoeba histolytica*, noncholera Vibrio species, and *Yersinia enterocolitica* caused by false positive results.[50] Some of these pseudo-outbreaks were among hospitalized and symptomatic immunocompromised patients. Other studies have shown false positives for *Salmonella* spp (lack of interassay agreement) with the Luminex xTAG GPP assay when compared with other multiplex assays.[51] False positive results can be particularly problematic for SOT patients given that an incorrect diagnosis of gastroenteritis may delay treatment of the primary disease and expose patients to unnecessary antibiotics.

In certain SOT patients, the cause of diarrhea can have a broad differential (ie, small bowel transplant patients).[52] One study showed that GI panels can increase the diagnostic yield of infectious causes of diarrhea among hematopoietic cell transplantation patients. Helping to distinguish between infectious and noninfectious causes of diarrhea may be particularly useful in small bowel transplant recipients when determining between infectious (viral gastroenteritis, *Clostridioides difficile*, norovirus, and so forth) and noninfectious (graft-versus-host disease, rejection, medication) causes of diarrhea. Given the high sensitivity of these assays and potential for false positive results (discussed above), further studies evaluating the utility and safety of using GI panels to distinguish between infectious and noninfectious causes would be useful.

These assays are an excellent adjunct to patient care, but clinicians should interpret results with caution when rare pathogens are detected and should not use these assays for screening asymptomatic patients.[53]

SUMMARY

When considering advanced molecular assays, clinicians should work with their clinical microbiology laboratory and Infectious Diseases specialists to assess optimal approaches to diagnosis and interpretation, with an eye toward diagnostic stewardship (see **Table 1** for a list of recommendations) to avoid waste of resources and potential harm through unnecessary or inappropriate testing. When clinicians are considering using mNGS especially, careful assessment of the clinical scenario, anatomic location or locations of potential specimens, and selection of routine testing up front is critical. Microbial cfDNA from plasma performs well for endovascular infections. It is less sensitive for deep-seated nonendovascular infections but may be an important adjunct for culture negative infections or when obtaining a specimen is contraindicated. Metagenomic NGS of CSF should not replace standard diagnostics but may be a useful adjunct when a rare pathogen is suspected or when traditional diagnostics do not yield a diagnosis. BRPCR is typically less sensitive than targeted PCR but detects a larger spectrum of organisms. BRPCR performs better in invasively collected specimens and performs poorly on blood and respiratory specimens. Syndromic panels are useful adjunct tests but cannot replace conventional diagnostic modalities, such as bacterial and fungal cultures. Clinicians should not use these panels for screening and should confirm any unexpected results with orthogonal tests.

CLINICS CARE POINTS

- Molecular diagnostics for bacteria and fungi cannot replace routine testing, including culture with susceptibility.

- Metagenomic next-generation sequencing of cerebrospinal fluid may be a useful adjunct for rare central nervous system infections or when routine testing is negative and the clinical suspicion for infection remains high.

- The microbial cell-free DNA test performs well for endovascular infections. It is less sensitive for deep-seated infections and does not include RNA viruses.

- Broad-range polymerase chain reaction has the most clinical impact for invasively collected tissue or sinus specimens. It does not perform well for blood or respiratory samples.

- Syndromic panels are widely available, relatively rapid, and highly sensitive.

- As with all diagnostic tests, caution should be used when molecular results do not fit the clinical picture.

REFERENCES

1. Lee R. Metagenomic next generation sequencing: How does it work and it is coming to your clinical microbiology lab? Nov 4, 2019. Available at: https://asm.org. Accessed September 14, 2022.
2. Schlaberg R, Chiu CY, Miller S, et al. Validation of metagenomic next–generation sequencing tests for universal pathogen detection. Arch Pathol Lab Med 2017; 141:776–86.
3. Miao Q, Ma Y, Wang Q, et al. Microbiological Diagnostic Performance of Metagenomic Next-generation Sequencing When Applied to Clinical Practice. Clin Infect Dis 2018;67(suppl_2):S231–40.
4. Flurin L, Wolf MJ, Mutchler MM, et al. Targeted Metagenomic Sequencing-based Approach Applied to 2146 Tissue and Body Fluid Samples in Routine Clinical Practice. Clin Infect Dis 2022;75(10):1800–8.
5. Simner PJ, Miller S, Carroll KC. Understanding the promises and hurdles of metagenomics next-generation sequencing as a diagnostic tool for infectious diseases. Clin Infect Dis 2018;66:778–88.
6. Miller S, Chiu C, Rodino KG, et al. Point-Counterpoint: Should We Be Performing Metagenomic Next-Generation Sequencing for Infectious Disease Diagnosis in the Clinical Laboratory? J Clin Microbiol 2020;58(3). 017399-e1819.
7. Sichtig H, Minogue T, Yan Yi, et al. FDA-ARGOS is a database with public quality-controlled reference genomes for diagnostic use and regulatory science. Nat Commun 2019;3313.
8. Blauwkamp TA, Thair S, Rosen MJ, et al. Analytical and clinical validation of a microbial cell-free DNA sequencing test for infectious disease. Nat Microbiol 2019; 4(4):663–74.
9. Lee RA, Al Dhaheri F, Pollock NR, et al. Assessment of the Clinical Utility of Plasma Metagenomic Next-Generation Sequencing in a Pediatric Hospital Population. J Clin Microbiol 2020;58(7):e00419–20.

10. Eichenberger EM, Degner N, Scott ER, et al. Microbial Cell-Free DNA Identifies the Causative Pathogen in Infective Endocarditis and Remains Detectable Longer Than Conventional Blood Culture in Patients with Prior Antibiotic Therapy. Clin Infect Dis 2022;ciac426. https://doi.org/10.1093/cid/ciac426.

11. Eichenberger EM, de Vries CR, Ruffin F, et al. Microbial Cell-Free DNA Identifies Etiology of Bloodstream Infections, Persists Longer Than Conventional Blood Cultures, and Its Duration of Detection Is Associated With Metastatic Infection in Patients With Staphylococcus aureus and Gram-Negative Bacteremia. Clin Infect Dis 2022;74(11):2020–7.

12. Hong DK, Blauwkamp TA, Kertesz M, et al. Liquid biopsy for infectious diseases: sequencing of cell-free plasma to detect pathogen DNA in patients with invasive fungal disease. Diagn Microbiol Infect Dis 2018;92(3):210–3.

13. Hill JA, Dalai SC, Hong DK, et al. Liquid Biopsy for Invasive Mold Infections in Hematopoietic Cell Transplant Recipients With Pneumonia Through Next-Generation Sequencing of Microbial Cell-Free DNA in Plasma. Clin Infect Dis 2021;73(11): e3876–83.

14. Shishido AA, Vostal A, Mayer R, et al. Diagnosis of central nervous system invasive aspergillosis in a liver transplant recipient using microbial cell-free next generation DNA sequencing. Transpl Infect Dis 2021;23(4):e13592.

15. Arrighi-Allisan AE, Vidaurrazaga MM, De Chavez VB, et al. Utility of liquid biopsy in diagnosing isolated cerebral phaeohyphomycosis: illustrative case. J Neurosurg Case Lessons 2022;3(5):CASE21557.

16. Vadhan JD, Melo AJ, Shogan JC, et al. Fast and Fusariosis: a systematic review and case report of a rapidly fatal central nervous system infection. Journal of Emerg Crit Care Med 2022. https://doi.org/10.21037/jeccm-21-125.

17. Hogan CA, Yang S, Garner OB, et al. Clinical Impact of Metagenomic Next-Generation Sequencing of Plasma Cell-Free DNA for the Diagnosis of Infectious Diseases: A Multicenter Retrospective Cohort Study. Clin Infect Dis 2021;72(2): 239–45.

18. Shishido AA, Noe M, Saharia K, et al. Clinical impact of a metagenomic microbial plasma cell-free DNA next-generation sequencing assay on treatment decisions: a single-center retrospective study. BMC Infect Dis 2022;22(1):372.

19. Wilson MR, Sample HA, Zorn KC, et al. Clinical Metagenomic Sequencing for Diagnosis of Meningitis and Encephalitis. N Engl J Med 2019;380(24):2327–40.

20. Debiasi RL, Tyler KL. Molecular methods for diagnosis of viral encephalitis. Clin Microbiol Rev 2004;17(4):903–25.

21. Miller S, Naccache SN, Samayoa E, et al. Laboratory validation of a clinical metagenomic sequencing assay for pathogen detection in cerebrospinal fluid. Genome Res 2019;29(5):831–42.

22. Piantadosi A, Mukerji SS, Ye S, et al. Enhanced Virus Detection and Metagenomic Sequencing in Patients with Meningitis and Encephalitis. mBio 2021;12(4): e0114321.

23. Shoskes A, Hassett C, Dani D, et al. Pearls & Oy-sters: Seronegative Eastern Equine Encephalitis in an Immunocompromised Stem Cell Transplant Recipient. Neurology 2022;99(22):1004–7.

24. Tschumi F, Schmutz S, Kufner V, et al. Meningitis and epididymitis caused by Toscana virus infection imported to Switzerland diagnosed by metagenomic sequencing: a case report. BMC Infect Dis 2019;19:591.

25. Kufner V, Plate A, Schmutz S, et al. Two Years of Viral Metagenomics in a Tertiary Diagnostics Unit: Evaluation of the First 105 Cases. Genes 2019;10(9):661.

26. Carpenter ML, Tan SK, Watson T, et al. Metagenomic Next-Generation Sequencing for Identification and Quantitation of Transplant-Related DNA Viruses. J Clin Microbiol 2019;57(12):e01113–9.

27. Sam SS, Rogers R, Gillani FS, et al. Evaluation of a Next-Generation Sequencing Metagenomics Assay to Detect and Quantify DNA Viruses in Plasma from Transplant Recipients. J Mol Diagn 2021;23(6):719–31.

28. Chen H, Yin Y, Gao H, et al. Clinical Utility of In-house Metagenomic Next-generation Sequencing for the Diagnosis of Lower Respiratory Tract Infections and Analysis of the Host Immune Response. Clin Infect Dis 2020;71(Suppl 4): S416–26.

29. Langelier C, Kalantar KL, Moazed F, et al. Integrating host response and unbiased microbe detection for lower respiratory tract infection diagnosis in critically ill adults. Proc Natl Acad Sci U S A 2018;115(52):E12353–62.

30. Ramachandran PS, Ramesh A, Creswell FV, et al. Integrating central nervous system metagenomics and host response for diagnosis of tuberculosis meningitis and its mimics. Nat Commun 2022;13(1):1675.

31. Azar MM, Turbett S, Gaston D, et al. A consensus conference to define the utility of advanced infectious disease diagnostics in solid organ transplant recipients. Am J Transplant 2022;22(12):3150–69.

32. Lieberman JA, Bryan A, Mays JA, et al. High Clinical Impact of Broad-Range Fungal PCR in Suspected Fungal Sinusitis. J Clin Microbiol 2021;59(11): e0095521.

33. Tkadlec J, Peckova M, Sramkova L, et al. The use of broad-range bacterial PCR in the diagnosis of infectious diseases: a prospective cohort study. Clin Microbiol Infect 2019;25(6):747–52.

34. Naureckas Li C, Nakamura MM. Utility of Broad-Range PCR Sequencing for Infectious Diseases Clinical Decision Making: a Pediatric Center Experience. J Clin Microbiol 2022;60(5):e0243721.

35. Fida M, Wolf MJ, Hamdi A, et al. Detection of Pathogenic Bacteria From Septic Patients Using 16S Ribosomal RNA Gene-Targeted Metagenomic Sequencing. Clin Infect Dis 2021;73(7):1165–72.

36. Sparks R, Balgahom R, Janto C, et al. Evaluation of the BioFire Blood Culture Identification 2 panel and impact on patient management and antimicrobial stewardship. Pathology 2021;53(7):889–95.

37. Peri AM, Ling W, Furuya-Kanamori L, et al. Performance of BioFire Blood Culture Identification 2 Panel (BCID2) for the detection of bloodstream pathogens and their associated resistance markers: a systematic review and meta-analysis of diagnostic test accuracy studies. BMC Infect Dis 2022;22(1):794.

38. Lutgring JD, Bittencourt C, McElvania TeKippe E, et al. Evaluation of the Accelerate Pheno System: Results from Two Academic Medical Centers. J Clin Microbiol 2018;56(4). 016722-e1717.

39. Drevinek P, Hurych J, Antuskova M, et al. Direct detection of ESKAPEc pathogens from whole blood using the T2Bacteria Panel allows early antimicrobial stewardship intervention in patients with sepsis. Microbiology Open Access 2021;10(3): e1210.

40. Nguyen MH, Clancy CJ, Pasculle AW, et al. Performance of the T2Bacteria Panel for Diagnosing Bloodstream Infections: A Diagnostic Accuracy Study. Ann Intern Med 2019;170(12):845–52.

41. Monday LM, Parraga Acosta T, Alangaden G. T2Candida for the Diagnosis and Management of Invasive *Candida* Infections. Journal of Fungi 2021;7(3):178.

42. Giannella M, Pankey GA, Pascale R, et al. Antimicrobial and resource utilization with T2 magnetic resonance for rapid diagnosis of bloodstream infections: systematic review with meta-analysis of controlled studies. Expert Rev Med Devices 2021;18(5):473–82.

43. Blankenship JR, Singh N, Alexander BD, et al. Cryptococcus neoformans isolates from transplant recipients are not selected for resistance to calcineurin inhibitors by current immunosuppressive regimens. J Clin Microbiol 2005;43(1):464–7.

44. O'Halloran JA, Franklin A, Lainhart W, et al. Pitfalls Associated With the Use of Molecular Diagnostic Panels in the Diagnosis of Cryptococcal Meningitis. Open Forum Infect Dis 2017;4(4):ofx242.

45. Farmakiotis D, Kontoyiannia DP. Emerging issues with diagnosis and management of fungal infections in solid organ transplant recipients. Am J Transplant 2015;15(5):1141–7.

46. Pandey U, Greninger AL, Levin GR, et al. Pathogen or bystander: Clinical significance of detecting human herpesvirus 6 in pediatric cerebrospinal fluid. J Clin Microbiol 2020;58(5):e00313–20.

47. Lee SH, Ruan SY, Pan SC, et al. Performance of a multiplex PCR pneumonia panel for the identification of respiratory pathogens and the main determinants of resistance from the lower respiratory tract specimens of adult patients in intensive care units. J Microbiol Immunol Infect 2019;52(6):920–8.

48. Collins ME, Popowitch EB, Miller MB. Evaluation of a Novel Multiplex PCR Panel Compared to Quantitative Bacterial Culture for Diagnosis of Lower Respiratory Tract Infections. J Clin Microbiol 2020;58(5):e02013–9.

49. Klein M, Bacher J, Barth S, et al. Multicenter Evaluation of the Unyvero Platform for Testing Bronchoalveolar Lavage Fluid. J Clin Microbiol 2021;59(3). 024977-e2520.

50. Robilotti E, Powell E, Usiak S, et al. The Perils of Multiplex Gastrointestinal Pathogen Panels: Pseudo-outbreaks of Salmonellae and Entamoeba histolytica in Immunocompromised Hosts. Infect Control Hosp Epidemiol 2018;39(7):867–70.

51. Yoo J, Park J, Lee HK, et al. Comparative Evaluation of Seegene Allplex Gastrointestinal, Luminex xTAG Gastrointestinal Pathogen Panel, and BD MAX Enteric Assays for Detection of Gastrointestinal Pathogens in Clinical Stool Specimens. Arch Pathol Lab Med 2019;143(8):999–1005.

52. Rogers WS, Westblade LF, Soave R, et al. Impact of a Multiplexed Polymerase Chain Reaction Panel on Identifying Diarrheal Pathogens in Hematopoietic Cell Transplant Recipients. Clin Infect Dis 2020;71(7):1693–700.

53. Hitchcock MM, Hogan CA, Budvytiene I, et al. Reproducibility of positive results for rare pathogens on the FilmArray GI Panel. Diagn Microbiol Infect Dis 2019; 95(1):10–4.

54. Rebecca Y, 2021. The genotype-to-phenotype dilemma: how should laboratories approach discordant susceptibility results? J Clin Microbiol, Vol. 59, No. 6.

55. The BioFire® FilmArray® Respiratory Panels (RP & RP2). BioFire Diagnostics. Published 2018. Available at: https://www.biofiredx.com/products/the-filmarray-panels/filmarrayrp/.

56. Respiratory Pathogen Panels | GenMark Diagnostics. Available at: www.genmarkdx.com. https://www.genmarkdx.com/panels/eplex-panels/respiratory-pathogen-panel/.

57. VERIGENE® Respiratory Pathogens Flex Test (RP Flex). Luminex EMEA/India. Available at: https://www.luminexcorp.com/eu/respiratory-pathogens-flex-test/#overview.

58. The BioFire® FilmArray® Pneumonia Panel. BioFire Diagnostics. Available at: https://www.biofiredx.com/products/the-filmarray-panels/filmarray-pneumonia/.

Antimicrobial Resistance in Organ Transplant Recipients

Maddalena Giannella, MD, PhD[a,b,*], Matteo Rinaldi, MD[a,b],
Pierluigi Viale, MD[a,b]

KEYWORDS

- Multidrug-resistant bacteria • Difficult to treat bacteria • Prevention • Surveillance
- Antibiotic prophylaxis • Early treatment • Graft failure • Mortality

KEY POINTS

- Solid organ transplant (SOT) candidates and recipients are highly susceptible to acquire multidrug-resistant organism (MDRO) colonization and/or infection with a significant impact on graft/patient survival.
- Optimal management of the MDRO burden in SOT patients should consist in individualized preventive strategies, fully integrated with infection control and antimicrobial stewardship activities with the goals of improving patient outcome and to minimize environmental damage.
- Infection control and antimicrobial stewardship activities (ie, surveillance screening for MDRO colonization, local guidelines for the management of main infectious syndromes, and/or perioperative antibiotic prophylaxis, implementation of rapid diagnostics to improve the time to appropriate therapy) should be adapted to the context of SOT according to local epidemiology.
- In this framework, patient risk stratification tools and rapid diagnostic tests may be useful in improving therapeutic management of MDRO in SOT population.

INTRODUCTION

In 2017, World health organization (WHO) released a list of 12 bacteria requiring new antibiotic treatments and classified as responsible of severe infections with high mortality rates. *Acinetobacter baumannii*, *Pseudomonas aeruginosa*, and Enterobacterales were identified as critical threats, whereas *Staphylococcus aureus* and *Enterococcus faecium* were considered as high priority. This global warning was due to a progressive widespread pattern of resistance in such bacteria, impacting

[a] Infectious Diseases, IRCCS Azienda Ospedaliero-Universitaria di Bologna, Bologna, Italy;
[b] Department of Medical and Surgical Sciences, Alma Mater Studiorum University of Bologna, Via Massarenti 11, Bologna 40137, Italy
* Corresponding author. Department of Medical and Surgical Sciences, University of Bologna, Via Massarenti 11, Bologna 40137, Italy.
E-mail address: maddalena.giannella@unibo.it

Infect Dis Clin N Am 37 (2023) 515–537
https://doi.org/10.1016/j.idc.2023.04.001
0891-5520/23/© 2023 Elsevier Inc. All rights reserved.

patient survival mainly among vulnerable populations. Indeed, multidrug-resistant organisms (MDRO) have a dramatic impact in solid organ transplant (SOT) recipients.

This review focuses on the most clinically relevant pathogens, such as methicillin-resistant *S aureus* (MRSA), vancomycin-resistant enterococci (VRE), extended-spectrum β-lactamase producing or extended-spectrum cephalosporin-resistant Enterobacterales (ESBL or ESCR-E), and carbapenem-resistant or carbapenemase-producing Enterobacterales (CRE or CPE), multidrug-resistant (MDR) *P aeruginosa*, and carbapenem-resistant *A baumannii* (CR-AB).

EPIDEMIOLOGY

Colonization and incidence rates of MDRO infections depend on local epidemiology, host factors, and selective pressure from antibiotic exposure. In SOT, the type of organ is a major determinant of the type of infection and associated pathogens, influencing the burden of specific MDR bacteria in each graft setting (**Table 1**). Indeed, cutaneous and/or upper respiratory colonizing bacteria such as *S aureus* and *P aeruginosa* more frequently cause infections in patients after heart and/or lung transplantation, whereas organisms colonizing gut microbiota such as enterococci and Enterobacterales more frequently cause infections after liver and/or kidney transplantation.

Regarding timeline, infections with MDR bacteria have traditionally been considered to most frequently occur within the early period (1–2 months) after SOT. However, recent studies have shown that the prevalence of bacterial infection remains high even later (>6 months) after SOT.[1,2] A recent report from the Swiss Transplant Cohort[1] including 2761 adult recipients (kidney 58%, liver 21%, lung 10%, heart 8%, and kidney-pancreas 3%), enrolled between 2008 and 2014, underlined that bacteria was responsible for 63% of post-SOT infections prevailing throughout the year with a predominance of Enterobacterales (54%), *Enterococcus* spp (20%), and *P aeruginosa* (9%). Owing to rising rates of antibiotic resistance among these pathogens, the investigators emphasized the need for new preventive strategies.

Deep surgical site infections (SSIs), lower respiratory tract infections (LRTIs), and central venous catheter bloodstream infections due to MDROs are relevant in all types of SOT. In the kidney transplant (KT) setting, the management of urinary tract infections (UTIs) due to MDRO can be challenging. In particular, uncertainties and heterogeneity exist in the approach to asymptomatic bacteriuria when MDROs are isolated.[3]

The incidence/prevalence of, the risk factors for, and the impact on clinical outcome of overall MDRO and of each clinically relevant MDR bacteria are summarized in **Table 1**.

Donor-Derived Multidrug-Resistant Organism Infections

The risk of bacterial transmission from donor to recipients is related to the presence of bloodstream infection and/or bacterial isolation at the graft level (eg, from urine in KT, from lower respiratory sample in lung transplant [Lu-T]).[4] A 2012 nationwide study investigated the rate of carbapenem-resistant gram-negative bacteria (CR-GNB) isolation in brain-dead donors from 190 Italian intensive care units (ICUs) over 4-month period. In one-third of donors a GNB was isolated from blood, urine, and/or lower respiratory tract (LRT) and 15% were CR-GNB. Such information was available and communicated before transplantation in only 15% of cases. Risk factors for isolation of CR-GNB included age less than 60 years, ICU stay $\geq$ 4 days, fever, and local epidemiology.[5]

When an MDRO is recognized in the donor, early management of the recipient is necessary to reduce the risk of infection, graft impairment, and mortality.[6,7] In fact,

Table 1
Incidence, risk factors, and outcome for multidrug-resistant organism infections in each type of solid organ transplant

Microorganism	Organ	Burden (Incidence/ Prevalence)	Risk Factors	Mortality	Outcome Graft Complications/loss
All MDRO	Liver	21.7%–25%	Hematoma, biloma, complicated intra-abdominal infection, cholangitis, and recurrent biliary infection	38.6%	NA
	Kidney	8.4%	Recurrent urinary tract infection Renal cyst infection Surgical site infection Peri-graft infected hematoma	NA	NA
	Lung	NA	Previous recipient-related colonization, previous exposure to broad-spectrum antibiotics, tracheostomy, ICU stay >14 d	NA	NA
	Heart	29.7%–37%	Deep surgical site infection, hospital-acquired pneumonia, diabetes, antibiotic treatment within 1 mo before transplant	30-d 14.3%	Early graft failure 21.4%
MRSA	Liver	4%–7.3%	Preoperative nasal carriage, alcoholic cirrhosis, decreased prothrombin ratio	0%–21%	0%
	Kidney	1.25%–1.9%	Preoperative nasal carriage, steroid treatment during the previous 4 wk	30-d 10%	10%
	Lung	14.8%–35%; 26% of early-onset pneumonia	Preoperative nasal carriage, mechanical ventilation for > 5 d	30-d 10%–17.6%	Acute rejection 13%–37% Chronic rejection 23%
	Heart	6.2%–38%	Preoperative nasal carriage	NA	NA

(continued on next page)

Table 1
(continued)

Microorganism	Organ	Burden (Incidence/Prevalence)	Risk Factors	Outcome	
				Mortality	Graft Complications/loss
VRE	Liver	0%–16%	Immunosuppression, antibiotic exposure, indwelling catheters, manipulation of the gastrointestinal tract, ERCP, anti-anaerobic antibiotics, reoperation	30-d: 9%–54% 1-y: 56%–80%	Rejection 20%
	Kidney	0%–13.6%	Continuous ambulatory peritoneal dialysis, vancomycin use	NA	NA
	Lung	0%–19%	Renal failure, diabetes	NA	NA
	Heart	0.8%–7%	Renal failure, diabetes	NA	NA
ESBL/ESCR-E	Liver	8%–13.2%	Previous 3 GC exposure, pretransplant colonization, prolonged tracheal intubation, long-term hospitalization, posttransplant renal replacement therapy, acute rejection, MELD $\geq$ 25, preoperative spontaneous bacterial peritonitis prophylaxis	2.6%	NA
	Kidney	26%–45%	Urinary tract obstruction and instrumentation, kidney-pancreas transplantation, recurrent urinary tract infection	2.9%–6.7%	NA
	Lung	2%–20.5%	Previous antibiotic exposure, pretransplant colonization, prolonged tracheal intubation	In-hospital: 18%–27%	NA
	Heart	5%–14.2%	Previous antibiotic exposure, pretransplant colonization, prolonged tracheal intubation	NA	NA

Organism	Organ	%	Risk factors	Mortality	Outcome
CRE/CPE	Liver	1%–16%	CRE carriage before/after transplant, high-MELD score, multiorgan transplant, reintervention, AKI or RRT, prolonged mechanical ventilation, graft rejection	45%–58%	NA
	Kidney	1%–11%	Ureteral stent, pretransplant CR-KP infection/colonization	28%	NA
	Lung	1%–8.1%	Length of hospital stay, deceased donor allograft, diabetes mellitus	30-d 36%, 1-y 64%	Re-transplantation 18.2%
	Heart	0.4%–6%	Carbapenem exposure, pretransplant CR-KP infection/colonization	NA	NA
CR-AB	Liver	2.2%–10.5%	Length of posttransplant ICU stay	30-d: 28.6%–66.7%	NA
	Kidney	1.1%–4.3%	NA	30-d: 12.5%–40.8%	66.7% graft loss
	Lung	NA	High blood urea nitrogen before LT, long duration of surgery, hypoalbuminemia	30-d: 5.9%, 90-d: 19.6%, 1-y: 66.7%	NA
	Heart	1.9%–3.1%	NA	30-d: 13%	NA
MDR P aeruginosa	Liver	0.3%–7.2%	Prior transplantation or ICU admission, nosocomial acquisition, septic shock	30-d: 30%	NA
	Kidney	0.9%	NA	NA	NA
	Lung	NA	Previous recipient-related colonization, empirical exposure to broad-spectrum antibiotics	NA	BOS in 22.7% of colonized Lu-T
	Heart	0.8%	NA	NA	NA

Abbreviations: BOS, bronchiolitis obliterans syndrome; CR-AB, carbapenem-resistant A baumannii; CRE/CPE, carbapenem-resistant/producing Enterobacterales; ESBL/ESCR-E, extended-spectrum beta-lactamase Enterobacterales; MDRO, multidrug-resistant organisms; MDR-PA, multidrug-resistant P aeruginosa; MRSA methicillin-resistant S aureus; NA, not available; RRT, renal replacement therapy; VRE, vancomycin-resistant enterococci.

several reports highlighted the importance of an early communication and the effectiveness of an appropriate targeted therapy in preventing transmission of MDRO infection in the recipients.[4,8] A recent review evaluated all published cases of MDRO donor-derived infections (DDIs).[6] For MRSA bacteremic donors, a 70% risk of infection transmission in the recipients without a targeted perioperative prophylaxis was reported with an associated mortality rate of 14%.[6] Seventeen of 33 (52%) recipients receiving graft from donors with prior isolation of MDR-GNB (mostly CRE or CR-AB) developed MDR-GNB infection after SOT. In most of the described cases, information about donor cultures was acquired after transplant, so a targeted perioperative prophylaxis was not performed. Regarding outcome, 59% of infected recipients either died or suffered allograft loss.

APPROACH TO PREVENTION AND MANAGEMENT

MDRO infection management in SOT recipients is largely based on prevention strategies aimed at reducing the risk of infection, and its consequences on graft/patient survival, in the most vulnerable patients (eg, carriers), settings (eg, high endemic and/or outbreaks), and periods (eg, early posttransplant period and/or ICU stay). Active surveillance for each type of MDRO pathogen, targeted antibiotic perioperative prophylaxis, decolonization, and early-targeted treatment are potential preventive strategies that are reviewed in this section.

Active Surveillance

Active surveillance consists of superficial cultures performed in asymptomatic patients to exclude colonization with an MDRO. Sites to be cultured vary according to the specific MDRO (ie, nasal swab for MRSA, rectal swab for VRE, ESBL-E, and CRE). Sampling multiple sites (ie, throat, axilla, inguinal in addition to nasal and rectal swabs) may improve screening accuracy, mainly for pathogens as MDR *P aeruginosa* and CR-AB.[9] The timing of surveillance is not standardized. It is usually performed before transplant at the inclusion in waiting list, at regular intervals during stay in waiting list, and/or at the moment of surgery. Few studies have investigated a relationship between timing of acquisition MDRO colonization before SOT and the risk of developing MDRO infection after SOT. In a recent series of 60 CRE, carriers undergoing different types of SOT, closer pretransplant carriage acquisition (0.9 vs 4.2 months), along with liver transplant (LT) as the type of SOT, were significantly associated with higher rate of posttransplant CRE infection.[10] Postoperative screening during the hospital stay is also encouraged as it revealed that more than two-thirds of CRE colonization acquisitions were detected after LT in a large multinational study.[11] Finally, an important issue to be considered is the local epidemiology. Any change in screening procedures should follow a careful assessment of the local prevalence of a specific MDRO colonization and infection in patients undergoing a specific graft transplantation. Although a prevalence threshold is not clearly defined to recommend the implementation of screening procedures, it is reasonable to consider a prevalence $\geq$10% as a cutoff for implementation evaluation according to previous recommendation.[12] The targets of surveillance efforts include MRSA, VRE, and MDR gram negatives, and surveillance efforts can be used to inform cohorting/infection control interventions and individual preventive strategies.

Methicillin-Resistant S aureus

As for MDR-gram-positive bacteria, current guidelines recommend active MRSA screening in centers with high prevalence or during outbreak settings.[13,14] However, in a study, Clancy and colleagues[15] using a computer simulation model to estimate the cost-effectiveness of routine *S aureus* screening and decolonization among lung and heart-Lu-T recipients showed that screening and decolonization were economically dominant for all scenarios tested, providing more cost savings and health benefits than no screening. The baseline rates of *S aureus* colonization and infection among carriers were 9.6% and 36.7%, respectively. Screening averted 6.7 *S aureus* infections (4.3 MRSA and 2.4 MSSA); 89 patients needed to be screened and decolonized to prevent one *S aureus* infection. Thus, some experts recommend careful consideration of MRSA screening in heart and Lu-T population.[16]

Vancomycin-Resistant Enterococci

Despite the strong correlation between VRE carriage and the risk of progression to VRE infection after SOT,[17,18] there are not specific indications about screening for VRE colonization in SOT candidates, and the approach varies across centers.[19,20]

Multidrug-Resistant Gram-Negative Bacteria

Three recent guidelines have addressed the issue of active screening for ESBL/ESCR-E, CRE/CPE, MDR *P aeruginosa*, and CR-AB in SOT (**Table 2**).[21–23] As for ESBL/ESCR-E, the American Society Transplantation (AST) guidelines consider screening necessary during outbreaks or periods of high prevalence to increase infection control activities,[22] whereas the European documents endorse ESBL/ESCR-E screening also to inform perioperative antibiotic prophylaxis and/or empirical treatment.[21,23] Such recommendation is principally based on six prospective studies evaluating abdominal surgery, three of them including LT recipients (LTRs).[24–29] Owing to a lack of evidence, the role of screening for ESBL-E in other types of SOT remains controversial and should be evaluated according to local epidemiology.[23] All available guidelines endorse active screening for CRE/CPE carriage in LTRs mainly in centers with high prevalence.[21–23] Such recommendation is based on several studies highlighting the relationship between CRE colonization at LT and increased risk of CRE infection in the posttransplant period with a significant impact on graft survival and mortality.[9,30–32] In other types of SOT, current guidelines consider good clinical practice (GCP) to perform an active screening before surgery, according to local epidemiology.[23] Few data are available regarding the effectiveness of multidrug-resistant *P aeruginosa* (MDR-PA) screening in SOT recipients. Major concerns raise from colonized Lu-T recipients, in which MDR-PA infection is associated with bronchiolitis obliterans syndrome development, the principal limitation for long-term survival after transplantation.[33] Although active screening through respiratory, rectal and urinary swab sampling may lead to earlier detection of carriers, a retrospective study failed to demonstrate an improvement in term of infection rates with carbapenem-resistant *P aeruginosa* before and after the implementation of screening measures, associated with contact isolation and cohorting of positive patients.[34] Thus, guidelines do not recommend an active screening of MDR-PA colonization. Such practice should be evaluated case-by-case, especially in Lu-T showing risk factors for severe MDR-PA infection as previous transplantation, history of nosocomial infection, and/or septic shock, previous ICU admission.[35–38] Considering that CR-AB has been identified in contaminated equipment or fomites of patients, leading to in-hospital outbreaks, an active surveillance should be used in settings with increased incidence.[22,39] In this context, European guidelines consider GCP to perform an active surveillance for CR-AB in all types of SOT.[23] Well-designed studies focusing on this topic are lacking, but two different studies conducted in LTRs showed a significant association between CR-AB colonization at transplantation and subsequent infection.[31,40] Therefore,

Table 2
Main recommendation statements for management of gram-negative colonization in solid organ transplant recipients

	GESITRA (2018)[21]	AST (2019)[22]	ESCMID (2022)[23]
ESBL-E/ESCR-E			
Screening	Yes	Controversial outside outbreaks	Yes in LT (conditional, low) GCP in all SOT[a] (expert opinion)
Targeted antibiotic prophylaxis	Yes, but avoid carbapenems	Undefined	Yes in LT (conditional, very low) GCP in all SOT[a] (expert opinion)
Decolonization	No	No	NA[b]
CRE/CPE			
Screening	Yes	Yes	Yes in LT (conditional, low) GCP in all SOT[a] (expert opinion)
Targeted antibiotic prophylaxis	No, but consider if high incidence of CPE SSI	Undefined	Insufficient evidence
Decolonization	No	No	NA[b]
MDR-PA			
Screening	No except in Lu-T recipients	NA	NA
Targeted antibiotic prophylaxis	No in non-Lu-T recipients	NA	NA
Decolonization	Nebulized antibiotics in Lu-T	NA	NA
CR-AB			
Screening	NA	In high-endemic settings or outbreak	Yes in LT[a] (conditional, low) GCP in all SOT[a] (expert opinion)
Targeted antibiotic prophylaxis	No	NA	Insufficient evidence
Decolonization	No	NA	NA

Abbreviations: CPE, carbapenem-resistant Enterobacterales; CR-AB, carbapenem-resistant *A baumannii*; ESBL-E, extended-spectrum Beta-lactamase Enterobacterales; GCP, good clinical practice; GESITRA, Group for the Study of Infection in Transplant Recipients; LT, liver transplant; Lu-T, lung transplant; MDR-PA, multidrug-resistant *P aeruginosa*; NA, not available; SOT, solid organ transplant.

[a] According to local epidemiology.
[b] Issue addressed in another ESCMID-EUCIC guideline.[91]

current guidelines conditionally recommend implementing active surveillance for CR-AB before LT according to local prevalence.[23]

Targeted Perioperative Antibiotic Prophylaxis

Targeted perioperative antibiotic prophylaxis (T-PAP) in MDRO carriers has been proposed as a strategy to reduce the risk of infection, especially SSIs, in the early post-transplant period. Similar to standard prophylaxis, T-PAP should be administered within 60 minutes before the incision (for fluoroquinolones and vancomycin, the infusion should be started 120 minutes before incision); intraoperative redosing may be necessary depending on the duration of the procedure, the half-life of the antibiotics used, and if significant blood loss during surgery occurs.[41] There is currently no formal consensus on standard PAP duration in transplant surgery due to a lack of comparative trials.[16] To minimize the risk of further resistance selection, in our opinion, T-PAP should not be prolonged more than the duration of standard PAP per each SOT type established at local level. In patients on treatment for an active well-controlled MDRO infection at the moment of transplant, this treatment should continue in the operating room and postoperatively as originally planned.[16]

Methicillin-resistant S aureus/vancomycin-resistant enterococci
Few data and no recommendation about T-PAP for MDR gram-positive bacteria are available, however, could be considered on a case by case basis known to be colonized.

Multidrug-resistant gram-negative bacteria
Recommendations exist for some MDR GNB, but these are based on low-quality evidence, are not endorsed by all professional societies, and are considered controversial. For example, AST guidelines do not recommend T-PAP for ESBL/ESCR-E colonization[42] and note potential for negative microbiologic impact secondary to carbapenem exposure.[22] In contrast, the European guidelines suggest the use of T-PAP in ESCR-E carriers with detection obtained within 1 month before transplant, possibly avoiding carbapenems if alternative molecules with in vitro activity against the colonizing ESCR-E are available.[21,23] This recommendation principally refers to LTRs and is based on the results from Logre and colleagues.[42] They analyzed 100 ESCR-E carriers undergoing LT in France, 35 developed a postoperative ESCR-E infection (11 SSIs, 10 UTIs, 9 pulmonary infections, and 5 sepses) at day 30. Only 68 patients could be assessed according to PAP, showing higher rates of ESCR-E postoperative infections among LTR receiving routine (7/11, 63%) compared with T-PAP (17/57, 30%) (P = .04). T-PAP included cefoxitin (40%), a carbapenem (31%), or piperacillin/tazobactam (29%). Although the results favored T-PAP, the quality of the study was low, with high risk of bias because of the retrospective nature, the limited sample size (with only 11 patients receiving routine prophylaxis), and the lack of outcome according to each regimen.

As for CRE/CPE and CR-AB, because the quality of published studies is low and the effectiveness of T-PAP remains unproven, current guidelines do not recommend for or against T-PAP in CRE/CPE and/or CR-AB carriers undergoing SOT.[21,23] In an 8-year retrospective study, after the first 4 years, standard PAP was implemented with amikacin in LTR at high risk for CR-GNB infection (colonization, exposure to antibiotics in the prior 30 days, model for end stage renal disease (MELD) >24, renal replacement therapy before LT).[31] The rate of SSIs caused by any CR-GNB (ie, Enterobacterales, *P aeruginosa, A baumannii*) decreased in the intervention period from 30% to 13%. However, in another study including different SOT, mainly LT, with a previous CRE colonization, T-PAP was more common in the group of patients who developed a

CRE infection after SOT.[10] In addition, a small single-center experience evaluating T-PAP versus standard PAP in seven LT pediatric recipients colonized with CRE observed a progressive restoration of gut microbiota in the standard group, meanwhile in the T-PAP (consisting in both intravenously and orally colistin-based regimens), group persistent dysbiosis was recorded even after 12 months of follow-up.[43]

Finally, colonization with MDR-PA is a concern in Lu-T candidates,[21] especially in those affected by cystic fibrosis where MDR-PA colonization could be as high as 75% and it has been associated with worse outcome.[44] Thus, in Lu-T, an extended T-PAP could be adopted awaiting donor and, if repeated, recipient culture results. There are no data to suggest an optimal duration of coverage, though most centers use at least 7 days of treatment postoperatively. This is based primarily on old reports of comparable outcomes among cystic fibrosis (CF) patients and non-CF patients when the CF patients were treated for 7 days based on their pretransplant cultures.[45]

Decolonization

Methicillin-resistant S aureus

The role of mupirocin for MRSA decolonization in SOT candidates remains controversial. A study conducted among LT candidates showed that decolonization procedures failed to prevent infection and almost 40% of decolonized carriers became recolonized.[46] Therefore, the long-term effectiveness of decolonization procedure in transplant candidates may be limited. However, the combination of active surveillance, decolonization with mupirocin, and the use of contact precautions was shown to significantly decrease MRSA infections and bacteremia during posttransplant hospital stay.[47] In addition, universal daily bathing with chlorhexidine 2% in hospitalized patients' pretransplant during the hospital stay; at the time of organ offer before going to the operating room and postoperatively, during the entire hospitalization is recommended to reduce colonization and infections with Gram-positive organisms including MRSA.[16]

Multidrug-resistant gram-negative bacteria

Several studies, including randomized trials, have evaluated the efficacy of a decolonization strategy in ESBL/ESCR-E or CRE/CPE carriers, especially in hematological and in ICU patients.[48–53] Although in some studies a reduction in infection rates has been reported, the long-term benefit of this intervention has yet to be defined[54] and selection of resistance is a concern.

In a multicenter randomized controlled trial conducted in Spain,[55] 768 SOT recipients were screened for MDR-Enterobacterales colonization (extended-spectrum β-lactamase or carbapenemase producing) before transplantation and +7 and + 14 days after transplantation; 105 were randomized 1:1 to receive oral treatment with colistin sulfate plus neomycin sulfate for 14 days (decolonization treatment [DT] group, $n = 53$) or no treatment (no DT [NDT] group, $n = 52$). No significant decrease in the risk of infection by MDR-E was observed in the DT group (9.4%, 5/53) compared with the NDT group (13.5%, 7/52) (relative risk 0.70; 95% confidence interval 0.24–2.08; p 0.517), but the number of events was small. Four patients (5.6%), three (5.6%) in the DT group and one (1.9%) in the NDT group, developed colistin resistance. Adverse events including diarrhea, skin rash, nausea, and vomiting were more common in the DT than NDT groups (27% vs 3.8%). Thus, as a net benefit in general and SOT population has not been determined, to date there is no evidence to support gut decolonization in SOT recipients colonized with MDR GNB.[27]

Airway colonization with CRE/CPE, MDR-PA, or CR-AB remains a significant issue after Lu-T. The efficacy of inhaled antibiotics, such as colistin or tobramycin, has been evaluated in small cohorts of non-SOT patients with discordant results.[56–60] As P

aeruginosa carriage in the immediate posttransplant period may lead to infection of the bronchial anastomosis and dehiscence of the suture, it is a common practice to prescribe nebulized antibiotics if such pathogen is isolated from respiratory secretions of an Lu-T recipient in the immediate posttransplant period. Conversely, inhaled antimicrobial therapy has not demonstrated any benefit in preventing infections caused by CR-AB in both colonized donors and Lu-T recipients.[21]

Preemptive Approach

As previous colonization is the main risk factor for MDRO infection in the posttransplant period, in the presence of signs/symptoms of infection, a prompt empirical treatment active against the colonizing strain is commonly adopted. In this regard, individual risk models and new rapid molecular tests may improve identification of patients at high risk and allows for early confirmation or exclusion of MDRO involvement at infection level optimizing the use of antibiotics, especially of the new drugs according to diagnostic and antimicrobial stewardship principles. Thus, along with the classical preemptive approach based on serial surveillance cultures and targeted antibiotic initiation on symptoms onset, we may improve patient management using tools able to stratify the individual risk of developing infection to guide the use of diagnostic procedures (imaging studies as well as microbiological investigations) and antimicrobial use.

With this aim, a recent study conducted among 840 LTRs, colonized with CRE before or after LT, in 15 different transplant centers investigated risk factors for developing CRE infection in the posttransplant period and further proposed a stratification tool including those variables independently associated with CRE infection.[11] The score was designed to be used in the immediate posttransplant period, ideally from the day of transplantation up to 3 to 4 weeks after transplantation. The cumulative risk of CRE infection within 30 to 60 days after liver transplant was assessed using a prediction model composed of the carriage status, the presence of multisite colonization after orthotopoic liver transplant (OLT), the need of prolonged mechanical ventilation (MV), the development of acute kidney injury (AKI), and/or the need of re-intervention. Exploring the potential clinical utility of this prediction model using a decision-curve analysis, a "net benefit" of applying model-directed interventions was found when the overall CRE infection threshold probability exceeded 10%. These interventions could consist of intensification in diagnostic investigations including imaging to identify an infectious focus potentially amenable to source control and the use of rapid molecular tests (ie, multiplex-polymerase chain reaction [PCR]) to rule out the presence of CRE in clinical specimens such as blood and/or lower respiratory samples. In addition, since in a further multistate analysis, the same score was also shown to predict mortality when the CRE infection risk approached 30%, it has been hypothesized that for threshold probabilities $\geq$30% initiation of empirical treatment waiting for the results of diagnostic investigations could be considered regardless of symptoms. However, the impact of such risk stratification tool in improving antimicrobial use, decreasing mortality, and further resistance selection is currently under investigation (NCT05594901).

Molecular diagnostic testing has gained attention in the last several years due to a rapid turnaround time and high sensitivity, potentially improving time to effective antibiotics and decreasing the duration unnecessarily broad therapy. Liang and colleagues highlighted the potential role of a multiplex PCR able to differentiate gram-positive from gram-negative bacterial DNA in a 3.5-hour time period in blood specimens.[61] Thereafter, different multiplexed PCR has been developed to rapidly detect specific resistance patterns such as genetic determinant of methicillin resistance (MEC), genetic determinant of vancomycin resistance (VAN), type of Beta-lactamase (CTX-M), Klebsiella pneumoniae carbapenemase (KPC), Verona Integron-encoded

Metallo-β-lactamase (type of carbapenemase) (VIM), and oxacillinase-48 (type of carbapenemase) (OXA-48) from blood cultures with a turnaround varying from 1 to 2.5 hours.[62,63] These novel tests showed a high concordance with the standard of care in overall 88.3% blood cultures, specifically in 92% and 96% of all samples growing gram-positive and gram-negative pathogens, respectively.[64] Although the presence of polymicrobial bacteremia could reduce sensitivity of these assays, concordance for detecting resistance mechanisms could reach 100%.[65] Furthermore, some new molecular assays have been developed considering specific syndromes, such as LRTIs. Indeed, several studies highlighted the potential role of syndromic molecular tests in improving antibiotic use mainly in the management of critically ill patients with hospital-acquired/ventilator-associated pneumonia[66,67] and in settings with high prevalence of MDROs. A recent study demonstrated an increase in detection of potential pneumonia pathogens compared with standard-of-care methods, pointing out the importance of semiquantification of bacterial load that ideally could assist physicians in understanding its clinical role.[68] Gram-negative resistance markers were detected in all cases. Considering the turnaround time of approximately 1 hour, it has the potential to improve antimicrobial stewardship. A randomized trial evaluating its benefit compared with standard of care is ongoing.[69] Thus, in immunosuppressed or critically ill patients, this approach may lead to a quasi-targeted treatment based on detecting or ruling out specific patterns of resistance.

THERAPEUTIC OPTIONS

Recommendations regarding antibiotic treatment for documented MDRO infection in SOT recipients do not differ from that for general population. The pivotal role of source control to improve graft/patient survival and reducing the risk of infection relapse should be emphasized.

Methicillin-Resistant S aureus

Infectious Diseases Society of America (IDSA) guidelines for the treatment of MRSA bloodstream infection have been published in 2011[70] and update of that document is ongoing with the collaboration of European Society of Clinical Microbiology and Infectious Diseases (ESCMID), whereas UK guidelines on the treatment of MRSA infections have been recently updated.[71] The choice of a specific treatment should be based on strain susceptibility and infection site. For MRSA bacteremia or endocarditis, intravenous vancomycin and daptomycin are considered first options. Linezolid, as well as ceftaroline and ceftobiprole, is considered good options for the treatment of MRSA pneumonia.[72,73]

Vancomycin-Resistant Enterococci

Linezolid and daptomycin are used for VRE infection treatment with several limitations. Linezolid has a bacteriostatic effect, and retrospective studies suggest an underexposure of daptomycin at standard dosage (4–6 mg/kg).[74–76] In fact, lower 30-day mortality rate and improved microbiological clearance in patients treated with high-dose (≥10 mg/Kg) daptomycin compared with medium or standard dose daptomycin were reported in one study.[77] Another study confirmed that the clinical response of daptomycin was dose-dependent.[78] Thus, the treatment options for VRE are limited, and mortality rates in historical cohorts remain high (up to 40%),[79] suggesting that new drugs are needed. In this regard, the long-acting lipoglycopeptide oritavancin, recently introduced in Europe for the treatment of Acute bacterial skin and skin structure infection (ABSSSI) in adults, was shown to have good in vitro activity against VRE strains (including those

Table 3
Main guidelines recommendations for multidrug-resistant organism treatment

IDSA[81,82]

	UTI	cUTI	Non-UTI	Notes
ESBL-E	Nitrofurantoin TMP-SMX	ERTA, MEM, IMP FQs, TMP-SMX	CARBAPENEM	If BL/BLI was initiated as empiric therapy for UTI with clinical improvement no change is necessary
CRE	FQs, TMP-SMX, single dose AG, HD MEM (or new drugs)	FQs, TMP-SMX, single-dose AG, HD MEM (or new drugs)	KPC: CAZ-AVI, MEM-VAB, IMP-REL OXA-48: CAZ-AVI MBL: CAZ-AVI + AZT, CFD	
DTR-PA	TOL/TZB, CAZ/AVI, IMP/REL, CFD	CFO/TZB, CAZ/AVI, IMP/REL, CFD	TOL/TZB, CAZ/AVI, IMP/REL	If strain is susceptible to multiple traditional beta-lactams or FQs carbapenem-sparing options are preferred
CR-AB		HD sulbactam (6–9 g/day) as monotherapy for mild infections	HD sulbactam (6–9 g/day) combined with other in vitro active drug (minocycline, tigecycline)	Cefiderocol should be limited to refractory infections and as a part of combination regimen.

ESCMID[83]

	Severe Infection	Non-severe Infection	cUTI	Notes
ESCR-E	CARBAPENEM, ERTAPENEM (if no septic shock)	BL/BLI, FQs, TMP-SMX	AG, IV fosfomycin	New BL/BLIs should be reserved for XDR bacteria
CRE	KPC: CAZ-AVI, MEM-VAB OXA-48: CAZ-AVI MBL: CAZ-AVI + AZT, CFD	Old antibiotics (combination)	AG	No evidence to recommend for or against IMP-REL

(continued on next page)

Table 3
(continued)

	ESCMID[83]			
	Severe Infection	Non-severe Infection	cUTI	Notes
CR-PA	TOL/TZB	Old antibiotics	Old antibiotics	No evidence to recommend for or against combination with new BL/BLIs Combination suggested for old antibiotics
CR-AB	Combination therapy including two *in vitro* active antibiotics	Ampicillin/sulbactam if susceptible If resistant, polymyxin or HD tigecycline	Ampicillin/sulbactam if susceptible If resistant, polymyxin or HD tigecycline	Cefiderocol is conditionally not recommended. If meropenem MIC ≤8 mg/L, consider carbapenem combination regimen

Abbreviations: 3GCephRE, third-generation cephalosporin-resistant Enterobacterales; AG, aminoglycosides; BL/BLI, beta-lactam/beta-lactamase inhibitor; CAZ-AVI, ceftazidime/avibactam; CFD, cefiderocol; CR-AB, carbapenem-resistant *A baumannii*; CRE, carbapenem-resistant Enterobacterales; cUTI, complicated UTI; DTR-PA, difficult-to-treat *P aeruginosa*; ERTA, ertapenem; ESBL, extended-spectrum beta-lactamase; FQs, fluoroquinolones; HD, high-dose; IMP, imipenem; IMP/REL, imipenem/relebactam; MEM, meropenem; MEM/VAB, meropenem/vaborbactam; TMP/SMX, trimethoprim/sulfamethoxazole; TOL/TZB, ceftolozane/tazobactam; UTIs, urinary tract infections.

resistant to daptomycin).[80] Clinical data on its efficacy and safety for the treatment of monomicrobial VRE SSN after SOT are needed.

Multidrug-Resistant Gram-Negative Bacteria

IDSA and ESCMID have been recently published guidance documents and guidelines, respectively, for the treatment of MDR-GNB infections.[81–83] Recommendations of such documents are summarized in **Table 3**. The main differences between the two documents include: (1) the application the Grading of Recommendations, Assessment, Development and Evaluations system in the European Guidelines thus limiting the indication for some drugs recently introduced in the clinical practice (ie, imipenem/relebactam), whereas the US guidance was based on a consensus of experts; (2) classification of resistance for *P aeruginosa,* European guidelines addressed the treatment of carbapenem resistant strains that could maintain in some cases susceptibility to piperacillin/tazobactam, ceftazidime, and cefepime. Although IDSA guidance adopted the more innovative definition of difficult-to-treat resistant (DTR) *P aeruginosa* more appropriate to depict strains with limited treatment options; and (3) recommendations regarding the drug of choice were declined according to clinical severity and to infection site in European and US documents, respectively.

Along with the choice of the drug, the dosage and the administration modality (ie, intermittent vs prolonged/continuous infusion) are the key to ensure pharmacokinetic/pharmacodynamic (PK/PD) target attainment. Indeed, even more real-life data underline that appropriate administration schedules (ie, loading dose followed by prolonged or continuous infusions of beta-lactams) supported by a therapeutic drug monitoring and the pharmacologic advice approach is associated with better microbiological and clinical outcome, especially in the management of immunocompromised patients with severe MDRO infections.[84–86]

Finally, it should be remarked that antibiotic resistance *per se* does not require a prolonged treatment duration,[81,82] this may be necessary only in case of inappropriate initial treatment and/or source control with delayed clinical and/or microbiological response.

FUTURE DIRECTIONS

Previous microbiome studies demonstrated that an increase in relative abundance of CPE is associated with subsequent bacteremia,[87] suggesting a crucial role for a dysregulated gut microbiota in infection development. Similarly, *Enterococcus* and Proteobacteria dominance has been correlated with an increased risk of bacteremia with VRE and GNB, respectively.[88] Fecal microbiota transplantation (FMT) has been proposed as a way to restore protective intestinal microbiome diversity. Indeed, it has been observed that patients undergoing FMT for recurrent *Clostridioides difficile* infection cleared also MDRO colonization. Food and Drug Administration (FDA) decided to allow its use for such purpose under an enforcement discretion policy. A recent systematic review focused on such issue.[89] Overall, 10 studies including one randomized open-label clinical trial were pooled. Among 112 FMT recipients colonized by CRE, decolonization was reported up to 60% and 79% at 1 and at 6 to 12 months, respectively. However, little is known about the efficacy and safety of FMT in SOT recipients, even if preliminary results, mainly regarding *C difficile* infection, seems promising.[90]

SUMMARY

The burden of MDRO infections in SOT may vary according to local prevalence and the type of SOT. Poorer impact on graft/patient outcome has been observed, in particular for CR-GNB infections where mortality rates were as high as 40% to 60% before the introduction of new drugs. New drugs have improved patient survival in the general population, but a significant percentage of microbiological failure with persistent or relapsing infection and/or emergence of further resistance has already been observed with their use. Thus, infection control and antimicrobial stewardship activities aimed at the reducing the spread and optimizing therapeutic management of MDRO in SOT recipients are needed. Screening strategies should be based on the careful assessment of local epidemiology. Protocols for T-PAP should consider the low level of evidence currently sustaining this approach and potential harmful consequences on gut dysbiosis. For the same reason, prolonged prophylaxis or treatment duration should be avoided. Predictive tools able to stratify patients according with their risk of developing MDRO infection and/or dying combined with the use of new rapid diagnostic tests may support clinicians in the appropriate use of antibiotic therapy. Finally, efficacy and safety of new nonantibiotic-based strategies, such as FMT, to reduce MDRO burden in SOT population should be investigated.

CLINICS CARE POINTS

- Solid organ transplant (SOT) candidates and recipients are highly susceptible to acquire multidrug-resistant organisms (MDRO) colonization and/or infection with a significant impact on graft/patient survival.
- Optimal management of the MDRO burden in SOT patients should consist in individualized preventive strategies, fully integrated with infection control and antimicrobial stewardship activities, with the goals of improving patient outcome as well as to minimize environmental damage.
- Patient risk stratification tools and rapid diagnostic tests may be useful in improving diagnostic and therapeutic management of MDRO in SOT population.
- New data should be acquired on the efficacy and safety of FMT in reducing the burden of MDRO in SOT patients.

DISCLOSURES

M. Rinaldi has not conflict of interest to declare; M. Giannella received grants as speaker or as advisor from Shionogi, MSD, Pfizer, Menarini, and Thermo Fisher.

REFERENCES

1. van Delden C, Stampf S, Hirsch HH, et al. Burden and Timeline of Infectious Diseases in the First Year After Solid Organ Transplantation in the Swiss Transplant Cohort Study. Clin Infect Dis 2020;71(7). e159–69.
2. Hamandi B, Husain S, Grootendorst P, et al. Clinical and microbiological epidemiology of early and late infectious complications among solid-organ transplant recipients requiring hospitalization. Transpl Int Off J Eur Soc Organ Transplant 2016;29(9):1029–38.
3. Coussement J, Maggiore U, Manuel O, et al. Diagnosis and management of asymptomatic bacteriuria in kidney transplant recipients: a survey of current practice in Europe. Nephrol Dial Transplant 2018;33(9):1661–8.
4. Mularoni A, Bertani A, Vizzini G, et al. Outcome of Transplantation Using Organs From Donors Infected or Colonized With Carbapenem-Resistant Gram-Negative

Bacteria. Am J Transplant Off J Am Soc Transplant Am Soc Transpl Surg 2015; 15(10):2674–82.

5. Procaccio F, Masiero L, Vespasiano F, Grossi PA, Gagliotti C, Pantosti A, et al. Organ donor screening for carbapenem-resistant gram-negative bacteria in Italian intensive care units: the DRIn study. Am J Transplant. 2020;20(1):262–73. Available at: https://onlinelibrary.wiley.com/doi/abs/10.1111/ajt.15566.

6. Lewis JD, Sifri CD. Multidrug-Resistant Bacterial Donor-Derived Infections in Solid Organ Transplantation. Curr Infect Dis Rep 2016;18(6):18.

7. Miller R, Covington S, Taranto S, et al. Communication gaps associated with donor-derived infections. Am J Transplant Off J Am Soc Transplant Am Soc Transpl Surg 2015;15(1):259–64.

8. Ariza-Heredia EJ, Patel R, Blumberg EA, et al. Outcomes of transplantation using organs from a donor infected with Klebsiella pneumoniae carbapenemase (KPC)-producing K. pneumoniae. Transpl Infect Dis Off J Transplant Soc 2012;14(3): 229–36.

9. Freire MP, Villela Soares Oshiro IC, Bonazzi PR, et al. Surveillance culture for multidrug-resistant gram-negative bacteria: Performance in liver transplant recipients. Am J Infect Control 2017;45(3):e40–4.

10. Taimur S, Pouch SM, Zubizarreta N, et al. Impact of pre-transplant carbapenem-resistant Enterobacterales colonization and/or infection on solid organ transplant outcomes. Clin Transplant 2021;35(4):e14239.

11. Giannella M, Freire M, Rinaldi M, et al. Development of a Risk Prediction Model for Carbapenem-resistant Enterobacteriaceae Infection After Liver Transplantation: A Multinational Cohort Study. Clin Infect Dis Off Publ Infect Dis Soc Am 2021; 73(4):e955–66.

12. World Health Organization. Global guidelines for the prevention of surgical site infection. World Health Organization; 2018. 184 p. Available from: https://apps.who.int/iris/handle/10665/277399.

13. Pereira MR, Rana MM, AST ID Community of Practice. Methicillin-resistant *Staphylococcus aureus* in solid organ transplantation-Guidelines from the American Society of Transplantation Infectious Diseases Community of Practice. Clin Transplant 2019;33(9):e13611.

14. Calfee DP, Salgado CD, Milstone AM, et al. Strategies to prevent methicillin-resistant *Staphylococcus aureus* transmission and infection in acute care hospitals: 2014 update. Infect Control Hosp Epidemiol 2014;35(7):772–96.

15. Clancy CJ, Bartsch SM, Nguyen MH, et al. A computer simulation model of the cost-effectiveness of routine *Staphylococcus aureus* screening and decolonization among lung and heart-lung transplant recipients. Eur J Clin Microbiol Infect Dis Off Publ Eur Soc Clin Microbiol 2014;33(6):1053–61.

16. Abbo LM, Grossi PA, AST ID Community of Practice. Surgical site infections: Guidelines from the American Society of Transplantation Infectious Diseases Community of Practice. Clin Transplant 2019;33(9):e13589.

17. Ziakas PD, Pliakos EE, Zervou FN, et al. MRSA and VRE colonization in solid organ transplantation: a meta-analysis of published studies. Am J Transplant Off J Am Soc Transplant Am Soc Transpl Surg 2014 Aug;14(8):1887–94.

18. Simkins J, Morris MI, Camargo JF, et al. Clinical outcomes of intestinal transplant recipients colonized with multidrug-resistant organisms: a retrospective study. Transpl Int 2017;30(9):924–31.

19. Nellore A, Huprikar S, AST ID Community of Practice. Vancomycin-resistant *Enterococcus* in solid organ transplant recipients: Guidelines from the American

Society of Transplantation Infectious Diseases Community of Practice. Clin Transplant 2019;33(9):e13549.

20. Malinis M, Boucher HW, AST Infectious Diseases Community of Practice. Screening of donor and candidate prior to solid organ transplantation-Guidelines from the American Society of Transplantation Infectious Diseases Community of Practice. Clin Transplant 2019;33(9):e13548.

21. Aguado JM, Silva JT, Fernández-Ruiz M, et al. Management of multidrug resistant Gram-negative bacilli infections in solid organ transplant recipients: SET/GESITRA-SEIMC/REIPI recommendations. Transplant Rev Orlando Fla 2018; 32(1):36–57.

22. Pouch SM, Patel G, Practice the AIDC of. Multidrug-resistant Gram-negative bacterial infections in solid organ transplant recipients—Guidelines from the American Society of Transplantation Infectious Diseases Community of Practice. Clin Transplant. 2019;33(9):e13594. Available from: https://onlinelibrary.wiley.com/doi/abs/10.1111/ctr.13594.

23. Righi E, Mutters NT, Guirao X, et al. ESCMID/EUCIC clinical practice guidelines on perioperative antibiotic prophylaxis in patients colonized by multidrug-resistant Gram-negative bacteria before surgery. Clin Microbiol Infect Off Publ Eur Soc Clin Microbiol Infect Dis 2022. S1198-743X(22)00632-2.

24. Apisarnthanarak A, Kondo S, Mingmalairak C, et al. Outcomes of extended-spectrum beta-lactamases producing Enterobacteriaceae colonization among patients abdominal surgery patients. Infect Control Hosp Epidemiol 2019; 40(11):1290–3.

25. Golzarri MF, Silva-Sánchez J, Cornejo-Juárez P, et al. Colonization by fecal extended-spectrum β-lactamase-producing Enterobacteriaceae and surgical site infections in patients with cancer undergoing gastrointestinal and gynecologic surgery. Am J Infect Control 2019;47(8):916–21.

26. Dubinsky-Pertzov B, Temkin E, Harbarth S, et al. Carriage of Extended-spectrum Beta-lactamase-producing Enterobacteriaceae and the Risk of Surgical Site Infection After Colorectal Surgery: A Prospective Cohort Study. Clin Infect Dis Off Publ Infect Dis Soc Am 2019;68(10):1699–704.

27. De Pastena M, Paiella S, Azzini AM, et al. Antibiotic Prophylaxis with Piperacillin-Tazobactam Reduces Post-Operative Infectious Complication after Pancreatic Surgery: An Interventional, Non-Randomized Study. Surg Infect 2021;22(5): 536–42.

28. Bert F, Larroque B, Paugam-Burtz C, et al. Pretransplant fecal carriage of extended-spectrum β-lactamase-producing Enterobacteriaceae and infection after liver transplant, France. Emerg Infect Dis 2012;18(6):908–16.

29. Bert F, Larroque B, Dondero F, et al. Risk factors associated with preoperative fecal carriage of extended-spectrum β-lactamase-producing Enterobacteriaceae in liver transplant recipients. Transpl Infect Dis Off J Transplant Soc 2014; 16(1):84–9.

30. Mazza E, Prosperi M, Panzeri MF, et al. Carbapenem-Resistant Klebsiella Pneumoniae Infections Early After Liver Transplantation: A Single-Center Experience. Transplant Proc 2017;49(4):677–81.

31. Freire MP, Song ATW, Oshiro ICV, et al. Surgical site infection after liver transplantation in the era of multidrug-resistant bacteria: what new risks should be considered? Diagn Microbiol Infect Dis 2021;99(1):115220.

32. Giannella M, Bartoletti M, Morelli MC, et al. Risk factors for infection with carbapenem-resistant Klebsiella pneumoniae after liver transplantation: the

importance of pre- and posttransplant colonization. Am J Transplant Off J Am Soc Transplant Am Soc Transpl Surg 2015;15(6):1708–15.

33. Weill D, Benden C, Corris PA, et al. A consensus document for the selection of lung transplant candidates: 2014–an update from the Pulmonary Transplantation Council of the International Society for Heart and Lung Transplantation. J Heart Lung Transplant Off Publ Int Soc Heart Transplant 2015;34(1):1–15.

34. Kochar S, Sheard T, Sharma R, et al. Success of an infection control program to reduce the spread of carbapenem-resistant Klebsiella pneumoniae. Infect Control Hosp Epidemiol 2009;30(5):447–52.

35. Johnson LE, D'Agata EMC, Paterson DL, et al. *Pseudomonas aeruginosa* bacteremia over a 10-year period: multidrug resistance and outcomes in transplant recipients. Transpl Infect Dis Off J Transplant Soc 2009;11(3):227–34.

36. Bodro M, Sabé N, Tubau F, et al. Extensively drug-resistant *Pseudomonas aeruginosa* bacteremia in solid organ transplant recipients. Transplantation 2015; 99(3):616–22.

37. Bodro M, Sabé N, Tubau F, et al. Risk factors and outcomes of bacteremia caused by drug-resistant ESKAPE pathogens in solid-organ transplant recipients. Transplantation 2013;96(9):843–9.

38. Tebano G, Geneve C, Tanaka S, et al. Epidemiology and risk factors of multidrug-resistant bacteria in respiratory samples after lung transplantation. Transpl Infect Dis Off J Transplant Soc 2016;18(1):22–30.

39. Enfield KB, Huq NN, Gosseling MF, et al. Control of simultaneous outbreaks of carbapenemase-producing enterobacteriaceae and extensively drug-resistant *Acinetobacter baumannii* infection in an intensive care unit using interventions promoted in the Centers for Disease Control and Prevention 2012 carbapenemase-resistant Enterobacteriaceae Toolkit. Infect Control Hosp Epidemiol 2014;35(7):810–7.

40. Freire MP, Pierrotti LC, Oshiro ICVS, et al. Carbapenem-resistant *Acinetobacter baumannii* acquired before liver transplantation: Impact on recipient outcomes. Liver Transplant Off Publ Am Assoc Study Liver Dis Int Liver Transplant Soc 2016;22(5):615–26.

41. Bratzler DW, Dellinger EP, Olsen KM, et al. Clinical practice guidelines for antimicrobial prophylaxis in surgery. Surg Infect 2013;14(1):73–156.

42. Logre E, Bert F, Khoy-Ear L, et al. Risk Factors and Impact of Perioperative Prophylaxis on the Risk of Extended-spectrum β-Lactamase-producing Enterobacteriaceae-related Infection Among Carriers Following Liver Transplantation. Transplantation 2021;105(2):338–45.

43. Cardile S, Del Chierico F, Candusso M, et al. Impact of Two Antibiotic Therapies on Clinical Outcome and Gut Microbiota Profile in Liver Transplant Paediatric Candidates Colonized by Carbapenem-Resistant Klebsiella pneumoniae CR-KP. Front Cell Infect Microbiol 2021;11:730904.

44. Hadjiliadis D, Steele MP, Chaparro C, et al. Survival of lung transplant patients with cystic fibrosis harboring panresistant bacteria other than Burkholderia cepacia, compared with patients harboring sensitive bacteria. J Heart Lung Transplant 2007;26(8):834–8.

45. Flume PA, Egan TM, Paradowski LJ, et al. Infectious complications of lung transplantation. Impact of cystic fibrosis. Am J Respir Crit Care Med 1994;149(6): 1601–7.

46. Paterson DL, Rihs JD, Squier C, Gayowski T, Sagnimeni A, Singh N. Lack of efficacy of mupirocin in the prevention of infections with *Staphylococcus aureus* in liver transplant recipients and candidates1. Transplantation. 2003;75(2):194.

Available from: https://journals.lww.com/transplantjournal/Fulltext/2003/01270/Lack_of_efficacy_of_mupirocin_in_the_prevention_of.6.aspx.

47. Singh N, Squier C, Wannstedt C, Keyes L, Wagener MM, Cacciarelli TV. Impact of an Aggressive Infection Control Strategy on Endemic Staphylococcus aureus Infection in Liver Transplant Recipients. Infect Control Hosp Epidemiol. 2006;27(2):122–6. Available from: https://www.cambridge.org/core/journals/infection-control-and-hospital-epidemiology/article/abs/impact-of-an-aggressive-infection-control-strategy-on-endemic-staphylococcus-aureus-infection-in-liver-transplant-recipients/CBACC922F6FF51F80B6B71F9D6FAA024.

48. Huttner B, Haustein T, Uçkay I, et al. Decolonization of intestinal carriage of extended-spectrum β-lactamase-producing Enterobacteriaceae with oral colistin and neomycin: a randomized, double-blind, placebo-controlled trial. J Antimicrob Chemother 2013;68(10):2375–82.

49. Jonsson AK, Larsson A, Tängdén T, et al. A trial with IgY chicken antibodies to eradicate faecal carriage of Klebsiella pneumoniae and Escherichia coli producing extended-spectrum beta-lactamases. Infect Ecol Epidemiol 2015;5:28224.

50. Buehlmann M, Bruderer T, Frei R, et al. Effectiveness of a new decolonisation regimen for eradication of extended-spectrum β-lactamase-producing Enterobacteriaceae. J Hosp Infect 2011;77(2):113–7.

51. Decré D, Gachot B, Lucet JC, et al. Clinical and Bacteriologic Epidemiology of Extended-Spectrum β-Lactamase-Producing Strains of Klebsiella pneumoniae in a Medical Intensive Care Unit. Clin Infect Dis 1998;27(4):834–44.

52. Abecasis F, Sarginson RE, Kerr S, et al. Is selective digestive decontamination useful in controlling aerobic gram-negative bacilli producing extended spectrum beta-lactamases? Microb Drug Resist Larchmt N 2011;17(1):17–23.

53. Troché G, Toly LM, Guibert M, Zazzo JF. Detection and Treatment of Antibiotic-Resistant Bacterial Carriage in a Surgical Intensive Care Unit: A 6-Year Prospective Survey. Infect Control Hosp Epidemiol. 2005;26(2):161–5. Available from: https://www.cambridge.org/core/journals/infection-control-and-hospital-epidemiology/article/abs/detection-and-treatment-of-antibioticresistant-bacterial-carriage-in-a-surgical-intensive-care-unit-a-6year-prospective-survey/8C22DB29FC89A9D0ADF1B9E332A1D87F.

54. Bar-Yoseph H, Hussein K, Braun E, et al. Natural history and decolonization strategies for ESBL/carbapenem-resistant Enterobacteriaceae carriage: systematic review and meta-analysis. J Antimicrob Chemother 2016;71(10):2729–39.

55. Fariñas MC, González-Rico C, Fernández-Martínez M, et al. Oral decontamination with colistin plus neomycin in solid organ transplant recipients colonized by multidrug-resistant Enterobacterales: a multicentre, randomized, controlled, open-label, parallel-group clinical trial. Clin Microbiol Infect Off Publ Eur Soc Clin Microbiol Infect Dis 2021;27(6):856–63.

56. Rattanaumpawan P, Lorsutthitham J, Ungprasert P, et al. Randomized controlled trial of nebulized colistimethate sodium as adjunctive therapy of ventilator-associated pneumonia caused by Gram-negative bacteria. J Antimicrob Chemother 2010;65(12):2645–9.

57. Lin CC, Liu TC, Kuo CF, et al. Aerosolized colistin for the treatment of multidrug-resistant *Acinetobacter baumannii* pneumonia: experience in a tertiary care hospital in northern Taiwan. J Microbiol Immunol Infect Wei Mian Yu Gan Ran Za Zhi 2010 Aug;43(4):323–31.

58. Hallal A, Cohn SM, Namias N, Habib F, Baracco G, Manning RJ, et al. Aerosolized tobramycin in the treatment of ventilator-associated pneumonia: A pilot study.

Surg Infect. 2007;8(1):73–81. Available from: http://www.scopus.com/inward/re-cord.url?scp=34247129544&partnerID=8YFLogxK.

59. Kofteridis DP, Alexopoulou C, Valachis A, et al. Aerosolized plus intravenous colistin versus intravenous colistin alone for the treatment of ventilator-associated pneumonia: a matched case-control study. Clin Infect Dis Off Publ Infect Dis Soc Am 2010;51(11):1238–44.

60. Michalopoulos A, Kasiakou SK, Mastora Z, Rellos K, Kapaskelis AM, Falagas ME. Aerosolized colistin for the treatment of nosocomial pneumonia due to multidrug-resistant Gram-negative bacteria in patients without cystic fibrosis. Crit Care. 2005;9(1):R53–9. Available at: https://www.ncbi.nlm.nih.gov/pmc/articles/PMC1065114/.

61. Liang F, Browne DJ, Gray MJ, et al. Development of a Multiplexed Microsphere PCR for Culture-Free Detection and Gram-Typing of Bacteria in Human Blood Samples. ACS Infect Dis 2018;4(5):837–44.

62. She RC, Bender JM. Advances in Rapid Molecular Blood Culture Diagnostics: Healthcare Impact, Laboratory Implications, and Multiplex Technologies. J Appl Lab Med 2019;3(4):617–630.

63. Peker N, Couto N, Sinha B, Rossen JW. Diagnosis of bloodstream infections from positive blood cultures and directly from blood samples: recent developments in molecular approaches. Clin Microbiol Infect. 2018;24(9):944–55. Available at: https://www.clinicalmicrobiologyandinfection.com/article/S1198-743X(18)30419-1/fulltext.

64. Berinson B, Both A, Berneking L, et al. Usefulness of BioFire FilmArray BCID2 for Blood Culture Processing in Clinical Practice. J Clin Microbiol 2021;59(8):e0054321.

65. García-Rivera C, Parra-Grande M, Merino E, Boix V, Rodríguez JC. Concordance of the filmarray blood culture identification panel 2 and classical microbiological methods in a bacteriemia diagnostic unit. Diagn Microbiol Infect Dis. 2022;104(4):115787. Available at: https://www.sciencedirect.com/science/article/pii/S0732889322001535.

66. Monard C, Pehlivan J, Auger G, et al. Multicenter evaluation of a syndromic rapid multiplex PCR test for early adaptation of antimicrobial therapy in adult patients with pneumonia. Crit Care Lond Engl 2020;24(1):434.

67. Peiffer-Smadja N, Bouadma L, Mathy V, et al. Performance and impact of a multiplex PCR in ICU patients with ventilator-associated pneumonia or ventilated hospital-acquired pneumonia. Crit Care Lond Engl 2020;24(1):366.

68. Ginocchio CC, Garcia-Mondragon C, Mauerhofer B, et al, the EME Evaluation Program Collaborative. Multinational evaluation of the BioFire® FilmArray® Pneumonia plus Panel as compared to standard of care testing. Eur J Clin Microbiol Infect Dis Off Publ Eur Soc Clin Microbiol 2021;40(8):1609–22.

69. High J, Enne VI, Barber JA, et al. INHALE: the impact of using FilmArray Pneumonia Panel molecular diagnostics for hospital-acquired and ventilator-associated pneumonia on antimicrobial stewardship and patient outcomes in UK Critical Care-study protocol for a multicentre randomised controlled trial. Trials 2021;22(1):680.

70. Liu C, Bayer A, Cosgrove SE, et al. Clinical Practice Guidelines by the Infectious Diseases Society of America for the Treatment of Methicillin-Resistant *Staphylococcus aureus* Infections in Adults and Children. Clin Infect Dis 2011;52(3). e18–55.

71. Brown NM, Brown EM, the Guideline Development Group. Treatment of methicillin-resistant *Staphylococcus aureus* (MRSA): updated guidelines from the UK. J Antimicrob Chemother 2021;76(6):1377–8.

72. Zhanel GG, Lam A, Schweizer F, et al. Ceftobiprole: a review of a broad-spectrum and anti-MRSA cephalosporin. Am J Clin Dermatol 2008;9(4):245–54.

73. Sotgiu G, Aliberti S, Gramegna A, et al. Efficacy and effectiveness of Ceftaroline Fosamil in patients with pneumonia: a systematic review and meta-analysis. Respir Res 2018;19(1):205.

74. Balli EP, Venetis CA, Miyakis S. Systematic review and meta-analysis of linezolid versus daptomycin for treatment of vancomycin-resistant enterococcal bacteremia. Antimicrob Agents Chemother 2014;58(2):734–9.

75. Whang DW, Miller LG, Partain NM, et al. Systematic review and meta-analysis of linezolid and daptomycin for treatment of vancomycin-resistant enterococcal bloodstream infections. Antimicrob Agents Chemother 2013;57(10):5013–8.

76. Britt NS, Potter EM, Patel N, et al. Comparison of the Effectiveness and Safety of Linezolid and Daptomycin in Vancomycin-Resistant Enterococcal Bloodstream Infection: A National Cohort Study of Veterans Affairs Patients. Clin Infect Dis Off Publ Infect Dis Soc Am 2015;61(6):871–8.

77. Britt NS, Potter EM, Patel N, et al. Comparative Effectiveness and Safety of Standard-, Medium-, and High-Dose Daptomycin Strategies for the Treatment of Vancomycin-Resistant Enterococcal Bacteremia Among Veterans Affairs Patients. Clin Infect Dis 2017;64(5):605–13.

78. Chuang YC, Lin HY, Chen PY, et al. Daptomycin versus linezolid for the treatment of vancomycin-resistant enterococcal bacteraemia: implications of daptomycin dose. Clin Microbiol Infect Off Publ Eur Soc Clin Microbiol Infect Dis 2016 Oct; 22(10):890.e1–7.

79. Edmond MB, Ober JF, Dawson JD, et al. Vancomycin-resistant enterococcal bacteremia: natural history and attributable mortality. Clin Infect Dis Off Publ Infect Dis Soc Am 1996;23(6):1234–9.

80. Carvalhaes CG, Sader HS, Streit JM, et al. Activity of Oritavancin against Gram-Positive Pathogens Causing Bloodstream Infections in the United States over 10 Years: Focus on Drug-Resistant Enterococcal Subsets (2010-2019). Antimicrob Agents Chemother 2022;66(2):e0166721.

81. Tamma PD, Aitken SL, Bonomo RA, et al. Infectious Diseases Society of America Guidance on the Treatment of Extended-Spectrum β-lactamase Producing Enterobacterales (ESBL-E), Carbapenem-Resistant Enterobacterales (CRE), and *Pseudomonas aeruginosa* with Difficult-to-Treat Resistance (DTR-P. aeruginosa). Clin Infect Dis Off Publ Infect Dis Soc Am 2021;72(7):e169–83.

82. Tamma PD, Aitken SL, Bonomo RA, et al. Infectious Diseases Society of America Guidance on the Treatment of AmpC β-Lactamase-Producing Enterobacterales, Carbapenem-Resistant *Acinetobacter baumannii*, and Stenotrophomonas maltophilia Infections. Clin Infect Dis Off Publ Infect Dis Soc Am 2022;74(12): 2089–114.

83. Paul M, Carrara E, Retamar P, et al. European Society of Clinical Microbiology and Infectious Diseases (ESCMID) guidelines for the treatment of infections caused by multidrug-resistant Gram-negative bacilli (endorsed by European society of intensive care medicine). Clin Microbiol Infect Off Publ Eur Soc Clin Microbiol Infect Dis 2022;28(4):521–47.

84. Gatti M, Giannella M, Rinaldi M, et al. Pharmacokinetic/Pharmacodynamic Analysis of Continuous-Infusion Fosfomycin in Combination with Extended-Infusion Cefiderocol or Continuous-Infusion Ceftazidime-Avibactam in a Case Series of

Difficult-to-Treat Resistant *Pseudomonas aeruginosa* Bloodstream Infections and/or Hospital-Acquired Pneumonia. Antibiot Basel Switz 2022;11(12):1739.

85. Gatti M, Pascale R, Cojutti PG, et al. A descriptive pharmacokinetic/pharmacodynamic analysis of continuous infusion ceftazidime-avibactam in a case series of critically ill renal patients treated for documented carbapenem-resistant Gram-negative bloodstream infections and/or ventilator-associated pneumonia. Int J Antimicrob Agents 2022;61(1):106699.

86. Gatti M, Fornaro G, Viale P, et al. Clinical efficacy of renal dosing adjustments of ceftazidime-avibactam in patients affected by carbapenem-resistant Gram-negative infections: A systematic review and meta-analysis of observational studies. Br J Clin Pharmacol 2023;89(2):617–29.

87. Shimasaki T, Seekatz A, Bassis C, et al. Increased Relative Abundance of Klebsiella pneumoniae Carbapenemase-producing Klebsiella pneumoniae Within the Gut Microbiota Is Associated With Risk of Bloodstream Infection in Long-term Acute Care Hospital Patients. Clin Infect Dis Off Publ Infect Dis Soc Am 2019; 68(12):2053–9.

88. Petersen AM, Mirsepasi-Lauridsen HC, Vester-Andersen MK, et al. High Abundance of Proteobacteria in Ileo-Anal Pouch Anastomosis and Increased Abundance of Fusobacteria Associated with Increased Pouch Inflammation. Antibiot Basel Switz 2020;9(5):237.

89. Macareño-Castro J, Solano-Salazar A, Dong LT, et al. Fecal microbiota transplantation for Carbapenem-Resistant Enterobacteriaceae: A systematic review. J Infect 2022;84(6):749–59.

90. Mehta N, Wang T, Friedman-Moraco RJ, et al. Fecal Microbiota Transplantation Donor Screening Updates and Research Gaps for Solid Organ Transplant Recipients. J Clin Microbiol 2022;60(2):e0016121.

91. Tacconelli E, Mazzaferri F, de Smet AM, et al. ESCMID-EUCIC clinical guidelines on decolonization of multidrug-resistant Gram-negative bacteria carriers. Clin Microbiol Infect Off Publ Eur Soc Clin Microbiol Infect Dis 2019;25(7):807–17.

Opportunities for Antimicrobial Stewardship Interventions Among Solid Organ Transplant Recipients

Erica J. Stohs, MD, MPH[a],*, Chelsea A. Gorsline, MD[b]

KEYWORDS

- Antimicrobial stewardship • Organ transplant • Diagnostic stewardship
- Antibiotic allergy

KEY POINTS

- Antimicrobial stewardship is needed to address rising rates of antimicrobial resistance, reduce antimicrobial-associated adverse events such as *Clostridioides difficile* infection, and optimize antimicrobial use in solid organ transplantation recipients.
- Over the past decade, diverse and rapidly evolving antimicrobial stewardship interventions have arisen in this field, including those at the patient level and health system level.
- Growing evidence supports delabeling antibiotic allergies in transplant candidates and recipients.
- Treatment of asymptomatic bacteriuria does not prevent progression to urinary tract infection and/or pyelonephritis in kidney recipients who are more than 1-2 months post-transplant.

INTRODUCTION

Antimicrobial stewardship is valuable to transplant programs to reduce the threat of antimicrobial resistance, improve patient outcomes, and attenuate risks of drug toxicities.[1,2] Antimicrobial stewardship interventions are designed to measure and improve appropriate use of antimicrobial agents by promoting the optimal antimicrobial drug regimen including dose, duration of therapy, and route of administration.[3,4] The importance of antimicrobial stewardship was nationally recognized following

[a] Division of Infectious Diseases, Department of Medicine, University of Nebraska Medical Center, 985400 Nebraska Medical Center, Omaha, NE 68198-5400, USA; [b] Division of Infectious Diseases, Department of Medicine, University of Kansas Medical Center, 3901 Rainbow Boulevard, Mailstop 1028, Kansas City, KS, USA
* Corresponding author.
E-mail address: erica.stohs@unmc.edu

Infect Dis Clin N Am 37 (2023) 539–560
https://doi.org/10.1016/j.idc.2023.04.005
0891-5520/23/© 2023 Elsevier Inc. All rights reserved.

the Centers for Diseases Control and Prevention (CDC)'s 2013 report detailing antibiotic resistance threats, which was since updated in 2019.[5,6] In the years that followed, the US health care facilities were required to implement antimicrobial stewardship programs (ASP), but they are not mandated specifically for transplant centers or programs.[7–9]

The need for transplant-specific antimicrobial stewardship is well recognized, both in United States and internationally.[1,10–24] Many emphasize transplant recipients are among those who would benefit most from ASP. Although transplantation has advanced significantly, complex surgeries, frequent antibiotic exposure, and immunosuppressive regimens place solid organ transplant recipients (SOTr) at disproportionately higher risk of infectious complications and antimicrobial resistance.[6] SOTr are at higher risk for colonization with and infection from multidrug-resistant organisms, such as methicillin-resistant *Staphylococcus aureus* (MRSA), vancomycin-resistant *Enterococci*, extended-spectrum beta-lactamase (ESBL)-producing *Enterobacterales*, multidrug-resistant *Pseudomonas aeruginosa* and carbapenemase-producing *Enterobacterales* (CRE).[6,25] SOTr are also subject to increased risk of drug toxicities due to polypharmacy and drug–drug interactions and often require special attention to antimicrobial selection and dosing in the setting of renal or hepatic dysfunction.[2] Utilization of costly prophylactic and therapeutic antimicrobials by transplant patients accounts for the top tier of hospital antimicrobial expenditures.[26] Other factors, such as physician's perceptions of patient complexity, anxiety regarding severity of illness, and variation in host risk factors, such as level of immunosuppression, recency of surgery, and potential for drug–drug interactions, present challenges in the implementation of ASP interventions.[1,25] Limited data inform ASP initiatives in the transplant population, but it is a field ripe with opportunities. There have been several calls to action published over the past decade which highlight the need for multidisciplinary approaches, collaboration with experts in transplantation, the use of early and appropriate diagnostics to guide therapy, and optimized duration.[10–13,17,27–29] We present current practices in ASP and discuss their applicability for use in SOT. We review (1) the metrics that ASP interventions target, (2) opportunities for diagnostic stewardship in transplant, and (3) syndrome- and systems-based targets for ASP interventions.

DEVELOPMENT OF ANTIMICROBIAL STEWARDSHIP PROGRAMS METRICS
Design of Interventions

The foundation for ASP interventions begins by establishing working relationships with transplant providers including medical transplant physicians, surgeons, advanced practice providers, pharmacists, and nursing staff. Such relationships build trust and ensure a mutual goal of improving patient care.[13] Multidisciplinary ASP interventions are supported by the Infectious Diseases Society of America[4,13] Therefore, collaboration with transplant infectious disease providers in ASP efforts is essential for its success as they are well positioned to obtain buy-in from multidisciplinary members of the transplant teams. In addition, it may be beneficial to perform an assessment of transplant providers' knowledge, attitudes, and practices surrounding antibiotic use to gauge what is needed for successful behavior change. This analysis could be formal, using a survey to understand prescribing practices,[30,31] or informal, through open discussion with transplant providers. There are several existing frameworks available to understand what is needed to shape the desired behavior change and may be useful tools when designing interventions.[32–35] One example is *The Behavior Change Wheel*, which offers a step-by-step guide to developing interventions through the lens of behavior change techniques.[35] Use of these strategies may help ASPs avoid incorrect assumptions about interventions.

Metrics

As ASP initiatives are a means of quality improvement, their development and implementation should use standardized and valid measures. The use of standardized metrics allows for streamlined development of interventions and provides a system to track progress during implementation. Measurements of quality improvement initiatives are typically grouped into outcome measures, process measures, and balancing measures.[1] Outcome measures usually relate to the type of intervention, such as cost analyses, mortality, or other adverse outcomes, but can also be specific to infections, like resistance rates or clearance of an infection. Process measures are used to assess whether an intervention has the desired effect and should be in line with outcome measures. These types of metrics may be more feasible than outcome measures as they can be less labor-intensive to collect. The most common process measures in ASP initiatives are antibiotic use rates, particularly for the use of agents such as intravenous vancomycin or high-risk antimicrobials, and cost analyses. Another process measure to consider is the assessment of guideline-concordant antibiotic prescribing. Balancing measures are those that seek to ensure unintended negative consequences do not occur with implementation of a new intervention. Balancing measures sometimes overlap with outcome measures, for instance, when evaluating mortality, readmission rates, or surgical site infections. Additional examples are provided in **Table 1**.

DIAGNOSTIC STEWARDSHIP OPPORTUNITIES

Diagnostic stewardship is the process of modifying the process of ordering, performing, and reporting diagnostic tests to improve patient care.[36] When used properly, diagnostic stewardship can lead to a reduction in inappropriate antimicrobial use and associated costs. Diagnostic stewardship often requires collaboration with the clinical laboratory and other clinicians to be successful. There are many opportunities for interventions across the spectrum of patient care, which include characterizing when a test is ordered, when a laboratory processes a specimen, or when results are reported (**Table 2**).

Many rapid diagnostic tools are available (**Table 3**), but optimal use in SOTr remains relatively unstudied.[37] Test performance, result interpretation, and costs associated with each test warrant collaboration with ASP with implementation. ASP can develop institutional guidance, inform diagnostic restrictions, and provide audit and feedback with associated antimicrobials. Examples of diagnostic stewardship for diarrheal illnesses and pneumonia are outlined in the syndromic target sections below.

Multiplex blood culture panels have been widely adopted in the past decade with numerous commercial options available. These panels are particularly helpful in the transplant population for their ability to detect resistance genes. In one study that included transplant recipients, a multiplex blood culture panel showed decreased time to appropriate antibiotic therapy, especially in the setting of high rates of resistant gram-negative organisms.[38] Use of multiplex blood culture panels should be employed in conjunction with ASP to aid in interpretation, promote early de-escalation of unnecessary agents, and improve time to effective therapy, length of stay, and mortality.[39,40] Although there are developments in the realm of metagenomic sequencing and broad-range polymerase chain reaction testing, ASP may choose to

Table 1
Measurements of quality improvement initiatives

Metric	Definition	Examples
Outcome measures	Outcome that is specific to the type of intervention	Primary outcomes[1] • Mortality • Length of stay • Appropriate use of antibiotics[119] Adverse events • Toxicity • Graft injury • Drug–drug interactions Infection specific[120–122] • Microbiologic cure • Resistance patterns • Antibiograms Infection prevention • *Clostridioides difficile* rates • Multidrug-resistant organism rates
Process measures	Assess whether intervention has intended effect and is congruent with outcome measures	Antibiotic use • Databases such as NHSN, Vizient, HEDIS[123] • Antibiotic use to Antimicrobial Resistance (AU/AR) ratio[124] Cost analysis
Balancing measures	Outcome to assess for unintended negative impacts • May overlap with outcome measures	• Length of stay • Readmission rates • Mortality • Recurrent or relapsed infection • Patient satisfaction • Surgical site infections (TransQIP)[125,126] • Desirability of outcome ranking[127,128]

restrict these due to the risk of false positive results and unclear utility in transplant recipients.

SYNDROMIC TARGETS FOR ANTIMICROBIAL STEWARDSHIP
Diarrheal Illnesses in Transplant

Antimicrobial stewardship opportunities for diarrheal illness in transplant recipients are largely diagnostic stewardship interventions. Diarrhea is a common complaint among transplant recipients and can cause significant morbidity in this population. The use of multiplex polymerase chain reaction (PCR) panels for the evaluation of diarrhea in transplant recipients increases the probability of identifying an infectious cause of diarrhea compared to ordering individual tests. Among liver transplant recipients, the use of multiplex PCR panels for diarrhea led to a change in antimicrobial therapy, reduction in length of stay, and a trend toward lower rates of colonoscopy and readmission within 30 days.[41] However, these panels offer the most benefit when used early in a hospitalization and may lead to false positive results due to high sensitivity of PCR. Use of diagnostic selection criteria such as reserved for those patients with liquid stool or only within 48 to 72 hours of admission to the hospital may mitigate some of the downsides of using multiplex PCR panels for diarrhea.[42]

Table 2
Diagnostic stewardship opportunities

Diagnostic Stewardship Opportunities	Examples
When a test is ordered	Order sets • Pneumonia bundle with recommended empiric antibiotic choices Clinical decision support tools • Embedded treatment algorithms for common diagnoses Electronic nudges • Timed reminders to reassess need for antimicrobial agent Requirements for ordering a test • Confirmation of > 3 liquid bowel movements for C difficile testing
When a specimen is processed	Use of specimen acceptance criteria • Laboratory rejection of formed stool for C difficile testing • Laboratory rejection of culture swabs for acid-fast bacilli cultures Reflex testing • Urinalysis with defined quantity of pyuria reflexes to urine culture • Positive hepatitis C antibody reflexes to quantitative PCR
When results are reported	Electronic nudges • Alert if receipt of laxative within 24 hours of C difficile testing Framing of results • Masking of antimicrobial susceptibility results to limit use of agents Cascading results • Stepwise unmasking of antimicrobial susceptibility results based on resistance pattern

Transplant recipients are at high risk for *Clostridioides difficile* infections (CDI), largely due to the collection of epidemiologic risk factors such as the need for empiric and prophylactic antibiotics, invasive surgery, intensive care, and immunosuppression.[43] Transplant recipients with CDI have worse outcomes in terms of 30-day readmission and mortality, underscoring the importance of antimicrobial stewardship to prevent CDI.[42,44] SOTr have higher rates of both colonization and disease due to *C. difficile* than the general population, often leading to overtreatment.[45] ASP can implement diagnostic criteria and multi-step laboratory testing for confirmation of toxins in stool. Diagnostic criteria may include documentation of at least three unformed stools, absence of a laxative receipt, and laboratory rejection of formed stool specimens to reduce testing on patients who have transient diarrhea.[46,47] One approach is to use a clinical support tool in the electronic medical record which requires the provider to answer a series of questions to order *C. difficile* testing. Kueht and colleagues implemented this strategy among SOTr and showed a significant decrease of 47% in *C. difficile* testing and a significant reduction in days of therapy (522 days of therapy per 1000 days compared to 300 days of therapy per 1000 patient days). This strategy did not alter the rate of negative tests.[48]

Antimicrobial stewardship teams may be tasked with developing local guidance or performing audit and feedback for CDI treatment of prophylaxis for high-risk patient

Table 3 Commercially available rapid diagnostic tools	
Panel	**Organism(s)**
Whole blood	
T2Biosystems	Bacteria and *Candida* panels
Growth from blood culture	
Accelerate Diagnostics: PhenoTest BC Kit	Gram-positive bacteria, gram-negative bacteria, and *Candida* panels
BioFire: FilmArray	Gram-positive bacteria, gram-negative bacteria, and *Candida* panels
Cepheid: Xpert	*Staphylococcus aureus*
GenMark Diagnostics: ePlex BCID	Gram-positive bacteria, gram-negative bacteria, and fungal panels
Luminex: Verigene	Gram-positive bacteria, gram-negative bacteria, and *Candida* panels
OpGen: AdvanDx	*Staphylococcus aureus* and coagulase-negative *Staphylococci* panel, gram-negative panel, and *Candida*
Respiratory specimens	
ARIES	Influenza A/B and RSV panel; *Bordetella parapertussis* and *pertussis*
BioFire: FilmArray	Upper and lower respiratory pathogens: viruses, bacteria
Cepheid: Xpert	SARS-CoV-2, Influenza A/B, and RSV panel; *Mycobacterium tuberculosis* and rifampin resistance
GenMark Diagnostics: Respiratory Patho	Upper and lower respiratory pathogens: viruses, bacteria
Luminex: Verigene and NxTAG	Viruses and *Bordetella* species or *Chlamydia pneumoniae* and *Mycoplasma pneumoniae*
OpGen: Unyvero System	Lower respiratory tract bacterial pathogens and *Pneumocystis jirovecii*
Stool	
ARIES	*Clostridioides difficile* and Norovirus
BioFire: FilmArray	Bacteria, viruses, and parasites
Cepheid: Xpert	*Clostridioides difficile* and Norovirus
Luminex: Verigene, xTAG, NxTAG	Bacteria, viruses, and parasites

Adapted from Vega AD, Abbo LM. Rapid molecular testing for antimicrobial stewardship and solid organ transplantation. Transpl Infect Dis. 2022;24(5):e13913; and Young BA, Hanson KE, Gomez CA. Molecular Diagnostic Advances in Transplant Infectious Diseases. Curr Infect Dis Rep. 2019;21(12); with permissions

populations such as SOTr due to their high burden of *C difficile* disease. However, more data are necessary to provide such guidance in SOTr. Although Infectious Disease Society of America (IDSA) guidelines recommend fidaxomicin as the preferred treatment of CDI, there are insufficient data comparing clinical outcomes from fidaxomicin and oral vancomycin therapy in SOTr specifically.[49,50] Therapies to prevent primary or recurrent CDI in SOTr is another area in need of further study. A meta-analysis of oral vancomycin prophylaxis showed a strong protective effect for primary and secondary *C. difficile* infections in over 900 patients, which included SOTr.[51] However, only 1 of 11 studies were randomized controlled trial (RCT), and dosing and duration strategy were variable. High-quality studies are needed on SOTr to support oral vancomycin prophylaxis. Similarly, the addition of bezlotoxumab to standard of care to prevent recurrent CDI in transplant recipients offers promise but larger studies are needed.[52]

Asymptomatic Bacteriuria in Renal Transplant

Screening and treating asymptomatic bacteriuria (ASB) in kidney transplant recipients is a "low-hanging fruit" for antimicrobial stewards in transplantation. The 2019 Infectious Disease Society of America's Clinical Practice Guidelines of ASB and the 2019 American Society of Transplantation Infectious Disease Community of Practice Guidelines for Urinary Tract Infection in Solid Organ Transplantation recommend against the treatment of ASB after 2 months post-kidney transplant because the risk of inducing drug resistance outweighs the benefit of treating ASB.[53,54] Some challenged these recommendations due to few studies with high-quality study designs.[55]

Gradually, more data emerged. A summary of supporting data among comparative trials is summarized in **Table 4**. Three RCTs demonstrated that ASB treatment does not prevent progression to urinary tract infection (UTI) and/or acute pyelonephritis.[56–58] Insufficient data exist within 2 months of transplant. Meanwhile, studies consistently reflect that ASB treatment is followed by the development of drug-resistant organisms.[56,57,59–61]

CMV Management Opportunities

Post-transplant cytomegalovirus (CMV) infection is common and represents an opportunity for ASP. CMV management can align with stewardship principles of the right drug (valganciclovir vs alternative antivirals for resistant, refractory CMV), dose (when CMV therapeutics require renal dose adjustment), duration (often based on serial CMV serum monitoring using highly sensitive assays), and de-escalation (back to prophylaxis or pre-emptive monitoring for example).

Antimicrobial stewardship-minded transplant providers should approach CMV management with specific targets. Antivirals directed at CMV are subject to overuse and misuse, which can lead to toxicities, CMV resistance, and poor patient outcomes including graft rejection and loss.[62,63] CMV-related stewardship activities can target not only these adverse events but also decrease the incidence of CMV disease, unnecessary testing, duration of therapy, hospital admission, lengths of stays, and associated costs.[62,64] With the availability of maribavir as an oral therapy for resistant and refractory CMV, a future ASP goal may be to limit the development of maribavir-resistant CMV and decrease foscarnet duration and its associated toxicities, hospital admissions, and costs.

Establishing local CMV management guidelines is the first step for transplant-specific ASP, which should be organ-specific and based on donor and recipient CMV risk profiles. The American Society of Transplantation guidance on prevention and management of CMV in solid transplant offers a primer for transplant clinicians,[65] and many transplant centers have adapted these locally. In a survey regarding stewardship strategies in the US transplant centers, 82% and 70% developed center-specific guidelines for CMV prophylaxis and treatment, respectively.[10] Local guidance may depend on the availability of highly sensitive CMV serum assays and could establish assay specific virologic thresholds for treatment of specific populations (eg, R+). Some centers may need to consider and address the appropriate use of CMV-specific T-cell immunity panels.

Table 4
Studies of ASB treatment versus no treatment in renal transplant recipients

Study	Timing of ASB	Clinical Outcomes
Coussement et al,[56] 2021 Multicenter RCT, n = 199	≥2 months post-transplant	No difference in UTI in subsequent 12 months. Antibiotic use 5x higher in treated group. Resistant organisms emerged in treated group.
Sabé et al,[57] 2021 Multicenter RCT, n = 87	≥1 month post-transplant	No difference in acute graft pyelonephritis during 12-month follow-up (primary outcome). No difference in graft rejection or dysfunction, hospitalization, or mortality. Antibiotic resistance developed more commonly in treated group than non-treated group.
Antonio et al,[58] 2022 Single center RCT, n = 80	≤2 months post-transplant	No difference in UTI and pyelonephritis during follow-up (up to 2 months post-transplant). Trend toward more recurrent UTIs in treated group. More hospitalizations in the treated group but no difference in UTI-related hospitalizations. High baseline ESBL *E. coli/ Klebsiella sp* but insufficient data regarding the emergence of resistance.
Origüen et al,[129] 2016 Single center RCT, n = 112	≥2 months post-transplant	No difference in acute graft pyelonephritis during 2-year follow-up (primary outcome). No differences in UTI incidence, graft function or rejection, all-cause mortality, *C diff* infection.
Moradi et al,[130] 2005 Prospective case control, n = 88	>1 year post-transplant	Treatment of ASB did not decrease the rate of UTIs during 1-year follow-up period.
Green et al,[131] 2013 Retrospective cohort; ages ≥16 y, n = 112	1–12 months post-transplant	No differences in hospitalization for UTI (primary outcome). More UTIs following treatment of ASB vs no treatment. More antibiotic resistance developed in treated group.

(continued on next page)

Table 4
(continued)

Study	Timing of ASB	Clinical Outcomes
El Amari et al,[60] 2011 Retrospective, n = 77	>1 month post-transplant	No differences in progression to UTI and graft function in treated vs untreated ASB patients. Following treatment of E coli and E faecalis ASB, 78% developed resistant organisms.
Bohn et al,[132] 2019 Retrospective observational, n = 64 with ASB	<12 months post-transplant	Treatment of AB was not associated with progression to UTI.
Bonnéric et al,[133] 2019 Retrospective pediatric, n = 37	2–24 months post-transplant	Acute pyelonephritis and UTIs occurred more commonly in the treated ASB group.
Kotagiri et al,[134] 2017 Retrospective, n = 75 with ASB	<12 months post-transplant	Treatment of ASB reduced the risk of UTI compared to untreated ASB.
Arencibia et al,[61] 2016 Prospective, n = 20 with ASB	Anytime post-transplant	Spontaneous clearance in 70% of untreated ASB. Bacterial clearance in 49% of treated ASB. Emergence of resistance in 48% of treated ASB patients.

Abbreviations: ASB, asymptomatic bacteriuria; ESBL, extended spectrum beta-lactamase producing; RCT, randomized controlled trial; UTI, urinary tract infection.
Studies above were conducted in adult kidney transplant recipients unless otherwise specified.

ASP strategies can be applied to CMV management in SOTr. Prospective audit and feedback and/or pre-authorization may be applied to the use of foscarnet, maribavir, and letermovir. Alternatively, transplant centers may restrict these agents to infectious disease consultation or approval.[62] Institutional ASP should be engaged with the addition of newer antiviral therapeutics as they necessitate formulary review and updates in local management. Some transplant centers have had success with pharmacist-driven antimicrobial stewardship interventions that utilize a combination of stewardship strategies, including local algorithms for serum CMV monitoring and treatment, standardized dosing algorithm for renal dose adjustment and monitoring, and prospective monitoring and feedback to name a few.[62,64]

Respiratory Infections

Bacterial pneumonia
Opportunities for antimicrobial stewardship interventions exist for health care-associated pneumonia in the early post-transplant period (<30 days) and community acquired pneumonia in the late post-transplant period (>6–12 months post-transplant) to direct diagnostic workup and duration of therapy. The national community acquired and health care-associated pneumonia guidelines excluded immunocompromised patients due to their increased risk for opportunistic infections,[66,67] but they represent a large proportion of pneumonia-associated hospitalizations.[68] Bacterial etiologies and clinical presentation in SOTr vary and empiric antibiotics require consideration of the following: individual's level of immunosuppression, time from transplant, history

of microorganisms, and local antibiograms. In SOTr, pneumonia occurs most commonly early post-transplant (<30 days post-transplant) and then >6 to 12 months post-transplant.[69] In the early post-transplant period, donor-derived and recipient airway colonization are important factors informing therapy in lung transplant recipients, whereas in liver transplant recipients, gram-negative bacterial etiologies predominate.[69] To date, there is no consensus for the appropriate duration of therapy, which remains an important target for antimicrobial stewardship.[1]

Determining the microbiologic etiology of pneumonia is important in SOTr to target therapy.[69] Access to rapid diagnostic platforms, such as the Biofire Filmarray Respiratory Panel or multiplex bacterial PCR panels, may allow for rapid identification for prespecified bacterial ± viral targets and subsequently targeted antimicrobial therapy.[70] Although no studies evaluated SOTr exclusively, early studies that included immunocompromised patients found earlier time-to-detection of a respiratory pathogen[71,72] and decreased duration of inappropriate antibiotic therapy.[71,73] One study examined the clinical impact of Biofire Pneumonia Plus (BPP), which includes viral, bacterial, and some resistance targets, in 60 lung transplant recipients with suspected lower respiratory tract infection who underwent bronchoscopy. The median time to result was 2.3 hours using BPP compared to 23.4 hours for viral detection using immune fluorescence testing and 25.2 hours for conventional cultures. Faster clinical decisions resulting in treatment modifications occurred in the BPP group (2.8 hours) compared to viral and traditional microbiologic methods (28.1 and 32.6 hours, respectively), which were statistically significant. There were six treatment modifications based on traditional lab methods missed by BPP, including three fungal pathogens.

Bronchoscopy delay may lead to increased antibiotic exposure. Azadeh and colleagues[74] compared Filmarray Respiratory Panel (17 viral and 3 bacterial targets) results from simultaneously collected bronchoalveolar lavage and nasopharyngeal specimens in immunocompromised patients, 27% of which were SOTr, and found 89% concordance between the samples, driven largely by shared negative results potentially offering more rapid identification of predominately viral pneumonia and antibiotic de-escalation.

Although rapid diagnostics for lower respiratory tract infections is promising, transplant providers and antimicrobial stewards need to consider diagnostic stewardship, limiting repeat testing within a short period as re-detection of targets is common and can result in overtreatment. In SOTr with a high likelihood of opportunistic infection or more than one pathogen, providers need to consider the presence of organisms not present on diagnostic panels, particularly fungal organisms. However, rapid molecular tests with high negative predictive values for methicillin-resistant *Staphylococcus aureus* (MRSA) and *Pseudomonas aeruginosa* can be helpful in ruling out these organisms, allowing discontinuation of vancomycin or de-escalating from anti-Pseudomonal agents.

Respiratory syncytial virus

In the past decade, antimicrobial stewards targeted the use of ribavirin to treat RSV in SOTr. Ribavirin is utilized to treat RSV upper and lower respiratory tract infections in SOTr based on conflicting evidence and is available in aerosolized, oral, and intravenous forms.[75] Aerosolized ribavirin is challenging to administer and costly, nearly 30,000 dollars per day.[2,75,76] Small observational studies offered efficacy with oral ribavirin including lung transplant recipients,[77–80] including in one comparing aerosolized and oral ribavirin with no significant differences in 6-month outcomes.[77] Therefore, due to both financial and administration constraints, many centers have elected to pursue oral ribavirin only, while others may permit inhaled ribavirin in only rare instances. Centers may offer local guidance for clinical circumstances for which ribavirin is considered or restrict use to certain transplant providers. Updated experience following the implementation of ribavirin guidance and restrictions, including clinical outcomes in lung transplant recipients with RSV, may add to the literature informing future antimicrobial stewardship interventions surrounding the use of ribavirin.

COVID-19

An evolving antimicrobial stewardship need during the COVID-19 pandemic surrounds antibiotic use in SOTr with COVID-19. Antibiotic overuse in hospitalized COVID-19 patients was common early in the pandemic.[81,82] SOTr were more likely to develop severe COVID-19 requiring hospitalization or leading to mortality,[83] which likely heightened pressure to add empiric antibiotics for secondary bacterial infections. A retrospective review found a higher prevalence of bacterial and fungal co-infections in SOTr with COVID-19, which was associated with prior hospitalization and the use of broad-spectrum antibiotics.[84] When clinicians have a high index of suspicion for secondary infections in SOTr with COVID-19, prompt diagnostic workup should be emphasized to allow targeted and/or de-escalation of antibiotic therapies.

Meanwhile, as antiviral guidance evolved during the pandemic, so too have ASP efforts surrounding COVID-19. The initial stewardship priorities included audit and feedback of therapies for appropriateness, managing and prioritizing limited antiviral supply, and ensuring compliance with Food and Drug Administration (FDA) emergency use authorizations.[85] More recent therapeutic advances offered outpatient treatment options for SOTr with mild–moderate COVID-19, including monoclonal antibodies, 3-day remdesivir infusions, and oral nirmatrelvir-ritonavir and molnupiravir.[86] Therefore, COVID-19-related ASP priorities have shifted over time toward updating therapeutic guidance based on newer COVID-19 variants, ordering and administration of outpatient therapeutics, and limiting toxicities and drug–drug interactions, such as oral nirmatrelvir-ritonavir's boosted effects of calcineurin-inhibitors and mTOR inhibitors.[87]

Invasive Fungal Infections

SOTr are at increased risk for invasive fungal infections (IFIs) and the use of antifungals is common. Invasive *Candida* and *Aspergillus* represent the most common IFIs in SOT.[88] The diagnosis of these infections may be difficult, which contributes to antifungal overuse. Prolonged antifungal therapy and prophylaxis account for 42% to 66% of antifungal overuse.[89] De-escalation from empiric therapy remains one of the most challenging aspects of antifungal stewardship.[90]

Use of fungal antigen tests is often employed. However, the performance of assays such as Aspergillus galactomannan (GM) and β-D-glucan (BDG) have variable sensitivity and specificity in solid organ overuse transplant recipients.[42] In this population, sensitivity of the serum GM for diagnosis of invasive Aspergillosis ranges from 22% to 68% across the different organ types.[91–93] Of particular concern is the low sensitivity of the assay to predict *Aspergillus tracheobronchitis* in lung transplant recipients.[42] Sensitivity and specificity for diagnosis of invasive Aspergillosis increase when GM is obtained on bronchoalveolar lavage specimens and when a higher cutoff of 1.0 is used, specificity improves.[94,95] BDG may also be used for diagnosis of invasive fungal infections (with the exception of *Mucorales* and *Cryptococcus*), but sensitivity and specificity in transplant recipients are much lower ranging from 57% to 80% and <50%, respectively,[96] though it is more useful in the diagnosis of *Pneumocystis jirovecii* pneumonia among SOTr.[97] The use of serum GM and BDG for the diagnosis of invasive fungal infections should be cautiously employed for compatible syndromes, but discouraged when used outside these parameters as it may lead to overdiagnosis and overtreatment. Other antifungal stewardship opportunities include guideline development, post-prescriptive review, and IV-to-oral antifungal conversion.[2,4,89,90]

SYSTEMS-BASED TARGETS FOR ANTIMICROBIAL STEWARDSHIP
Antibiotic Allergies

Antibiotic allergy labels (AAL) are defined as antibiotic allergies that are a part of the patient's medical record. AAL are common among SOTr and prevalence ranges from 16% to 17% in the literature.[98-100] The most common types of AAL are beta-lactams and sulfamethoxazole-trimethoprim (SMX-TMP). Beta-lactam allergies pose significant challenges to SOTr as they may negatively impact surgical prophylaxis, lead to the use of unnecessary broad-spectrum agents, and increase the use of antibiotics in the immediate post-transplant setting.[100,101] SMX-TMP allergies pose a significant risk with the inability to use first-line prophylaxis for *P jirovecii* and *Nocardia* infections. The use of broader spectrum antibiotics in those with beta-lactam allergies may lead to the development of multidrug-resistant organisms[102-105] while the use of second- or third-line prophylaxis agents in those with SMX-TMP allergy may be more costly.[106]

AAL delabeling is the practice of removing AAL from a patient's chart either by testing or medical reconciliation.[107] Delabeling is associated with increased use of narrow spectrum agents, reduced length of hospital stay[107], and improved prescribing with guideline-preferred regimen[101] making it an ideal target for ASP. Delabeling of AAL has been shown to be safe in the pre-transplant setting for those with AAL to vancomycin, SMX-TMP, beta-lactams, and fluoroquinolones and cost-effective in the setting of SMX-TMP delabeling.[106] AAL delabeling begins with an assessment of the severity of the reaction. Those with suspected non-immune reactions, that is, non-allergic symptoms, or those who have documented tolerance to the drug, may have the AAL removed without testing.

Delabeling of penicillin AAL begins with risk stratification (**Table 5**).[108] For penicillin allergy risk stratification at the point of care, consider the use of PEN-FAST, a clinical decision rule which was validated in a diverse population including SOTr.[109] The American Academy of Allergy, Asthma and Immunology (AAAAI) recommends direct oral amoxicillin challenge without preceding skin testing for patients with low-risk penicillin allergy features, while skin testing is reserved for those patients with a history of high-risk features.[110] For those with SMX-TMP allergy, desensitization is no longer recommended by the AAAAI. Instead, direct oral challenge in one or two steps may be considered for most patients.[110] In a recent study, 17 SOTr patients underwent direct oral challenge with SMX-TMP with 16 successfully passing the challenge, which suggests that the AAAAI's recommendation extends to use in SOTr.[111] Direct oral challenge now plays a role in the assessment of AAL for cephalosporins, fluoroquinolones, and macrolides as well.[110]

Perioperative stewardship

Surgical site infections (SSI) in SOTr lead to longer hospitalizations, higher costs, increased graft failure, and mortality.[112,113] Targeting antimicrobial SSI perioperative prophylaxis serves both stewardship and infection prevention goals. Perioperative SSI guidance in SOTr exists,[114,115] but additional antimicrobial stewardship opportunities remain. Institutions may be reluctant to follow guidelines based on local SSI history or established practices. Data based on local data may be reassuring. For example, Allen and colleagues[116] narrowed their left ventricular assist device (LVAD) SSI prophylaxis from a four-drug regimen (vancomycin, rifampin, ciprofloxacin, and

Table 5
Risk stratification of reported antibiotic allergies

Non-Allergic Symptoms	Low-Risk Symptoms	Severe Immediate Symptoms	Severe Delayed Symptoms
Gastrointestinal symptoms	Remote history (>5–10 years ago) of non-severe symptoms	Diffuse hives or urticaria	Oral or eye ulcerations
Family history of allergy	Delayed onset of urticaria	Angioedema	Skin or mucosal sloughing
Fear of allergy	Remote history (>5–10 years ago) of urticaria	Dyspnea, wheezing, cough	Immune mediate kidney or liver injury
		Shock	Stevens-Johnsons syndrome
		Comatose	Toxic epidermal necrolysis
			Drug reaction with eosinophilia and systemic symptoms
			Acute generalized exanthematous pustulosis

Adapted from Stone CA, Trubiano J, Coleman DT, Rukasin CRF, Phillips EJ. The challenge of de-labeling penicillin allergy. Allergy: European Journal of Allergy and Clinical Immunology. 2020;75(2):273-288; with permission.

fluconazole) to anti-*Staphylococcal* coverage only (vancomycin and cefazolin) without changes in 30- or 90-day mortality. Some argue for individualized perioperative antimicrobial use based on organ-specific guidelines, donor and recipient microbial colonization, antibiotic allergies, and PK/PD dosing parameters surrounding SOTr's end-organ failure.[117,118] Antibiotic allergy delabeling could also optimize transplant SSI prophylaxis.[100] Other opportunities in peritransplant prophylaxis include optimizing intra-operative antimicrobial dosing and clarifying post-operative dose duration.[118]

SUMMARY

Transplant recipients benefit from antimicrobial stewardship program interventions. We reviewed ASP metrics and designs upon which current and future interventions can build. Diagnostic stewardship opportunities include *C. difficile* testing and many rapid diagnostic platforms, which should be paired with antimicrobial stewardship guidance for optimal use in transplant recipients. Among syndromic and systems-based antimicrobial stewardship opportunities, growing evidence supports delabeling antibiotic allergies in transplant candidates and recipients and withholding treatment of ASB in patients who received renal transplantation more than 2 months ago. Larger studies are needed to build on observational and retrospective antimicrobial stewardship studies in transplant recipients.

CLINICS CARE POINTS

- Clinicians can target *C. difficile* infections in transplant recipients through diagnostic testing stewardship and comparative trials of therapeutic and prophylactic agents.
- Renal transplant recipients do not benefit from treatment of ASB when greater than 2 months from transplant.
- Solid organ transplant recipients benefit from antibiotic allergy delabeling, allowing receipt of narrowed, targeted antibiotics.

DISCLOSURES

E.J. Stohs received grant funding from Merck & Co, United States and bioMerieux, Inc. C.A. Gorsline has no disclosures to report.

REFERENCES

1. So M, Hand J, Forrest G, et al. White paper on antimicrobial stewardship in solid organ transplant recipients. Am J Transplant 2022;22(1):96–112.
2. Liu C, Stohs EJ. Antimicrobial stewardship for transplant candidates and recipients. In: Morris MI, Kotton CN, Wolfe CR, editors. Emerging transplant infections. Cham Switzerland: Springer Nature Switzerland AG; 2021. p. 131–54.
3. Fishman N. Policy statement on antimicrobial stewardship by the society for healthcare epidemiology of America (SHEA), the infectious diseases society of America (IDSA), and the pediatric infectious diseases society (PIDS). Infect Control Hosp Epidemiol 2012;33(4):322–7.
4. Barlam TF, Cosgrove SE, Abbo LM, et al. Implementing an antibiotic stewardship program: guidelines by the infectious diseases society of america and the society for healthcare epidemiology of America. Clin Infect Dis 2016; 62(10):e51–77.

5. Centers for Disease Control and Prevention. Antibiotic Resistance Threats in the United States, 2013. Available at: https://www.cdc.gov/drugresistance/pdf/ar-threats-2013-508.pdf. Accessed May 25, 2023.
6. Centers for Disease Control and Prevention. Antibiotic Resistance Threats in the United States, 2019. Available at: https://www.cdc.gov/drugresistance/pdf/threats-report/2019-ar-threats-report-508.pdf. Accessed May 25, 2023.
7. The Joint Commission. Antimicrobial Stewardship in Ambulatory Health Care. R3 Report | Requirement, Rationale, Reference. Published 2019. Available at: https://www.jointcommission.org/standards/r3-report/r3-report-issue-23-antimicrobial-stewardship-in-ambulatory-health-care/. Accessed May 25, 2023.
8. The Joint Commission. New Antimicrobial Stewardship Standard. R3 Report | Requirement, Rationale, Reference. Published 2016. Available at: https://www.jointcommission.org/standards/r3-report/r3-report-issue-8-new-antimicrobial-stewardship-standard/. Accessed May 25, 2023.
9. Centers for Medicare and Medicaid Services (CMS). Omnibus Burden Reduction (Conditions of Participation). Final Rule CMS-3346-F. Final Rule. Published 2019. Available at: https://www.cms.gov/newsroom/fact-sheets/omnibus-burden-reduction-conditions-participation-final-rule-cms-3346-f. Accessed May 25, 2023.
10. Seo SK, Lo K, Abbo LM. Current state of antimicrobial stewardship at solid organ and hematopoietic cell transplant centers in the United States. Infect Control Hosp Epidemiol 2016;37(10):1195–200.
11. Aitken SL, Palmer HR, Topal JE, et al. Call for antimicrobial stewardship in solid organ transplantation. Am J Transplant 2013;13(9):2499.
12. Hand JM. The time is now: antimicrobial stewardship in solid organ transplantation. Curr Opin Organ Transplant 2021;26(4):405–11.
13. Abbo LM, Ariza-Heredia EJ. Antimicrobial stewardship in immunocompromised hosts. Infect Dis Clin North Am 2014;28(2):263–79.
14. Silva JT, Aguado JM. Current state of antimicrobial stewardship and organ transplantation in Spain. Transpl Infect Dis 2022;24(5):e13851.
15. Bielicki JA, Manuel O, Study (STCS) Swiss Transplant Cohort. Antimicrobial stewardship programs in solid-organ transplant recipients in Switzerland. Transpl Infect Dis 2022;24(5):e13902.
16. Kitaura S, Jindai K, Okamoto K. Japan perspective on antimicrobial stewardship and solid organ transplantation. Transpl Infect Dis 2022;24(5):e13939.
17. Ioannou P, Karakonstantis S, Schouten J, et al. Importance of antimicrobial stewardship in solid organ transplant recipients: An ESCMID perspective. Transpl Infect Dis 2022;24(5):e13852.
18. Almaziad S, Bosaeed M. Current state of antimicrobial stewardship and organ transplantation in Saudi Arabia. Transpl Infect Dis 2022;24(5):e13891.
19. Porto APM, Tavares BM, de Assis DB, et al. Brazilian perspective: antimicrobial stewardship in solid organ transplant. Transpl Infect Dis 2022;24(5):e13874.
20. Chotiprasitsakul D, Bruminhent J, Watcharananan SP. Current state of antimicrobial stewardship and organ transplantation in Thailand. Transpl Infect Dis 2022;24(5):e13877.
21. Chung SJ, Liew Y, Lee WHL, et al. Current state of antimicrobial stewardship in organ transplantation in Singapore. Transpl Infect Dis 2022;24(5):e13886.
22. Stewart AG, Isler B, Paterson DL. An Australian perspective on antimicrobial stewardship programs and transplantation. Transpl Infect Dis 2022;24(5):e13912.

23. Kitano T, Allen U. Antimicrobial stewardship in pediatric solid organ transplantation: Is it possible? Transpl Infect Dis 2022;24(5):e13928.

24. Robilotti E, Holubar M, Seo SK, et al. Feasibility and applicability of antimicrobial stewardship in immunocompromised patients. Curr Opin Infect Dis 2017;30(4): 346–53.

25. So M, Walti L. Challenges of antimicrobial resistance and stewardship in solid organ transplant patients. Curr Infect Dis Rep 2022;24(5):63–75.

26. Dela-Pena J, Kerstenetzky L, Schulz L, et al. Top 1% of inpatients administered antimicrobial agents comprising 50% of expenditures: a descriptive study and opportunities for stewardship intervention. Infect Control Hosp Epidemiol 2017;38(3):259–65.

27. So M, Yang DY, Bell C, et al. Solid organ transplant patients: are there opportunities for antimicrobial stewardship? Clin Transplant 2016;30(6):659–68.

28. Forrest GN, So M, Hand J, et al. Antimicrobial stewardship in solid organ transplantation—A call for action. Transpl Infect Dis 2022;24(5). https://doi.org/10. 1111/tid.13938.

29. Imlay H, Spellberg B. Shorter is better: The case for short antibiotic courses for common infections in solid organ transplant recipients. Transpl Infect Dis 2022; 24(5):e13896.

30. Salsgiver E, Bernstein D, Simon MS, et al. Knowledge, attitudes, and practices regarding antimicrobial use and stewardship among prescribers at acute-care hospitals. Infect Control Hosp Epidemiol 2018;39:316–22. https://doi.org/10. 1017/ice.2017.317. Cambridge University Press.

31. Gorsline CA, Staub MB, Nelson GE, et al. Antimicrobial de-escalation in patients with high-risk febrile neutropenia: Attitudes and practices of adult hospital care providers. Antimicrobial Stewardship and Healthcare Epidemiology 2021;1(1). https://doi.org/10.1017/ash.2021.185.

32. Michie S, Johnston M, Abraham C, et al. Making psychological theory useful for implementing evidence based practice: a consensus approach. Qual Saf Health Care 2005;14:26–33.

33. Michie S, van Stralen MM, West R. The behaviour change wheel: A new method for characterising and designing behaviour change interventions. Implement Sci 2011;6(1). https://doi.org/10.1186/1748-5908-6-42.

34. Michie S, West R, Campbell R, et al. ABC of behaviour change theories. Sutton, UK: Silverback Publishing; 2014.

35. Michie S, Atkins L, West R. The behaviour change wheel: a guide to designing interventions. Sutton, UK: Silverback Publishing; 2014.

36. Morgan DJ, Malani P, Diekema DJ. Diagnostic stewardship - leveraging the laboratory to improve antimicrobial use. JAMA, J Am Med Assoc 2017;318(7): 607–8.

37. Young BA, Hanson KE, Gomez CA. Molecular diagnostic advances in transplant infectious diseases. Curr Infect Dis Rep 2019;21(12). https://doi.org/10.1007/ s11908-019-0704-7.

38. Graff KE, Palmer C, Anarestani T, et al. Clinical impact of the expanded biofire blood culture identification 2 panel in a U.S. Children's hospital. Microbiol Spectr 2021;9(1). https://doi.org/10.1128/SPECTRUM.00429-21.

39. Timbrook TT, Morton JB, Mcconeghy KW, et al. The effect of molecular rapid diagnostic testing on clinical outcomes in bloodstream infections: a systematic review and meta-analysis. Clin Infect Dis 2017;64(1):15–23.

40. Banerjee R, Teng CB, Cunningham SA, et al. Randomized trial of rapid multiplex polymerase chain reaction-based blood culture identification and susceptibility testing. Clin Infect Dis 2015;61(7):1071–80.
41. Ching CK, Nobel YR, Pereira MR, et al. The role of gastrointestinal pathogen polymerase chain reaction testing in liver transplant recipients hospitalized with diarrhea. Transpl Infect Dis 2022;24(4):e13873.
42. Husson J, Bork JT, Morgan D, et al. Is diagnostic stewardship possible in solid organ transplantation? Transpl Infect Dis 2022;24(5). https://doi.org/10.1111/tid.13899.
43. Antonelli M, Martin-Loeches I, Dimopoulos G, et al. Clostridioides difficile (formerly Clostridium difficile) infection in the critically ill: an expert statement. Intensive Care Med 2020;46(2):215–24.
44. Amjad W, Qureshi W, Malik A, et al. The outcomes of Clostridioides difficile infection in inpatient liver transplant population. Transpl Infect Dis 2022;24(1). https://doi.org/10.1111/TID.13750.
45. Revolinski SL, Munoz-Price LS. Clostridium difficile in immunocompromised hosts: a review of epidemiology, risk factors, treatment, and prevention. Clin Infect Dis 2019;68(12):2144–53.
46. Pouch SM, Friedman-Moraco RJ. Prevention and treatment of clostridium difficile-associated diarrhea in solid organ transplant recipients. Infect Dis Clin North Am 2018;32(3):733–48.
47. Truong CY, Gombar S, Wilson R, et al. Real-time electronic tracking of diarrheal episodes and laxative therapy enables verification of Clostridium difficile clinical testing criteria and reduction of Clostridium difficile infection rates. J Clin Microbiol 2017;55(5):1276–84.
48. Kueht M, Kharsa A, Mujtaba M, et al. Antibiotic stewardship and inpatient clostridioides difficile testing in solid organ transplant recipients: the need for multi-level checks and balances. Transplant Proc 2022;54(3):605–9.
49. Johnson S, Lavergne V, Skinner AM, et al. Clinical practice guideline by the infectious diseases society of America (IDSA) and society for healthcare epidemiology of America (SHEA): 2021 focused update guidelines on management of clostridioides difficile infection in adults. Clin Infect Dis 2021;73(5):e1029–44.
50. Mullane KM, Dubberke ER. Management of Clostridioides (formerly Clostridium) difficile infection (CDI) in solid organ transplant recipients: guidelines from the American society of transplantation community of practice. Clin Transplant 2019;33(9). https://doi.org/10.1111/ctr.13564.
51. Maraolo AE, Mazzitelli M, Zappulo E, et al. Oral vancomycin prophylaxis for primary and secondary prevention of clostridioides difficile infection in patients treated with systemic antibiotic therapy: a systematic review, meta-analysis and trial sequential analysis. Antibiotics 2022;11(2). https://doi.org/10.3390/antibiotics11020183.
52. Johnson TM, Howard AH, Miller MA, et al. Effectiveness of bezlotoxumab for prevention of recurrent clostridioides difficile infection among transplant recipients. Open Forum Infect Dis 2021;8(7):1–8.
53. Nicolle LE, Gupta K, Bradley SF, et al. Clinical practice guideline for the management of asymptomatic bacteriuria: 2019 update by the infectious diseases society of Americaa. Clin Infect Dis 2019;68(10):1611–5.
54. Goldman JD, Julian K. Urinary tract infections in solid organ transplant recipients: guidelines from the american society of transplantation infectious diseases community of practice. Clin Transplant 2019;e13507. https://doi.org/10.1111/ctr.13507. Epub.

55. Coussement J, Scemla A, Abramowicz D, et al. Management of asymptomatic bacteriuria after kidney transplantation: what is the quality of the evidence behind the Infectious Diseases Society of America Guidelines? Clin Infect Dis 2020;70(5):987–8.

56. Coussement J, Kamar N, Matignon M, et al. Antibiotics versus no therapy in kidney transplant recipients with asymptomatic bacteriuria (BiRT): a pragmatic, multicentre, randomized, controlled trial. Clin Microbiol Infection 2021;27(3):398–405.

57. Sabé N, Cruzado JM, Carratalà J. Asymptomatic bacteriuria in kidney transplant recipients: to treat or not to treat—that is the question. Clin Microbiol Infect 2021;27(3):319–21.

58. Antonio MEE, Cassandra BGC, Emiliano RJD, et al. Treatment of asymptomatic bacteriuria in the first 2 months after kidney transplant: A controlled clinical trial. Transpl Infect Dis 2022;(July):1–9. https://doi.org/10.1111/tid.13934.

59. Green H, Rahamimov R, Gafter U, et al. Antibiotic prophylaxis for urinary tract infections in renal transplant recipients: a systematic review and meta-analysis. Transpl Infect Dis 2011;13(5):441–7.

60. el Amari EB, Hadaya K, Bühler L, et al. Outcome of treated and untreated asymptomatic bacteriuria in renal transplant recipients. Nephrol Dial Transplant 2011;26(12):4109–14.

61. Arencibia N, Agüera ML, Rodelo C, et al. Short-term outcome of untreated versus treated asymptomatic bacteriuria in renal transplant patients. Transplant Proc 2016;48(9):2941–3.

62. Jorgenson MR, Descourouez JL, Kleiboeker H, et al. Cytomegalovirus antiviral stewardship in solid organ transplant recipients: a new gold standard. Transpl Infect Dis 2022;24(5). https://doi.org/10.1111/tid.13864.

63. Rolling KE, Jorgenson MR, Descourouez JL, et al. Ganciclovir-resistant cytomegalovirus infection in abdominal solid organ transplant recipients: case series and review of the literature. Pharmacotherapy 2017;37(10):1258–71.

64. Wang N, Athans V, Neuner E, et al. A pharmacist-driven antimicrobial stewardship intervention targeting cytomegalovirus viremia in ambulatory solid organ transplant recipients. Transpl Infect Dis 2018;20(6):e12991.

65. Razonable RR, Humar A. Cytomegalovirus in solid organ transplant recipients—guidelines of the American society of transplantation infectious diseases community of practice. Clin Transplant 2019;33(9). https://doi.org/10.1111/ctr.13512.

66. Metlay JP, Waterer GW, Long AC, et al. Diagnosis and treatment of adults with community-acquired pneumonia. Am J Respir Crit Care Med 2019;200(7):E45–67.

67. Kalil AC, Metersky ML, Klompas M, et al. Management of Adults With Hospital-acquired and Ventilator-associated Pneumonia: 2016 clinical practice guidelines by the infectious diseases society of America and the American thoracic society. Clin Infect Dis 2016;63(5):e61–111.

68. Hayes BH, Haberling DL, Kennedy JL, et al. Burden of pneumonia-associated hospitalizations: United States, 2001-2014. Chest 2018;153(2):427–37.

69. Dulek DE, Mueller NJ. Pneumonia in solid organ transplantation: Guidelines from the American society of transplantation infectious diseases community of practice. Clin Transplant 2019;33(9):1–11.

70. Vega AD, Abbo LM. Rapid molecular testing for antimicrobial stewardship and solid organ transplantation. Transpl Infect Dis 2022;24(5):e13913.

71. Darie AM, Khanna N, Jahn K, et al. Fast multiplex bacterial PCR of bronchoalveolar lavage for antibiotic stewardship in hospitalised patients with pneumonia

at risk of Gram-negative bacterial infection (Flagship II): a multicentre, randomised controlled trial. Lancet Respir Med 2022;10(9):877–87.

72. Kayser MZ, Seeliger B, Valtin C, et al. Clinical decision making is improved by BioFire Pneumonia Plus in suspected lower respiratory tract infection after lung transplantation: results of the prospective DBATE-IT* study. Transpl Infect Dis 2022;24(1). https://doi.org/10.1111/tid.13725.

73. Buchan BW, Windham S, Balada-Llasat JM, et al. Practical comparison of the BioFire FilmArray pneumonia panel to routine diagnostic methods and potential impact on antimicrobial stewardship in adult hospitalized patients with lower respiratory tract infections. J Clin Microbiol 2020;58(7). https://doi.org/10.1128/JCM.00135-20.

74. Azadeh N, Sakata KK, Saeed A, et al. Comparison of respiratory pathogen detection in upper versus lower respiratory tract samples using the BioFire FilmArray respiratory panel in the immunocompromised host. Can Respir J 2018;2018. https://doi.org/10.1155/2018/2685723.

75. Manuel O, Estabrook M. RNA respiratory viral infections in solid organ transplant recipients: guidelines from the American society of transplantation infectious diseases community of practice. Clin Transplant 2019;33(9). https://doi.org/10.1111/ctr.13511.

76. Chemaly RF, Aitken SL, Wolfe CR, et al. Aerosolized ribavirin: the most expensive drug for pneumonia. Transpl Infect Dis 2016;18(4):634–6.

77. Li L, Avery R, Budev M, et al. Oral versus inhaled ribavirin therapy for respiratory syncytial virus infection after lung transplantation. J Heart Lung Transplant 2012;31(8):839–44.

78. Pelaez A, Lyon GM, Force SD, et al. Efficacy of oral ribavirin in lung transplant patients with respiratory syncytial virus lower respiratory tract infection. J Heart Lung Transplant 2009;28(1):67–71.

79. Trang TP, Whalen M, Hilts-Horeczko A, et al. Comparative effectiveness of aerosolized versus oral ribavirin for the treatment of respiratory syncytial virus infections: a single-center retrospective cohort study and review of the literature. Transpl Infect Dis 2018;20(2). https://doi.org/10.1111/tid.12844.

80. Burrows FS, Carlos LM, Benzimra M, et al. Oral ribavirin for respiratory syncytial virus infection after lung transplantation: Efficacy and cost-efficiency. J Heart Lung Transplant 2015;34(7):958–62.

81. Langford BJ, So M, Raybardhan S, et al. Bacterial co-infection and secondary infection in patients with COVID-19: a living rapid review and meta-analysis. Clin Microbiol Infection 2020;26(12):1622–9.

82. Vaughn VM, Gandhi TN, Petty LA, et al. Empiric antibacterial therapy and community-onset bacterial coinfection in patients hospitalized with Coronavirus disease 2019 (COVID-19): a multi-hospital cohort study. Clin Infect Dis 2021;72(10):533–74.

83. Jering KS, McGrath MM, Mc Causland FR, et al. Excess mortality in solid organ transplant recipients hospitalized with COVID-19: a large-scale comparison of SOT recipients hospitalized with or without COVID-19. Clin Transplant 2022;36(1):1–9.

84. Shafiekhani M, Shekari Z, Boorboor A, et al. Bacterial and fungal co-infections with SARS-CoV-2 in solid organ recipients: a retrospective study. Virol J 2022;19(1):1–7.

85. Pierce J, Stevens MP. COVID-19 and antimicrobial stewardship: lessons learned, best practices, and future implications. Int J Infect Dis 2021;113:103–8.

86. Avery RK. Update on COVID-19 therapeutics for solid organ transplant recipients, including the omicron surge. Transplantation 2022;106(8):1528–37.

87. Fishbane S, Hirsch JS, Nair V. Special considerations for paxlovid treatment among transplant recipients with SARS-CoV-2 infection. Am J Kidney Dis 2022;79(4):480–2.

88. Schwartz IS, Patterson TF. The emerging threat of antifungal resistance in transplant infectious diseases. Curr Infect Dis Rep 2018;20(3). https://doi.org/10.1007/s11908-018-0608-y.

89. Urbancic KF, Thursky K, Kong DCM, et al. Antifungal stewardship: developments in the field. Curr Opin Infect Dis 2018;31(6):490–8.

90. Ananda-Rajah MR, Slavin MA, Thursky KT. A case for antifungal stewardship. Curr Opin Infect Dis 2012;25(1):107–15.

91. Hoyo I, Sanclemente G, de la Bellacasa JP, et al. Epidemiology, clinical characteristics, and outcome of invasive aspergillosis in renal transplant patients. Transpl Infect Dis 2014;16(6):951–7.

92. López-Medrano F, Fernández-Ruiz M, Silva JT, et al. Clinical Presentation and Determinants of Mortality of Invasive Pulmonary Aspergillosis in Kidney Transplant Recipients: A Multinational Cohort Study. Am J Transplant 2016;16(11):3220–34.

93. Pfeiffer CD, Fine JP, Safdar N. Diagnosis of invasive aspergillosis using a galactomannan assay: a meta-analysis. Clin Infect Dis 2006;42(10):1417–27.

94. Husain S, Paterson DL, Studer SM, et al. Aspergillus galactomannan antigen in the bronchoalveolar lavage fluid for the diagnosis of invasive aspergillosis in lung transplant recipients. Transplantation 2007;83(10):1330–6.

95. Clancy CJ, Jaber RA, Leather HL, et al. Bronchoalveolar lavage galactomannan in diagnosis of invasive pulmonary aspergillosis among solid-organ transplant recipients. J Clin Microbiol 2007;45(6):1759–65.

96. Lamoth F, Akan H, Andes D, et al. Assessment of the role of 1,3-β-d-glucan testing for the diagnosis of invasive fungal infections in adults. Clin Infect Dis 2021;72:S102–8.

97. Borstnar S, Lindic J, Tomazic J, et al. Pneumocystis Jirovecii pneumonia in renal transplant recipients: a national center experience. Transplant Proc 2013;45:1614–7.

98. Khumra S, Chan J, Urbancic K, et al. Antibiotic allergy labels in a liver transplant recipient study. Antimicrob Agents Chemother 2017;61(5). https://doi.org/10.1128/AAC.00078-17.

99. Imlay H, Krantz EM, Stohs EJ, et al. Reported β-lactam and other antibiotic allergies in solid organ and hematopoietic cell transplant recipients. Clin Infect Dis 2020;71(7):1587–94.

100. Mowrer C, Lyden E, Matthews S, et al. Beta-lactam allergies, surgical site infections, and prophylaxis in solid organ transplant recipients at a single center: a retrospective cohort study. Transpl Infect Dis 2022;24(5). https://doi.org/10.1111/tid.13907.

101. Trubiano JA, Grayson ML, Thursky KA, et al. How antibiotic allergy labels may be harming our most vulnerable patients HHS Public Access. Med J Aust 2018;208(11):469–70.

102. Safdar N, Maki DG. The commonality of risk factors for nosocomial colonization and infection with antimicrobial-resistant Staphylococcus aureus, enterococcus, gram-negative bacilli, Clostridium difficile, and Candida. Ann Intern Med 2002;136(11):834–44.

103. Patel G, Huprikar S, Factor SH, et al. Outcomes of carbapenem-resistant klebsiella pneumoniae infection and the impact of antimicrobial and adjunctive therapies. Infect Control Hosp Epidemiol 2008;29(12):1099–106.

104. Reddy P, Zembower TR, Ison MG, et al. Carbapenem-resistant Acinetobacter baumannii infections after organ transplantation. Transpl Infect Dis 2010;12(1): 87–93.

105. Linares L, Cervera C, Cofán F, et al. Epidemiology and outcomes of multiple antibiotic–resistant bacterial infection in renal transplantation. Transplant Proc 2007;39(7):2222–4.

106. Gorsline CA, Afghan AK, Stone CA, et al. Safety and value of pretransplant antibiotic allergy delabeling in a quaternary transplant center. Transpl Infect Dis 2022;24(5):e13885.

107. Waldron JL, Trubiano JA. Antibiotic allergy labels in immunocompromised populations. Transpl Infect Dis 2022;24(5). https://doi.org/10.1111/tid.13955.

108. Stone CA, Trubiano J, Coleman DT, et al. The challenge of de-labeling penicillin allergy. Allergy: European Journal of Allergy and Clinical Immunology 2020; 75(2):273–88.

109. Trubiano JA, Vogrin S, Chua KYL, et al. Development and validation of a penicillin allergy clinical decision rule. JAMA Intern Med 2020;180(5):745–52.

110. Khan DA, Banerji A, Blumenthal KG, et al. Drug allergy: a 2022 practice parameter update. J Allergy Clin Immunol 2022. https://doi.org/10.1016/j.jaci.2022. 08.028.

111. Krantz MS, Stone CA, Abreo A, et al. Oral challenge with trimethoprim-sulfamethoxazole in patients with "sulfa" antibiotic allergy. J Allergy Clin Immunol Pract 2020;8(2):757–60.e4.

112. Anesi JA, Blumberg EA, Abbo LM. Perioperative antibiotic prophylaxis to prevent surgical site infections in solid organ transplantation. Transplantation 2018;102(1):21–34.

113. Bartoletti M, Giannella M, Tedeschi S, et al. Multidrug-resistant bacterial infections in solid organ transplant candidates and recipients. Infect Dis Clin North Am 2018;32(3):551–80.

114. Bratzler DW, Dellinger EP, Olsen KM, et al. Clinical practice guidelines for antimicrobial prophylaxis in surgery. Surg Infect 2013;14(1):73–156.

115. Abbo LM, Antonio Grossi P. Surgical site infections: guidelines from the american society of transplantation infectious diseases community of practice. Clin Transplant 2019;33(9):e13589.

116. Allen L, Bartash R, Minamoto GY, et al. Impact of narrowing perioperative antibiotic prophylaxis for left ventricular assist device implantation. Transpl Infect Dis 2022;24(5):e13900.

117. Graziano E, Peghin M, Grossi PA. Perioperative antibiotic stewardship in the organ transplant setting. Transpl Infect Dis 2022;24(5):e13895.

118. Kinn PM, Ince D. Outpatient and peri-operative antibiotic stewardship in solid organ transplantation. Transpl Infect Dis 2022;24(5):e13922.

119. So M, Morris AM, Nelson S, et al. Antimicrobial stewardship by academic detailing improves antimicrobial prescribing in solid organ transplant patients. Eur J Clin Microbiol Infect Dis 2019;38(10):1915–23.

120. López-Medrano F, San Juan R, Lizasoain M, et al. A non-compulsory stewardship programme for the management of antifungals in a university-affiliated hospital. Clin Microbiol Infection 2013;19(1):56–61.

121. Shah DN, Yau R, Weston J, et al. Evaluation of antifungal therapy in patients with candidaemia based on susceptibility testing results: implications for antimicrobial stewardship programmes. J Antimicrob Chemother 2011;66(9):2146–51.

122. Rosa R, Simkins J, Camargo JF, et al. Solid organ transplant antibiograms: an opportunity for antimicrobial stewardship. Diagn Microbiol Infect Dis 2016; 86(4):460–3.

123. Greenlee SB, Acosta TJP, Makowski CT, et al. Bridging the gap: an approach to reporting antimicrobial stewardship metrics specific to solid organ transplant recipients. Transpl Infect Dis 2022;24(5):e13944.

124. Chang SY, Santos CAQ. Could cell-free DNA and host biomarkers assist in antimicrobial stewardship with organ transplant recipients? Transpl Infect Dis 2022; 24(5):e13971.

125. Shwaartz C, Reichman TW. Transplant surgeons' perspective on antimicrobial stewardship: experience with TransQIP. Transpl Infect Dis 2022;24(5). https://doi.org/10.1111/tid.13950.

126. Frenette C, Sperlea D, Leharova Y, et al. Impact of an infection control and antimicrobial stewardship program on solid organ transplantation and hepatobiliary surgical site infections. Infect Control Hosp Epidemiol 2016;37(12):1468–74.

127. Evans SR, Rubin D, Follmann D, et al. Desirability of outcome ranking (DOOR) and response adjusted for duration of antibiotic risk (RADAR). Clin Infect Dis 2015;61(5):800–6.

128. Doernberg SB. Desirability of outcome ranking and quality life measurement for antimicrobial research in organ transplantation. Transpl Infect Dis 2022;24(5). https://doi.org/10.1111/tid.13888.

129. Origüen J, López-Medrano F, Fernández-Ruiz M, et al. Should asymptomatic bacteriuria be systematically treated in kidney transplant recipients? Results from a randomized controlled trial. Am J Transplant 2016;16(10):2943–53.

130. Moradi M, Abbasi M, Moradi A, et al. Effect of antibiotic therapy on asymptomatic bacteriuria in kidney transplant recipients. Urol J 2005;2(1):32–5.

131. Green H, Rahamimov R, Goldberg E, et al. Consequences of treated versus untreated asymptomatic bacteriuria in the first year following kidney transplantation: Retrospective observational study. Eur J Clin Microbiol Infect Dis 2013; 32(1):127–31.

132. Bohn BC, Athans V, Kovacs CS, et al. Impact of asymptomatic bacteriuria incidence and management post-kidney transplantation. Clin Transplant 2019; 33(6):e13583.

133. Bonnéric S, Maisin A, Kwon T, et al. Asymptomatic bacteriuria in pediatric kidney transplant recipients: to treat or not to treat? A retrospective study. Pediatr Nephrol 2019;34(6):1141–5.

134. Kotagiri P, Chembolli D, Ryan J, et al. Urinary tract infections in the first year post-kidney transplantation: potential benefits of treating asymptomatic bacteriuria. Transplant Proc 2017;49(9):2070–5.

Update on Epidemiology and Outcomes of Infection in Pediatric Organ Transplant Recipients

Daniel E. Dulek, MD

KEYWORDS

- Solid organ transplant • Infection • Cytomegalovirus • Adenovirus • Fungus
- Multidrug-resistant bacteria

KEY POINTS

- Recent development of cytomegalovirus-active antivirals provides new opportunities for preventing and treating cytomegalovirus in pediatric solid organ transplant recipients.
- Invasive fungal infection is an infrequent but clinically significant infection in pediatric organ transplant recipients.
- Multidrug-resistant bacterial infections occur frequently in some cohorts of pediatric liver transplantation.
- Multicenter studies of infection prevention, treatment, and risk stratification are needed in pediatric organ transplant recipients to further improve transplant related outcomes.

INTRODUCTION

Pediatric organ transplant recipients have many of the same infectious complications as adults solid organ transplant (SOT) recipients. However, key differences exist in the epidemiology, prevention, and treatment of infections in pediatric SOT recipients compared with their adult counterparts. Oftentimes, children have fewer comorbidities than adults by the time of transplantation, which likely alter infection risk, especially for bacterial and invasive fungal infections. However, risk of other infections such as adenovirus and Epstein-Barr virus (EBV) is higher in children than adults. In addition, given the smaller number of pediatric organ transplants performed each year, few randomized controlled trials of prevention and treatment strategies for infections in pediatric SOT have been performed. Thus, many knowledge gaps and opportunities for further investigation exist to improve the care of pediatric SOT recipients.

Vanderbilt University Medical Center, Monroe Carell Jr. Children's Hospital at Vanderbilt, Nashville, TN, USA
E-mail address: daniel.dulek@vumc.org

Infect Dis Clin N Am 37 (2023) 561–575
https://doi.org/10.1016/j.idc.2023.06.002
0891-5520/23/© 2023 Elsevier Inc. All rights reserved.
id.theclinics.com

This article highlights recently published data for prevention and treatment of infections in pediatric SOT recipients. Selected viral, fungal, and bacterial infections are addressed. Where major recent developments have been made in adult SOT, implications for pediatric SOT recipients are discussed.

VIRAL INFECTIONS
Cytomegalovirus

As in adults, cytomegalovirus (CMV) is a well-defined infectious complication of SOT in children. However, few pediatric-specific SOT CMV-focused studies exist to provide data for recommendations in this population.[1] Recent studies have further characterized CMV epidemiology and have highlighted ongoing challenges with regard to optimal antiviral prophylaxis dosing in children. Important differences between children and adults include the increased frequency of CMV D + R-serostatus in children, the importance of accounting for weight and/or body surface area (BSA) for valganciclovir dosing, and the limited number of prospective studies evaluating prophylaxis and treatment strategies in children.[1]

Several retrospective single-center studies have enhanced understanding of the incidence and impact of CMV infection in pediatric organ transplantation in the current era[2–7](**Table 1**). Two of these studies assessed the impact of a standardized CMV prevention protocol.[6,7] These studies vary with regard to inclusion of multiorgan and lung transplant recipients and durations of follow up. However, they still provide useful information to guide future prevention and treatment interventions in pediatric SOT recipients. Overall, these studies demonstrate an incidence of CMV DNAemia/infection ranging from 11% to 34%, with a low rate of CMV tissue invasive disease ranging from 1% to 2%. Among these studies, breakthrough infection occurring while on CMV prophylaxis was identified in 4% to 34% of patients. Although breakthrough infections on prophylaxis in these cohorts were typically asymptomatic CMV DNAemia, the high frequency of breakthrough infection in some of these cohorts raises important questions about optimal valganciclovir prophylaxis dosing and monitoring. Current areas of uncertainty include the relative benefits and risks of weight-based versus BSA-based dosing, the utility of CMV polymerase chain reaction (PCR) monitoring while on prophylaxis, and the clinical and immunologic impact of breakthrough infection.

Optimal prophylaxis dosing in pediatric SOT recipients remains a key question requiring further study.[8,9] Significant clinical practice variation exists regarding valganciclovir dosing in pediatric SOT recipients.[10] Some centers use either weight-based or BSA-based dosing while other centers use weight-based dosing for certain age/weight categories and BSA-based dosing for other age/weight categories. Generally, weight-based dosing results in lower blood ganciclovir levels and is theorized to impart less risk of valganciclovir-associated adverse events. However, a recent single-center study in which weight-based dosing was exclusively employed for pediatric SOT recipients demonstrated a high rate of neutropenia and breakthrough infection, suggesting that universal weight-based dosing may not be an optimal strategy for CMV prevention.[2] Notably, initiation of and adherence to an institution-based CMV prevention protocol primarily focused on decreased prophylaxis duration compared with the pre-intervention period, which was shown in 1 study to decrease the frequency of multiple neutropenia episodes in pediatric SOT recipients.[7] Given the debates surrounding optimal dosing of valganciclovir for CMV prophylaxis, the potential benefit of therapeutic drug monitoring (TDM) has been raised.[11,12] Prospective evaluation of adult transplant recipients has shown significant intra- and interpatient variability in ganciclovir pharmacokinetics, especially in the setting of dialysis

Table 1
Single-center studies on the incidence and impact of cytomegalovirus infection in pediatric organ transplantation in the current era

Year/Citation	Years of Data	Organs Transplanted/ Cohort Size	Prophylaxis Dosing	CMV DNAemia or Infection	Overall CMV Disease Rate	Ae during Prophy	Breakthrough Infection Rate
Ganapathi etal,[7] 2019	2009–2014	Kidney, heart, liver, lung, multiorgan	Weight-based or BSA dosing	Overall DNAemia– 11% Kidney – 6.7% Liver – 16.3% Heart – 16.3% Lung – 22.2% Multi – 66.7%	2%	Neutropenia any – 56.4% >1 episode – 21.2% BSI – 1.2%	Not reported
Pangonis et al,[6] 2020	2009–2017	Total, n = 380 Kidney – 157 Liver – 153 Heart – 70	Weight-based or BSA dosing	Overall infection – 17.3% Kidney – 7.6% Liver – 24.1% Heart – 24.3%	2.1%	Prophylaxis stopped because of neutropenia – 2.6%	5%
Das[5] 2020	2010–2016	Heart, n = 97	Weight-based	Overall infection[a] - 34% D + R- 71.4% R+ 40% D-R- 18%	1.0%	Not reported	Overall 12% D + R- 14% R+ 10%
Valencia et al,[4] 2022	2011–2018	Total, n = 687 Kidney - 175 Liver - 259 Heart - 152 Lung – 87 Multiorgan - 14	Not reported	Overall DNAemia[b] – 23% Kidney – 10% Liver – 29% Heart – 20% Lung – 33.3% Multi – 28.5%	1.0%	Not reported	34%
Downes et al,[3] 2022	2012–2018	Total, n = 271 Kidney – 81 Liver – 97 Heart – 63 Lung – 30	Not reported	Overall infection – 15.9% Kidney – 16% Liver 12.4% Heart – 20.6% Lung 16.7%	1.8%	Not reported	4.8%
Liverman et al,[2] 2023	2010–2018	Total, n = 393 Kidney – 180 Liver – 117 Heart – 96	Weight-based	Overall DNAemia – 20.6% Kidney – 18.9% Liver – 19.7% Heart 25%	Not reported	Neutropenia – 25.8%	14.5%

[a] Follow-up period variable with median of 3 years post-transplant follow-up and range of 12 months to 7.6 years.
[b] Median (IQR) follow-up time post-transplant was 1133 (620–2007) days after transplant.

and/or fluctuating renal function.[13] This variability is likely to be higher in pediatric transplant recipients given the additional variability that weight-/BSA-adjusted dosing introduces.[11,14] Given the many variables that impact valganciclovir/ganciclovir dosing in children and the high frequency of breakthrough infection, it is likely that valganciclovir/ganciclovir TDM will be of benefit to pediatric organ transplant recipients. As with other areas of uncertainty, prospective studies are critical for quantifying these benefits and determining whether they outweigh the costs and challenges of additional monitoring.

A recent retrospective, single-center study provides more detailed information about renal and hematologic toxicities associated with valganciclovir in pediatric SOT recipients.[15] In this study, patients receiving valganciclovir compared with those receiving no antiviral therapy had increased frequency of kidney injury (27.0% vs 18.1%, $P=.04$), leukopenia (52.1% vs 24.8%, $P<.001$), and neutropenia (29.4% vs 15.9%, $P=.001$). Of note, the rationale for no antiviral receipt was not defined in this study and could potentially have been because of low/no risk for viral infection or because of use of a pre-emptive monitoring approach. In the multivariable analysis, valganciclovir prophylaxis was significantly associated with neutropenia (relative risk [RR] 4.82; 95% confidence interval [CI] 3.08–7.55, $P<.001$) and kidney injury (RR 1.79; 95% CI 1.22–2.65, $P=.008$). In addition to valganciclovir receipt, occurrence of non-CMV viral infection was also significantly associated with neutropenia in the multivariable analysis. Interestingly, in this study valganciclovir dose was not associated with either hematologic or kidney toxicity. These findings highlight the importance of further evaluation for risk factors for VGC-associated adverse events and the importance of evaluating novel CMV antivirals for prevention in pediatric SOT recipients.

Letermovir, a CMV-specific antiviral with novel mechanism of action, is an intriguing alternative to valganciclovir-based CMV prophylaxis.[16] Following key clinical trials and US Food and Drug Administration (FDA) approval of letermovir for use in adult hematopoietic cell transplant (HCT) recipients,[17] there has been widespread interest in determining the safety and efficacy of letermovir in pediatric transplant populations. Preliminary abstract data from a phase 3 trial of letermovir versus valganciclovir for CMV prevention in adult kidney transplant recipients demonstrated that letermovir prophylaxis was associated with similar CMV disease frequency but decreased overall drug -related adverse events, neutropenia, and adverse event-related prophylaxis discontinuation compared with valganciclovir prophylaxis.[18] Several case series have reported prophylactic use of letermovir in pediatric HCT recipients.[19–22] However, published data in pediatric SOT recipients remain limited to small case reports and series of letermovir as secondary prophylaxis or as part of salvage combination therapy.

Advances have been made in CMV treatment in addition to CMV prevention. Maribavir was approved in 2021 by the FDA for treatment of resistant and/or refractory CMV infections in SOT and HCT recipients. In the phase 3, randomized open-label multicenter study that led to licensure, maribavir treatment was associated with significantly increased CMV DNAemia clearance and symptom control compared with investigator-assigned therapy.[23] Importantly, although children 12 years of age and older were eligible for this study, no pediatric patients were enrolled. Importantly, a study to evaluate safety and tolerability of maribavir in children as young as 6 years of age is in development.[24] Both clinical trial and real-world data will be essential for guiding resistant CMV treatment in pediatric SOT recipients.

Over the past several years, increased attention has been given to the potential for CMV T cell immunity measurement to inform CMV prevention and treatment strategies. As with other interventions, the major studies have been performed in adult transplant recipients. Several large, prospective studies have evaluated CMV T cell immunity measurement in adult organ transplant recipients.[25–27] In general, these studies have shown that the presence of detectable CMV specific immunity is highly predictive of protection from postprophylaxis CMV infection and/or disease. Notably, performance characteristics for these assays are less robust in the setting of antithymocyte globulin-based induction[28] and in the setting of D + R- CMV serostatus.[26]

Pediatric data evaluating the ability of CMV-specific immunity assays to predict the occurrence of post-transplant CMV infection are limited to small single-center cohort studies. An early study defined the feasibility of measuring CMV-specific immunity by ELISPOT and cytokine supernatant measurement.[29] In this small cohort of 9 pediatric SOT recipients measured serially and 14 pediatric SOT recipients measured at single time points, CMV-specific interferon (IFN)-γ expression was reduced in organ transplant recipients up to 3 months after transplant compared with healthy controls, yet no different from healthy controls at later time points. In a larger cohort of 28 pediatric heart transplant recipients that measured CMV-specific multifunctional (tumor necrosis factor [TNF]-α, interleukin [IL]-2, and IFN-γ) cytokine expression, IFN-γ expression correlated with presence of recipient seropositivity and occurrence of CMV DNAemia.[30] Most recently, a prospective study of liver or intestinal transplant recipients was performed that included 109 children.[31] In this study, CMV-specific T cells expressing elevated frequencies of CD154 expression were found to be associated with absence of CMV viremia. Similarly, in a subset of CMV seronegative recipients, elevated pretransplant CD154 expression frequency on T cells following ex vivo CMV peptide stimulation was associated with protection from post-transplant CMV infection.[31] Despite these encouraging results, no large prospective study has been performed to validate the ability of CMV-specific immunity to predict post-transplant CMV infection and inform CMV prevention strategies. If larger studies identify effective cutoffs to predict risk of post-SOT CMV, next steps include determining the impact of immunologic monitoring on antiviral utilization, CMV infection, and associated costs.

Although the previously mentioned studies have improved understanding of CMV epidemiology in children, much work remains to be done to improve CMV prevention strategies and ensure that novel antiviral ages are well-studied in and available for pediatric SOT recipients.

Epstein Barr Virus/Post-Transplant Lymphoproliferative Disorder

Post-transplant lymphoproliferative disorder (PTLD) remains a major infectious complication of SOT in pediatric recipients with frequencies of PTLD ranging from 1% to 2% for kidney transplantation, to as high as 32% in small intestinal transplant.[32] Many single-center studies have been published in the past 5 years. [33–38] Despite extensive single-center publications, few new developments have significantly advanced the prevention and treatment of PTLD in children. Consensus conference guidelines on the monitoring, prevention, and treatment of PTLD in children have recently been published that highlight the current state of the PTLD literature and focus on key areas for focused study moving forward.[39,40] EBV D + R-serostatus, younger age, higher immunosuppression, and receipt of lung or intestinal transplant are all significant risk factors for PTLD occurrence in pediatric SOT recipients. Given the challenges of predicting which patients are at higher risk for PTLD both within and outside of the previously mentioned categories, pediatric centers typically rely on EBV PCR monitoring in addition to monitoring of clinical symptoms and examination findings. Reducing immunosuppression remains a key intervention when EBV

DNAemia is identified and even in the setting of polymorphic PTLD. However, lack of a clear threshold for EBV DNAemia that allows for prediction of current or future risk for PTLD has continued to hamper prevention strategies. In addition to immunosuppression reduction, administration of rituximab is a potential pre-emptive strategy for decreasing PTLD risk in the setting of EBV DNAemia. However, as of yet this has not been adequately studied, and a prospective study large enough to demonstrate benefit and delineate risks has not yet been performed. Finally, a large, multicenter National Institutes of Health (NIH)-funded trial to identify biomarkers for PTLD in children has completed enrollment, with published data eagerly anticipated.[41] Recent pediatric studies have addressed the chronic high viral load EBV state, EBV-negative PTLD, and the potential role of virus-specific T cells and chimeric antigen T cell therapy for PTLD treatment.

The chronic high viral load EBV (CHL) state has been associated with significant risk of PTLD in pediatric heart recipients,[42] but not in pediatric liver[43] or intestinal[44] transplant recipients. The reasons for these organ-specific differences remain undefined. More recently, the occurrence of the CHL carrier state was defined in a single institution study of pediatric kidney transplant patients.[45] Similar to pediatric liver and intestinal transplant recipients, the CHL state was not associated with occurrence of PTLD but rather with eventual spontaneous resolution.[45] In addition, in this study, there was no impact of ganciclovir exposure on the EBV viral load in the blood. Similarly, in a study from Norway of pediatric liver transplant recipients, there was no impact of ganciclovir treatment on occurrence or duration of EBV viremia.[46]

Although approximately 80% to 90% of PTLD in children is EBV+,[32] EBV-negative PTLD occurs in children but has so far been mostly defined through case reports and single institutions studies. A recent multicenter study described the clinical characteristics and outcomes of monomorphic PTLD at 12 centers in the United States and United Kingdom.[47] This cohort included 36 patients with EBV-negative PTLD, most of whom were kidney or heart recipients. Most importantly, similar to published adult data , 3-year event-free survival and overall survival rates were similar to those seen in EBV + PTLD, although theywere inferior to those seen in non-Hodgkin lymphoma in nontransplant pediatric patients. Thus, large multicenter studies will be needed for further inform and improve treatment for EBV-negative PTLD in pediatric SOT recipients.

Chimeric antigen T cell receptor therapy and increasing availability of EBV -specific T cells represent 2 key advances that hold significant potential for improving outcomes in pediatric SOT recipients. Although numerous case reports exist, further study of these treatment approaches is needed to optimize outcomes and determine best strategies for their more widespread use.[48–52]

Adenovirus

As adenovirus infections occur frequently overall in children, it is not surprising that they are a common viral infection seen in pediatric SOT recipients.[53] Adenovirus infection in pediatric SOT recipients can occur either early or late after transplant, reflecting reactivation of endogenous/recent recipient infection, donor-derived infection, or community-acquired infection.[54] Ranges of reported adenovirus infection incidence in pediatric transplant patients suggest higher incidence in intestinal (4%–57%) and thoracic (7%–50%) transplant recipients followed by liver (3.5%–38%), and kidney (11%) recipients.[53] As community-acquired exposure is likely similar between organ recipients; these differential incidences may reflect increased immunosuppression levels in intestinal and lung transplant recipients as well as increased monitoring and potentially increased risk of severe infection.

Older studies, case reports, and small case series suggest that adenovirus is associated with significant morbidity and mortality in pediatric SOT recipients.[53,55,56] More recently, a large single-center retrospective study of adenovirus infection in pediatric SOT recipients highlighted the infrequent detection of adenovirus overall in SOT recipients (10.6% of total cohort with at least 1 positive test) in the first 180 days after transplantation.[57] Adenovirus infection incidence in this cohort was highest in liver recipients (15.3%) with heart, kidney, and liver recipients having 8.6%, 8.3%, and 4.2% incidence, respectively. In addition, in this cohort there was a low frequency of either adenovirus disease (defined as organ-specific radiologic and/or laboratory abnormalities) at initial detection or progression to adenovirus disease after initial virus detection. Finally, there was no all-cause mortality in the adenovirus-positive patients during the study follow-up period. Therefore, although an important cause of post-transplant infection in children, adenovirus appears to not be associated with significant mortality in children. Despite this conclusion, case reports of adenovirus infection in pediatric SOT recipients illustrate patients in whom significant morbidity or even mortality occurred. Thus, determining patient-related and virus-related risk factors for poor outcomes associated with adenovirus infection in pediatric SOT are needed to guide monitoring and treatment approaches.

Although not FDA-approved for the treatment of adenovirus infections, cidofovir treatment is reported and used in many centers for adenovirus treatment in pediatric transplant recipients.[58–60] Importantly, no prospective randomized clinical trials exist to define the impact of antiviral therapy on adenovirus infection in SOT recipients. Despite these limitations, cidofovir treatment may be of benefit in the setting of disseminated adenovirus infection, rising adenovirus DNAemia, and/or severe end organ infection. Any consideration for the use of cidofovir to treat adenovirus infection in a pediatric SOT recipient should take into account the risk for nephrotoxicity (as high as 30% to 50% in some studies) as well and the potential for resolution without antiviral therapy. Considerable uncertainty exists with regard to identifying pediatric SOT patients most likely to benefit from cidofovir treatment.

Potential additional or alternative therapies for adenovirus treatment include brincidofovir and adenovirus-specific T cells. A recent case series described the use of brincidofovir, a lipid ester prodrug of cidofovir, in 4 pediatric SOT recipients.[61] However, brincidofovir is no longer available outside of the clinical trial setting. Finally, virus-specific T cells are increasingly available and used to treat adenovirus infection in the setting of HCT.[62] However, there are few reports of their use in pediatric SOT patients.

A recent prospective study used quantification of adenovirus-specific T cells (along with CMV- and HSV-specific T cells) to guide immunosuppression levels in pediatric kidney transplant recipients.[63] Data from this study suggest that this strategy may allow for safe reduction in decreasing overall immunosuppression exposure. Further studies of this approach are needed.

An additional topic of recent importance is the is the role of adenovirus as a cause of acute liver failure in children. Previously rarely reported, recent clusters of adenovirus-associated acute hepatitis in children were identified in the United States and Europe with a high frequency of progression to liver failure and subsequent liver transplant.[64,65] Many, but not all, of these cases had detection of adenovirus from liver tissue or blood.[65,66] This association raised questions related to whether adenovirus was truly causal for acute hepatitis in these cases. Intriguingly, a case control study from the United Kingdom identified a strong association of adeno-associated virus 2 (AAV2) with acute hepatitis in cases from this outbreak.[67] The study compared 38 acute hepatitis cases with 66 age-matched immunocompetent controls and 21 immunocompromised comparator subjects. High levels of AAV2 DNA were detected in cases compared with infrequent and low-level detection in immunocompetent and immunocompromised controls respectively. The authors posited that high-level AAV2 replication led to immune-mediated hepatic disease. A similar association was noted in a US cohort study.[68] Reports of successful liver transplantation in this setting inform decisions to move forward with transplantation and strategies for transplantation in critically ill pediatric acute liver failure patients.[66]

FUNGAL INFECTIONS

Given the potential for frequent hospitalization and antibiotic exposure, surgical complications, and prolonged exposure to immunosuppression, invasive fungal infections (IFI) are a major concern in SOT recipients. Publications describing the burden of IFI in adult SOT recipients demonstrate that invasive candidiasis and invasive aspergillosis are the most frequently identified IFI in this setting.[69,70] In a large multicenter study determining incidence of IFI in adult SOT recipients, 1-year incidence of invasive candidiasis and invasive aspergillosis were 1.95% and 0.65%, respectively.[71]

In contrast to adult SOT recipients, the incidence of IFI in pediatric SOT recipients is generally low. Highlighting this, a single-institution retrospective cohort of pediatric SOT recipients from 2000 to 2013 demonstrated an overall incidence of 2.2%, with highest incidence in heart/lung and lung transplant recipients followed by liver transplant recipients.[72] As with adult series, most IFI infections in this cohort were *Candida spp.* In this series, no cases of IFI were identified in heart or kidney recipients. Deaths likely attributable to IFI occurred in lung and heart/lung transplant recipients.

Few studies have rigorously identified risk factors for IFI in pediatric SOT recipients. In a 2-center retrospective study of invasive candidiasis in pediatric liver transplant recipients, 2.5% of 397 liver recipients developed invasive candidiasis. Eight of these infections were candidemia, with 1 episode each of hepatic abscess and peritoneal infection. Bivariate analysis demonstrated that intensive care unit (ICU) admission before transplant, prolonged operating time, high intraoperative volume infusion, and exposure to broad-spectrum antibiotics were significantly associated with occurrence of invasive candidiasis. However, in the multivariate analysis, only ICU admission before transplant remained significantly associated.[73]

A prospective study of 59 pediatric lung transplant patients identified pulmonary fungal infection in 17% of patients over the 2-year follow-up period.[74] In this study, older age was significantly associated with occurrence of pulmonary fungal infection. Notably, there were no deaths attributed to pulmonary fungal infections. In contrast, in a larger multicenter cohort, pulmonary fungal infection was independently associated with decreased 12-month survival.[75]

The previously mentioned studies indicate that, although infrequent, IFI occurs and can significantly impact outcomes of SOT in pediatric patients. As discussed previously, future large multicenter studies are needed to further identify risk factors, outcomes, and subsets of patients who would benefit from targeted prevention and/or more intensive evaluation for IFI. Moreover, epidemiologic monitoring for emergence of fungi with broad-spectrum resistance, such as *Candida auris*, will be critical.[76]

MULTIDRUG-RESISTANT BACTERIA

Antibiotic-resistant bacterial infections, including multidrug-resistant gram-negative bacteria (MDR-GNB), significantly impact the care of SOT recipients.[77,78] Some adult studies suggest increasing incidence of bacterial bloodstream infections including MDR-GNB.[79,80] Although a fair amount of adult SOT data has been published on this topic, studies evaluating the incidence and impact of MDR infection in pediatric SOT are limited. A large multicenter international study of adult SOT recipients evaluated clinical score-based morality prediction in the setting of carbapenemase-producing bloodstream infections (CPE-BSI).[81] In this cohort of 216 patients with CPE-BSI, CMV infection and lymphopenia were associated with CPE-BSI associated mortality. Inclusion of each of these factors into a previously validated mortality prediction score improved overall predictive performance. A retrospective study of adult heart transplant recipients identified high frequency of MDR and extensively drug-resistant (XDR) pathogens in their cohort in the first-year after transplant, with XDR infection significantly associated with mortality.[82]

Studies defining the epidemiology of MDR-GNB infection in pediatric SOT recipients have primarily been performed in the setting of liver transplantation.[83–86] In a single-center retrospective study of pediatric liver transplant recipients in Thailand, 62% of gram-negative isolates were multidrug resistant, with 10% of these isolates being carbapenem resistant.[83] In this cohort, third-generation cephalosporin exposure, operative time, and ICU duration were significantly associated with MDR-GNB infection risk. In a cohort of pediatric liver transplant recipients from France, 11% of gram-negative isolates were MDR.[84] Notably, in this cohort, colonization with MDR bacteria was a risk factor for overall bacterial infection as well as severe sepsis and surgical site infection. Finally, in a cohort from London, 27% of 96 pediatric liver recipients were colonized with MDR-GNB, with 16.6% of the overall cohort having MDR-GNB infection.[85] Patients with MDR infection in this cohort had significantly longer total hospitalization duration as well as ICU stay duration. Few studies address MDR bacterial infection in other pediatric organ transplants.[87] Thus, MDR gram-negative infections are prevalent in pediatric liver transplant patients, with some data demonstrating an impact on hospital utilization. Importantly, as incidence and epidemiology of MDR infections vary significantly by institution, prospective multicenter studies are necessary to better understand the incidence, impact, and optimal prevention and treatment of these infections in pediatric organ transplant recipients. In the setting of this uncertainty, use of institution-specific antibiograms is critical to guide empiric therapy and monitor trends in antimicrobial resistance. Where feasible, development of transplant-specific antibiograms may provide further granularity to guide empiric treatment.[88] Finally, in recent years newer broad-spectrum antibiotics with activity against many MDR-GNR pathogens have become available.[89,90] Several of these novel β-lactams and β-lactam/β-lactamase inhibitor combinations, including ceftazidime-avibactam and ceftolazone-tazobactam, have had sufficient clinical and efficacy data to receive FDA approval for specific indications.[89] However, few data exist to demonstrate the impact that use of these novel antibiotics has on pediatric SOT outcomes.

SUMMARY

Key recent publications have provided important data on the epidemiology and outcomes of viral, fungal, and bacterial infections in pediatric SOT recipients. However, significant needs exist for large, multicenter studies comparing prevention and treatment strategies for infection in these vulnerable patients.

CLINICS CARE POINTS

- Valganciclovir remains the primary CMV active antiviral for prophylaxis in pediatric organ transplant recipients despite uncertainties related to dosing and clear risk for neutropenia.

- Adenovirus Virus Specific T cell formulations are increasingly available for off the shelf use in treatment of severe adenovirus infection in pediatric organ transplant recipients.
- Novel β-lactams and β-lactam/β-lactamase inhibitor combinations, including ceftazidime-avibactam and ceftolazone-tazobactam, are available for treatment of multidrug resistant gram negative bacterial infections in pediatric organ transpalnt recipients.

DISCLOSURE

Dr D.E. Dulek receives nonsalary research support for study supplies from Eurofins Viracor.

REFERENCES

1. Razonable RR, Humar A. Cytomegalovirus in solid organ transplant recipients-guidelines of the American Society of Transplantation infectious diseases community of practice. Clin Transplant 2019;33(9):e13512.
2. Liverman R, Serluco A, Nance G, et al. Incidence of cytomegalovirus dnaemia in pediatric kidney, liver, and heart transplant recipients: efficacy and risk factors associated with failure of weight-based dosed valganciclovir prophylaxis. Pediatr Transplant 2023;27:e14493.
3. Downes KJ, Sharova A, Boge CLK, et al. CMV infection and management among pediatric solid organ transplant recipients. Pediatr Transplant 2022;26(3):e14220.
4. Valencia Deray KG, Hosek KE, Chilukuri D, et al. Epidemiology and long-term outcomes of cytomegalovirus dnaemia and disease in pediatric solid organ transplant recipients. Am J Transplant 2022;22(1):187–98.
5. Das BB, Prusty BK, Niu J, et al. Cytomegalovirus infection and allograft rejection among pediatric heart transplant recipients in the era of valganciclovir prophylaxis. Pediatr Transplant 2020;24(8):e13750.
6. Pangonis S, Paulsen G, Andersen H, et al. Evaluation of a change in cytomegalovirus prevention strategy following pediatric solid organ transplantation. Transpl Infect Dis 2020;22(2):e13232.
7. Ganapathi L, Blumenthal J, Alawdah L, et al. Impact of standardized protocols for cytomegalovirus disease prevention in pediatric solid organ transplant recipients. Pediatr Transplant 2019;23(7):e13568.
8. Villeneuve D, Brothers A, Harvey E, et al. Valganciclovir dosing using area under the curve calculations in pediatric solid organ transplant recipients. Pediatr Transplant 2013;17(1):80–5.
9. Dulek DE, Ardura MI. "Weight-ing" For an answer on optimal valganciclovir prophylaxis dosing in pediatric solid organ transplantation recipients. Pediatr Transplant 2023;e14494.
10. Shaikh S, Jasiak-Panek N, Park JM. A national survey of valganciclovir dosing strategies in pediatric organ transplant recipients. Clin Transplant 2018;32(9):e13369.
11. Nguyen T, Oualha M, Briand C, et al. Population pharmacokinetics of intravenous ganciclovir and oral valganciclovir in a pediatric population to optimize dosing regimens. Antimicrob Agents Chemother 2021;65(3).
12. Märtson AG, Edwina AE, Kim HY, et al. Therapeutic drug monitoring of ganciclovir: where are we? Ther Drug Monit 2022;44(1):138–47.
13. Märtson AG, Edwina AE, Burgerhof JGM, et al. Ganciclovir therapeutic drug monitoring in transplant recipients. J Antimicrob Chemother 2021;76(9):2356–63.

14. Murphy M, Chamberlain A, Tang P, et al. Paediatric ganciclovir dosing in extracorporeal membrane oxygenation: is standard dosing good enough? J Clin Pharm Ther 2020;45(1):218–20.
15. Hayes M, Boge CLK, Sharova A, et al. Antiviral toxicities in pediatric solid organ transplant recipients. Am J Transplant 2022;22(12):3012–20.
16. Saullo JL, Miller RA. Cytomegalovirus therapy: role of letermovir in prophylaxis and treatment in transplant recipients. Annu Rev Med 2023;74:89–105.
17. Marty FM, Ljungman P, Chemaly RF, et al. Letermovir prophylaxis for cytomegalovirus in hematopoietic-cell transplantation. N Engl J Med 2017;377(25): 2433–44.
18. Limaye AP, Budde K, Humar A, et al. Safety and efficacy of letermovir (let) versus valganciclovir (vgcv) for prevention of cytomegalovirus (cmv) disease in kidney transplant recipients (ktrs): a phase 3 randomized study. vol Abstract #LB2307). Washington, DC: ID Week; 2022.
19. Körholz KF, Füller MA, Hennies M, et al. Letermovir for prophylaxis and preemptive therapy of cytomegalovirus infection in paediatric allogeneic haematopoietic cell transplant patients. Paediatr Drugs 2023;25(2):225–32.
20. Kuhn A, Puttkammer J, Madigan T, et al. Letermovir as cytomegalovirus prophylaxis in a pediatric cohort: a retrospective analysis. Transplant Cell Ther 2023; 29(1):62.e1–4.
21. P Daukshus N, Cirincione A, Siver M, et al. Letermovir for cytomegalovirus prevention in adolescent patients following hematopoietic cell transplantation. J Pediatric Infect Dis Soc 2022;11(7):337–40.
22. Richert-Przygonska M, Jaremek K, Debski R, et al. Letermovir prophylaxis for cytomegalovirus infection in children after hematopoietic cell transplantation. Anticancer Res 2022;42(7):3607–12.
23. Avery RK, Alain S, Alexander BD, et al. Maribavir for refractory cytomegalovirus infections with or without resistance post-transplant: results from a phase 3 randomized clinical trial. Clin Infect Dis 2022;75(4):690–701.
24. Available at: https://www.clinicaltrials.gov/ct2/show/NCT05319353. Accessed April 18, 2023.
25. Jarque M, Crespo E, Melilli E, et al. Cellular immunity to predict the risk of cytomegalovirus infection in kidney transplantation: a prospective, interventional, multicenter clinical trial. Clin Infect Dis 2020;71(9):2375–85.
26. Kumar D, Chin-Hong P, Kayler L, et al. A prospective multicenter observational study of cell-mediated immunity as a predictor for cytomegalovirus infection in kidney transplant recipients. Am J Transplant 2019;19(9):2505–16.
27. Kumar D, Chernenko S, Moussa G, et al. Cell-mediated immunity to predict cytomegalovirus disease in high-risk solid organ transplant recipients. Am J Transplant 2009;9(5):1214–22.
28. Fernández-Ruiz M, Rodríguez-Goncer I, Parra P, et al. Monitoring of cmv-specific cell-mediated immunity with a commercial elisa-based interferon-γ release assay in kidney transplant recipients treated with antithymocyte globulin. Am J Transplant 2020;20(8):2070–80.
29. Patel M, Stefanidou M, Long CB, et al. Dynamics of cell-mediated immune responses to cytomegalovirus in pediatric transplantation recipients. Pediatr Transplant 2012;16(1):18–28.
30. Jacobsen MC, Manunta MDI, Pincott ES, et al. Specific immunity to cytomegalovirus in pediatric cardiac transplantation. Transplantation 2018;102(9):1569–75.
31. Ashokkumar C, Green M, Soltys K, et al. CD154-expressing cmv-specific T cells associate with freedom from DNAemia and may be protective in seronegative

recipients after liver or intestine transplantation. Pediatr Transplant 2020;24(1): e13601.

32. Allen UD, Preiksaitis JK, Practice AIDCo. Post-transplant lymphoproliferative disorders, epstein-barr virus infection, and disease in solid organ transplantation: Guidelines from the american society of transplantation infectious diseases community of practice. Clin Transplant 2019;33(9):e13652.

33. Quintero Bernabeu J, Juamperez J, Mercadal-Hally M, et al. Epstein-Barr virus-associated risk factors for post-transplant lymphoproliferative disease in pediatric liver transplant recipients. Pediatr Transplant 2022;26(6):e14292.

34. Ramos-Gonzalez G, Crum R, Allain A, et al. Presentation and outcomes of post-transplant lymphoproliferative disorder at a single institution pediatric transplant center. Pediatr Transplant 2022;26(5):e14268.

35. L'Huillier AG, Dipchand AI, Ng VL, et al. Posttransplant lymphoproliferative disorder in pediatric patients: characteristics of disease in ebv-seropositive recipients. Transplantation 2019;103(11):e369–74.

36. L'Huillier AG, Dipchand AI, Ng VL, et al. Posttransplant lymphoproliferative disorder in pediatric patients: survival rates according to primary sites of occurrence and a proposed clinical categorization. Am J Transplant 2019;19(10):2764–74.

37. West SC, Friedland-Little JM, Schowengerdt KO, et al. Characteristics, risks, and outcomes of post-transplant lymphoproliferative disease >3 years after pediatric heart transplant: a multicenter analysis. Clin Transplant 2019;33(5):e13521.

38. Schultze-Florey RE, Tischer S, Kuhlmann L, et al. Dissecting Epstein-Barr virus-specific t-cell responses after allogeneic EBV-specific T-cell transfer for central nervous system posttransplant lymphoproliferative disease. Front Immunol 2018;9:1475.

39. Wilkinson JD, Allen U, Green M, et al. The IPTA Nashville Consensus Conference on post-transplant lymphoproliferative disorders after solid organ transplantation in children: I-methodology for the development of consensus practice guidelines. Pediatr Transplant 2022;e14333.

40. Green M, Squires JE, Chinnock RE, et al. The ipta nashville consensus conference on post-transplant lymphoproliferative disorders after solid organ transplantation in children: Ii-consensus guidelines for prevention. Pediatr Transplant 2022;e14350.

41. Available at: https://clinicaltrials.gov/ct2/show/NCT02182986. Accessed April 18, 2023.

42. Bingler MA, Feingold B, Miller SA, et al. Chronic high Epstein-Barr viral load state and risk for late-onset posttransplant lymphoproliferative disease/lymphoma in children. Am J Transplant 2008;8(2):442–5.

43. Green M, Soltys K, Rowe DT, et al. Chronic high Epstein-Barr viral load carriage in pediatric liver transplant recipients. Pediatr Transplant 2009;13(3):319–23.

44. Lau AH, Soltys K, Sindhi RK, et al. Chronic high Epstein-Barr viral load carriage in pediatric small bowel transplant recipients. Pediatr Transplant 2010;14(4): 549–53.

45. Yamada M, Nguyen C, Fadakar P, et al. Epidemiology and outcome of chronic high Epstein-Barr viral load carriage in pediatric kidney transplant recipients. Pediatr Transplant 2018;22(3):e13147.

46. Østensen AB, Sanengen T, Holter E, et al. No effect of treatment with intravenous ganciclovir on Epstein-Barr virus viremia demonstrated after pediatric liver transplantation. Pediatr Transplant 2017;21(6):1–8.

47. Afify ZAM, Taj MM, Orjuela-Grimm M, et al. Multicenter study of pediatric epstein-barr virus-negative monomorphic post solid organ transplant lymphoproliferative disorders. Cancer 2023;129(5):780–9.

48. Portuguese AJ, Gauthier J, Tykodi SS, et al. CD19 car-T therapy in solid organ transplant recipients: case report and systematic review. Bone Marrow Transplant 2023;58(4):353–9.

49. Oren D, DeFilippis EM, Lotan D, et al. Successful car T cell therapy in a heart and kidney transplant recipient with refractory ptld. JACC CardioOncol 2022;4(5):713–6.

50. de Nattes T, Camus V, François A, et al. Kidney transplant T cell-mediated rejection occurring after anti-CD19 car T-cell therapy for refractory aggressive Burkitt-like lymphoma with 11q aberration: a case report. Am J Kidney Dis 2022;79(5):760–4.

51. Keam SJ. Tabelecleucel: first approval. Mol Diagn Ther 2023;27:425–43.

52. Prockop S, Doubrovina E, Suser S, et al. Off-the-shelf EBV-specific T cell immunotherapy for rituximab-refractory EBV-associated lymphoma following transplantation. J Clin Invest 2020;130(2):733–47.

53. Florescu DF, Schaenman JM, Practice AIDCo. Adenovirus in solid organ transplant recipients: guidelines from the American Society of Transplantation Infectious Diseases Community of Practice. Clin Transplant 2019;33(9):e13527.

54. Lion T. Adenovirus infections in immunocompetent and immunocompromised patients. Clin Microbiol Rev 2014;27(3):441–62.

55. Hoffman JA. Adenovirus infections in solid organ transplant recipients. Curr Opin Organ Transplant 2009;14(6):625–33.

56. Engen RM, Huang ML, Park GE, et al. Prospective assessment of adenovirus infection in pediatric kidney transplant recipients. Transplantation 2018;102(7):1165–71.

57. Boge CLK, Fisher BT, Petersen H, et al. Outcomes of human adenovirus infection and disease in a retrospective cohort of pediatric solid organ transplant recipients. Pediatr Transplant 2019;23(6):e13510.

58. Guerra Sanchez CH, Lorica CD, Arheart KL, et al. Virologic response with 2 different cidofovir dosing regimens for preemptive treatment of adenovirus dnaemia in pediatric solid organ transplant recipients. Pediatr Transplant 2018;22:e13231.

59. Engelmann G, Heim A, Greil J, et al. Adenovirus infection and treatment with cidofovir in children after liver transplantation. Pediatr Transplant 2009;13(4):421–8.

60. Ganapathi L, Arnold A, Jones S, et al. Use of cidofovir in pediatric patients with adenovirus infection. F1000Res 2016;5:758.

61. Londeree J, Winterberg PD, Garro R, et al. Brincidofovir for the treatment of human adenovirus infection in pediatric solid organ transplant recipients: a case series. Pediatr Transplant 2020;24(7):e13769.

62. Leen AM, Bollard CM, Mendizabal AM, et al. Multicenter study of banked third-party virus-specific t cells to treat severe viral infections after hematopoietic stem cell transplantation. Blood 2013;121(26):5113–23.

63. Ahlenstiel-Grunow T, Liu X, Schild R, et al. Steering transplant immunosuppression by measuring virus-specific T cell levels: the randomized, controlled ivist trial. J Am Soc Nephrol 2021;32(2):502–16.

64. Gutierrez Sanchez LH, Shiau H, Baker JM, et al. A case series of children with acute hepatitis and human adenovirus infection. N Engl J Med 2022;387(7):620–30.

65. Cates J, Baker JM, Almendares O, et al. Interim analysis of acute hepatitis of unknown etiology in children aged <10 years - United States, October 2021-June 2022. MMWR Morb Mortal Wkly Rep 2022;71(26):852–8.
66. Banc-Husu AM, Moulton EA, Shiau H, et al. Acute liver failure and unique challenges of pediatric liver transplantation amidst a worldwide cluster of adenovirus-associated hepatitis. Am J Transplant 2023;23(1):93–100.
67. Morfopoulou S, Buddle S, Montaguth OET, et al. Genomic investigations of unexplained acute hepatitis in children. Nature 2023;617:564–73.
68. Servellita V, Gonzalez AS, Lamson DM, et al. Adeno-associated virus type 2 in us children with acute severe hepatitis. Nature 2023;617:574–80.
69. Husain S, Camargo JF. Invasive aspergillosis in solid-organ transplant recipients: Guidelines from the American Society of Transplantation Infectious Diseases Community of Practice. Clin Transplant 2019;33(9):e13544.
70. Aslam S, Rotstein C, Practice AIDCo. *Candida* infections in solid organ transplantation: guidelines from the American Society of Transplantation Infectious Diseases Community of Practice. Clin Transplant 2019;33(9):e13623.
71. Pappas PG, Alexander BD, Andes DR, et al. Invasive fungal infections among organ transplant recipients: results of the Transplant-Associated Infection Surveillance Network (Transnet). Clin Infect Dis 2010;50(8):1101–11.
72. Saxena S, Gee J, Klieger S, et al. Invasive fungal disease in pediatric solid organ transplant recipients. J Pediatric Infect Dis Soc 2018;7(3):219–25.
73. De Luca M, Green M, Symmonds J, et al. Invasive candidiasis in liver transplant patients: incidence and risk factors in a pediatric cohort. Pediatr Transplant 2016; 20(2):235–40.
74. Ammerman E, Sweet SC, Fenchel M, et al. Risk and outcomes of pulmonary fungal infection after pediatric lung transplantation. Clin Transplant 2017; 31(11):1–8.
75. Danziger-Isakov LA, Worley S, Arrigain S, et al. Increased mortality after pulmonary fungal infection within the first year after pediatric lung transplantation. J Heart Lung Transplant 2008;27(6):655–61.
76. Berrio I, Caceres DH, Coronell RW, et al. Bloodstream infections with candida auris among children in colombia: clinical characteristics and outcomes of 34 cases. J Pediatric Infect Dis Soc 2021;10(2):151–4.
77. Pouch SM, Patel G, Practice AIDCo. Multidrug-resistant gram-negative bacterial infections in solid organ transplant recipients-guidelines from the american society of transplantation infectious diseases community of practice. Clin Transplant 2019;33(9):e13594.
78. Pereira MR, Rana MM, Practice AICo. Methicillin-resistant *Staphylococcus aureus* in solid organ transplantation-guidelines from the American Society of Transplantation Infectious Diseases Community of Practice. Clin Transplant 2019;33(9):e13611.
79. Berenger BM, Doucette K, Smith SW. Epidemiology and risk factors for nosocomial bloodstream infections in solid organ transplants over a 10-year period. Transpl Infect Dis 2016;18(2):183–90.
80. Pilmis B, Weiss E, Scemla A, et al. Multidrug-resistant enterobacterales infections in abdominal solid organ transplantation. Clin Microbiol Infect 2023;29(1):38–43.
81. Pérez-Nadales E, Gutiérrez-Gutiérrez B, Natera AM, et al. Predictors of mortality in solid organ transplant recipients with bloodstream infections due to carbapenemase-producing enterobacterales: the impact of cytomegalovirus disease and lymphopenia. Am J Transplant 2019;20:1629–41.

82. Bhatt PJ, Ali M, Rana M, et al. Infections due to multidrug-resistant organisms following heart transplantation: epidemiology, microbiology, and outcomes. Transpl Infect Dis 2020;22(1):e13215.
83. Phichaphop C, Apiwattanakul N, et al. High prevalence of multidrug-resistant gram-negative bacterial infection following pediatric liver transplantation. Medicine (Baltim) 2020;99(45):e23169.
84. Dohna Schwake C, Guiddir T, Cuzon G, et al. Bacterial infections in children after liver transplantation: a single-center surveillance study of 345 consecutive transplantations. Transpl Infect Dis 2020;22(1):e13208.
85. Verma A, Vimalesvaran S, Dhawan A. Epidemiology, risk factors and outcome due to multidrug resistant organisms in paediatric liver transplant patients in the era of antimicrobial stewardship and screening. Antibiotics (Basel) 2022; 11(3):387.
86. Sun Y, Yu L, Gao W, et al. Investigation and analysis of the colonization and prevalence of carbapenem-resistant. Infect Drug Resist 2021;14:1957–66.
87. Cruz AT, Tanverdi MS, Swartz SJ, et al. Frequency of bacteremia and urinary tract infection in pediatric renal transplant recipients. Pediatr Infect Dis J 2022;41(12): 997–1003.
88. Kitano T, Science M, Nalli N, et al. Solid organ transplant-specific antibiogram in a tertiary pediatric hospital in canada. Pediatr Transplant 2021;25(4):e13980.
89. Olney KB, Thomas JK, Johnson WM. Review of novel β-lactams and β-lactam/β-lactamase inhibitor combinations with implications for pediatric use. Pharmacotherapy 2023.
90. Marner M, Kolberg L, Horst J, et al. Antimicrobial activity of ceftazidime-avibactam, ceftolozane-tazobactam, cefiderocol, and novel darobactin analogs against multidrug-resistant pseudomonas aeruginosa isolates from pediatric and adolescent cystic fibrosis patients. Microbiol Spectr 2023;11(1):e0443722.

Mycobacteria in Organ Transplant Recipients

Niyati Narsana, MD[a],*, María Alejandra Pérez, MD[b],
Aruna Subramanian, MD[c]

KEYWORDS

- *Mycobacterium tuberculosis* • Non-tuberculous mycobacteria
- Solid organ transplant • Latent tuberculosis

KEY POINTS

- Organ transplant recipients are at higher risk of tuberculosis (TB) reactivation than the general population.
- All recipients must be screened for their risk of TB before transplantation by taking an appropriate history, imaging, and with screening tests such as interferon gamma release assays or tuberculin skin test .
- The drugs for treatment of TB have significant interactions with immunosuppressants, hence, they must be monitored very closely.
- The incidence of non-tuberculous mycobacteria (NTM) infections is higher in lung and heart transplant patients compared to abdominal organ transplants. *M abscessus* and mycobacterium avium complex (MAC) are the most common NTM species that cause infections in organ transplant.

MYCOBACTERIUM TUBERCULOSIS
Epidemiology and Risk Factors

The prevalence of tuberculosis (TB) in solid organ transplantation (SOT) is reported between 1.24% and 6.4% in non-endemic countries and 7.32% and 13.72% in endemic countries.[1,2] The incidence of TB has been reported to be 4- to 30-fold higher in SOT compared to the general population.[3] In a cohort of 4388 SOT recipients, the highest incidence of TB was seen in lung transplant recipients, with a relative risk of 5.6 compared to non-lung SOT recipients, and recipient age was also associated with increased risk.[4] The other risk factors for active TB after transplant that have been described in the literature are detection of latent TB infection (LTBI) before transplant, pre-transplant diabetes mellitus, cirrhosis, need for hemodialysis, hepatitis C virus

[a] UC Davis School of Medicine, 4150 V Street, G500, Sacramento, CA 95817, USA; [b] ICESI University, Street 18 number 122 - 135, Cali, Colombia; [c] Stanford University School of Medicine, 300 Pasteur Drive, Lane Building Suite 134, Stanford, CA 94305, USA
* Corresponding author.
E-mail address: nnarsana@ucdavis.edu

Infect Dis Clin N Am 37 (2023) 577–591
https://doi.org/10.1016/j.idc.2023.04.004
0891-5520/23/© 2023 Elsevier Inc. All rights reserved.

infection, intensity of immunosuppression (higher risk reported with antithymocyte globulin and azathioprine, but lower with basiliximab), and allograft rejection.[4-7]

Active TB in SOT can occur via three different mechanisms—reactivation of latent TB (which is the most common mechanism), transmission from the donor, or acquisition of a new infection in the recipient. To understand the risk factors for donor transmission, the Organ Procurement and Transplantation Network ad hoc disease transmission committee, evaluated the transmission of TB from nine donors to six lung and five non-lung recipients. Of these, six donors were born in an endemic country, five had traveled to a TB endemic region, three were incarcerated and three had LTBI.[8]

Prevention of Tuberculosis

Pre-transplant evaluation of recipients

Factors to consider pre-transplant are listed in **Box 1**. A thorough evaluation of the recipient's history including prior exposure, previous LTBI test results, stay in or travel to endemic areas, incarceration, and homelessness is important before transplantation. All transplant candidates must undergo screening for latent TB. Latent TB can be diagnosed by tuberculin skin test (TST) or interferon-gamma release assays (IGRA); both detect the host's cellular response. In a systematic review and meta-analysis of 12 studies that directly compared TST with IGRA in patients with organ transplantation, both tests were strongly associated with clinical risk factors and radiological signs of prior TB. Relative comparisons indicated that IGRA positivity was more strongly associated with radiologic signs of prior TB compared to TST positivity (Relative OR 3.24, CI [1.1–9.56]). A systematic review that assessed the performance of LTBI tests in patients with end stage renal disease (ESRD), in countries with low to moderate TB prevalence, found that compared to a positive TST result, a positive ELISA-based IGRA was four times more likely to be associated with radiologic evidence of past TB (ROR, 3.36; 95% CI, 1.61–7.01; P =.001).[9,10] These tests must be interpreted with caution in patients with impaired cellular immunity, as they can result as falsely negative or indeterminate. One study demonstrated that IGRA testing was better than TST in patients with advanced liver disease with MELD scores of >18.[9] In a single-center study in New York, an indeterminate Quantiferon TB test (QFT) was 16 times more likely in a patient with a model for end stage liver disease (MELD) score >25. None of the patients who developed active TB had a positive QFT. All of them were born outside of the United States or had a pre-transplantation CT chest demonstrating granulomatous disease.[11] In another study of patients with advanced liver disease, the rate of indeterminate QFT results was 7.8%. Low lymphocyte count

---

Box 1
Factors to consider for risk evaluation pre-transplantation in transplant recipients

History evaluation—prior exposure, prior LTBI results, stay in or travel to an endemic area, incarceration, or homelessness

Screening test for latent TB (TST or IGRA)—interpret negative/indeterminate tests with caution in patients with impaired cellular immunity

Screening with imaging—CXR or CT chest, review prior imaging

If patient has symptoms—rule out active TB pre-transplant

Abbreviations: CT, computed tomography; IGRA, interferon-gamma release assay; LTBI, latent tuberculosis infection; TB, tuberculosis; TST, tuberculin skin test.

and high MELD score were significant factors that were associated with indeterminate results.[12]

All patients with epidemiologic risk for TB should undergo chest imaging to screen for any lesions that are suggestive of prior TB. Chest x-ray (CXR) can be useful in detecting prior scars, calcifications, and other signs of old healed TB, however, chest CT may be preferred when feasible. A retrospective study of liver transplant patients showed that pre-transplant CT chest with abnormal lesions was predictive of development of TB post-transplant, even in patients with normal CXR. However, there were 15 (60%) patients without any pre-transplant CT changes, who developed TB following transplant.[13] Another retrospective study of lung transplant recipients demonstrated that patients with residual lesions on pre-transplant CT chest were at higher risk for development of TB.[14] CT chest may be helpful and could be considered for evaluation in patients who have a high risk for TB but with negative or indeterminate LTBI testing. For every patient, the decision to treat for latent TB must be individualized based on their risk factors. All living donors must also be screened in the same way as the recipients.

Transmission of TB from deceased donors has also been reported. IGRA and TST testing have their limitations in deceased patients. TST is not feasible due to the need for a reading 48 to 72 hours after placement. A study of 105 deceased donors in low TB prevalence area compared cell-mediated immunity assays in deceased donors— the performance of the T cell assays was variable and there was a high rate of indeterminate test results. Another study of 38 deceased donors from Iran showed a high rate of indeterminate Quantiferon TB gold test results.[15–17] Hence, a careful history for risk exposure must be obtained from the donor's family. If there are risk factors, chest imaging with CXR or CT chest must be considered. Respiratory samples must be obtained for acid fast bacilli (AFB) smear and cultures for further evaluation, to rule out active TB. If active TB is diagnosed postmortem in the donor, the recipient should be treated for active TB.[1] The risk of transmission of TB is likely higher in lung transplantation, however, transmission through abdominal organs has also been reported.[8]

Treatment of latent tuberculosis

A systematic review of 41 observational studies of TB in SOT candidates from Europe, USA, and South America showed that active TB developed in 36 of 2010 patients (1.8%) compared to (2.5%) 250 of 9750 who did not receive prophylaxis. The patients received prophylaxis before transplant in 13 studies and post-transplant in 19 studies. However, there was considerable heterogeneity in these studies and a meta-analysis could not be performed.[9]

The various first-line and alternative treatments for LTBI are listed in **Table 1**.

A retrospective review of renal transplant candidates with LTBI showed a high treatment completion rate with 12 weekly isoniazid and rifapentine (INH + RPT) combination compared to 9 months of INH, and no hepatotoxicity was observed in the INH + RPT group, unlike the 9-month INH group.[18]

In general, for patients who are 3 to 6 months pre-transplant, any of the shorter regimens (rifampin [RIF] for 4 months, INH + RPT for 12 weeks, or INH + RIF for 3 months) can be considered. Rifamycin-based regimens should generally be avoided in the post-transplant setting to minimize the risk of drug-drug interactions (DDI).

Management of Latent Tuberculosis Infection in Liver Transplant

The management of LTBI in patients with liver cirrhosis or chronic liver disease can be challenging due to risk of hepatotoxicity from anti-TB drugs such as INH and

Table 1
Treatments for latent tuberculosis infection in solid organ transplantation recipients

Regimen	Comments
Isoniazid (INH) daily for 6 or 9 months	1. Does not have any major drug interactions, can be used post-transplant 2. Risk of hepatotoxicity, liver enzymes must be monitored at baseline and then monthly
Rifampin daily for 4 months	1. Shorter regimen 2. Preferable for use in the pre-transplant setting 3. Can lead to drug–drug interactions (DDI), hence, should be avoided in the post-transplant setting
INH and rifapentine weekly for 12 weeks	1. Shorter regimen 2. Preferable for use in the pre-transplant setting 3. Monitor for DDI
Isoniazid and rifampin daily for 3 months	1. Preferable in pre-transplant setting 2. Shorter regimen 3. Monitor for rifampin DDI 4. Monitor for risk of hepatotoxicity

rifamycins. The reported incidence of hepatotoxicity with anti-tubercular drugs is 2% to 28%.[19,20] In a meta-analysis by Holty and colleagues, 6% of 139 liver transplant patients developed INH-related hepatotoxicity.[21] Another meta-analysis of 6105 patients found the incidence of toxic hepatitis was 2.55% in patients taking INH + rifampin and 1.6% in those taking INH alone.[22] Another retrospective study among 55 liver transplant candidates who were treated with INH showed no evidence of hepatotoxicity.[23]

In patients with elevation of liver enzymes (aspartate transaminase [AST] and ALT) > 5 times the upper limit of normal, the decision to treat LTBI must be made very carefully after weighing the risks and benefits. Our approach is to defer treatment of LTBI in patients with decompensated liver cirrhosis or acute hepatitis until after liver transplant and normalization of the liver enzymes. In patients with compensated cirrhosis, LTBI treatment can be started before transplantation with very close monitoring of liver enzymes. Another option for treatment of LTBI is fluoroquinolones such as levofloxacin. A multicenter randomized trial compared treatment with levofloxacin for LTBI pre-transplant to isoniazid 3 to 6 months post-transplantation. This study was suspended early due to the occurrence of tenosynovitis in 18% of patients in the levofloxacin arm. None of the 64 patients from both arms developed active TB.[24]

Clinical Manifestations of Tuberculosis

The classical signs of TB such as fevers, night sweats, and weight loss may not be present in SOT patients as the inflammatory response may be blunted in the setting of immunosuppression. In SOT patients, TB commonly presents as a disseminated disease with extrapulmonary manifestations.[1,25] The median time for development of TB is 6 to 26 months post-transplantation, with donor-derived infection accounting for earlier cases post-transplant.[1,3] The different radiographic findings noted on chest imaging in SOT were focal infiltrates, nodules, miliary pattern, diffuse infiltrates, and cavitary lesions. Other uncommon sites were skin, lymph node, bone and joint, eyes, and pericardium.[25]

Diagnosis

The diagnosis of active TB requires a high index of suspicion, and examination of respiratory samples, either sputum or bronchoalveolar lavage or sampling of any tissue/

fluid of the involved site. The specimens must be tested for smear, culture for acid-fast bacilli, and also for histopathological examination. Mycobacterial culture remains the gold standard for diagnosis of mycobacterium tuberculosis (MTB). There are three types of culture media (Lowenstein-Jensen), agar-based (Middlebrook 7H10 or 7H11), and liquid (Middlebrook 7H12). The growth in liquid media is usually faster (1–3 weeks) compared to solid media (3–7 weeks).

There are molecular assays that are available and widely used for detection of MTB DNA and genes with mutations that confer drug resistance. Nucleic acid amplification testing uses a nucleic acid probe to detect specific nucleic acid sequences for MTB and helps provide a rapid diagnosis (24–48 hours). The MTB Xpert/RIF assay can detect *M tuberculosis* and also mutations in the rpoB gene that determines rifampin resistance.

Various studies have investigated host response to TB with a microarray based gene expression profiling from peripheral blood. Although these are still in development, they may be helpful in future. For example, a three gene set to predict active TB was identified and validated in independent cohorts. The three gene test performed well in diagnosis of LTBI and active TB in patients with human immunodeficiency virus (HIV) co-infection.[26] This three gene TB score was able to identify progression from latent to active TB 6 months before sputum conversion, and identified patients with active TB with 90% sensitivity, and 70% specificity at 4% prevalence.[27] There are no data on the performance of this test in other immunocompromised populations.

Treatment of Active Tuberculosis

The treatment of TB in SOT is largely like immunocompetent patients. The first line of therapy includes four drugs for the initial 2 months—isoniazid, a rifamycin (rifampin or rifabutin), pyrazinamide, and ethambutol. Drug interactions pose a major challenge in the treatment as rifamycins can reduce the levels of calcineurin and mammalian target of rapamycin (mTOR) inhibitors such as tacrolimus, sirolimus, everolimus, and cyclosporine. Rifampin is a potent inducer of the cytochrome P 450 enzymes, which decreases the levels of these immunosuppressants. Rifabutin is a less potent inducer, causes lesser drug interaction, and hence, may be used as a substitute for rifampin. Rifamycins also lead to interactions with azole antifungals. In a cohort of 41 Thai patients who were receiving fluconazole concomitantly with rifampin, the fluconazole AUC decreased by 22% by day 8.[28] Mold-active azoles such as voriconazole and isavuconazole are also substrates of the CYP3A4 system. Rifampin can decrease the AUC of both drugs by 90%. A case report showed a 50% decrease in AUC when posaconazole was administered with rifampin.[29] Despite these drug interactions, rifamycin-based therapies are still the first line of recommended treatment of TB in this population.

Fluoroquinolones such as levofloxacin and moxifloxacin are second-line agents for treatment of TB. They can be used as alternate options in patients who have hepatotoxicity from the first-line agents, especially in liver transplant patients.[1] The second line of drugs that are available for treatment of MDR TB are cycloserine, ethionamide, amikacin, capreomycin, linezolid, clofazimine, bedaquiline, and delamanid.

Treatment of TB carries a significant morbidity in SOT patients. A review of 2082 cases of SOT that were treated for TB, showed a rate of 19% hepatotoxicity and 15% allograft loss. They were not associated with increased mortality. It was not reported if this was related to the use of rifamycin containing regimen; 75% of patients with rifamycin-sparing regimens were successfully treated and one died from a TB-related cause.[30] The duration of treatment is similar to non-transplant candidates, however, it may need to be prolonged if the clinical response is slow or second line agents need to be utilized.

NON-TUBERCULOUS MYCOBACTERIA IN SOLID ORGAN TRANSPLANTATION
Epidemiology and Risk Factors

Non-tuberculous mycobacteria (NTM) are a group of bacteria found in soil and water. They have been associated with health care-related infections and outbreaks and can cause contamination in operating rooms and cosmetic procedures such as tattoos, mesotherapy, or pedicures.[31–33]

In the United States, the annual prevalence of NTM varies from 1.4 to 13.9 per 100,000 persons, with a higher number of patients in the states of Florida, Texas, and California.[31,34] In studies involving non-transplant patients with comorbidities such as chronic obstructive pulmonary disease (COPD), cystic fibrosis, and diabetes mellitus, it was found that pulmonary involvement (75.1%) was more frequent than extrapulmonary involvement (24.9%).[31]

The incidence rates vary depending on the type of organ transplanted. The highest reported rate is in lung transplant recipients at 0.46% to 4.4%, followed by heart transplant at 0.24% to 2.80%, and then, kidney transplant 0.16% to 0.55%, and liver transplant patients at 0.1%.[35] Within transplant patients, several risk factors coincide, such as anatomical alteration and iatrogenic immunosuppression due to depressed cell immunity. The lung transplant patients are at a higher risk due to direct exposure to the environment. In a multinational retrospective case control study of SOT recipients, the various factors that were associated with increased risk of NTM infection were older age, hospital admission within 90 days, and receipt of antifungals and anti-lymphocyte antibodies.[36] In lung transplant, the risk is due to a combination of immunosuppression, alteration in the anatomy, compromise of the ciliary function and post-transplant lymphatic insufficiency.[7] In a systematic review carried out by Marty and colleagues, it was found that cystic fibrosis and pre-transplant isolation of NTM were associated with increased risk of NTM disease. The NTM disease was associated with increased mortality and chronic lung allograft dysfunction (CLAD).[24]

The common species that cause human infections are listed in **Table 2**. The NTM are classified based on their growth pattern into rapidly growing if they take < 7 days from subculture to grow and slow growing if they take > 7 days.

Table 2
Common species of non-tuberculous mycobacteria that cause human infections

Rapidly Growing Mycobacteria	Slow-Growing Mycobacteria
M abscessus	M avium complex
M fortuitum	M kansasii
M chelonae	M marinum
M mucogenicum	M xenopi
	M scrofulaceum
	M gordonae (this is rarely a true pathogen)
	M ulcerans
	M szulgai
	M asiaticum
	M haemophilum

RAPIDLY GROWING NON-TUBERCULOUS MYCOBACTERIA

In a retrospective cohort study of 33 SOT patients by Longworth and colleagues,[37] it was found that the most common organism was M abscessus in 44% of the infections, followed by MAC in 41%. Among the transplanted patients, a history of lung transplantation was associated with a higher risk (OR 9.45) in a single transplant and (OR 16.22) in a bilateral transplant.[37]

The presence of external devices such as cardiac implants, as well as peritoneal dialysis catheters, has been reported in cases of infections caused by Mycobacterium chelonae, M fortuitum, and Mycobacterium avium complex.[38] Nosocomial outbreaks of M abscessus from a contaminated water source in the hospital have been reported.[39] Mycobacterium chimaera outbreaks have been associated with the contamination of heater-cooler units of cardiac bypass machines.[40] A particular risk among pre-transplant patients are those diagnosed with structural lung disease such as cystic fibrosis, COPD, bronchiectasis, patients on anti-tumor necrosis factor (TNF) agents, and those with genetic defects in the interleukin -12 (IL-12) and interferon-gamma pathways. The reported incidence of NTM infection is 13% to 28% in patients with cystic fibrosis (CF) and 3% to 10% with bronchiectasis.[41]

In a cohort of 36 patients, 9 had NTM disease, whereas 27 were colonized. It was found that both infection and colonization by non-tuberculous mycobacteria were associated with an increased risk of mortality after lung transplantation.[42] In a study of 20 patients by Ebisu and colleagues, seven were thought to be colonized and were not treated, two of these died of a cause unrelated to infection, and the remaining five survived without infection at 1-year follow-up.[43] In a cohort of 30 lung transplant patients with NTM infections, the NTM cohort was more likely to develop bronchiolitis obliterans syndrome, however, it was not independently associated with it.[44] In the report by Osmani and colleagues[45] from the Mayo Clinic in Florida, the infection among those with pulmonary M abscessus was diagnosed within 7.5 months after transplant with later complications of bronchiolitis obliterans in those who survived in 50% of cases.

SLOW-GROWING NON-TUBERCULOUS MYCOBACTERIA

In patients with SOT, the most frequently reported species of NTM is MAC (M avium complex) followed by fast-growing NTM such as M chelonae, M fortuitum, and M kansasii within the slow-growing NTM.[25,46] MAC now contains 12 species, the most common being M avium, M intracellulare, and M chimaera.[47] Prolonged exposure to soil has been associated as a risk factor for MAC infection in the United States.[48] In a study of 38 lung transplant patients with NTM infections, 55% were due to MAC. The 5-year mortality was higher in patients with NTM compared to those who did not have an infection (P 0.016). It did not significantly increase the risk of CLAD.[42]

Pre-lung Transplant Evaluation

NTM colonization before transplant increases the risk of development of disease post-transplantation. Lung transplant for patients who are colonized with M abscessus spp, has been a topic of debate, as there is a high chance of recurrence, and treatment is prolonged with multiple drugs which limit tolerability due to side effects. Historically, this infection was considered a contra-indication to transplant. Several single-center studies have reported morbidities, and favorable survival outcomes in patients with pre-transplant NTM infections in lung transplant.[49–51] The ideal duration of treatment of M abscessus infection prior and post-transplantation is unknown. The patients must be able to tolerate the multidrug therapy and show clinical response before proceeding with transplant. These patients must have surveillance cultures via bronchoscopy at routine intervals post-transplantation, as defined by individual institutional protocols. Post-operative surgical site and pulmonary infections are common.[49,51]

All patients with pre-transplant NTM infection must be treated pre-transplant to reduce the bacterial burden. The decision to continue with treatment post-transplantation depends on the type of organism, extent of disease, and bacterial burden.

CLINICAL MANIFESTATIONS

The time of disease occurrence has been reported from 2.2 months to 7.5 years post-transplantation.[37] Most common site of involvement is pleuropulmonary and the symptoms include chronic cough, dyspnea, pain, pleuritic pain, fever, and chills.[37,40] Among lung transplant patients, there is a possibility of infection at the anastomosis during the post-operative period. It can present from 1 to 72 months post-transplantation.[52] It can cause bronchiectasis, nodular opacities, and cavities in the lungs. Other presentations include skin and soft tissue, musculoskeletal, catheter-associated, and disseminated disease.

Most patients do not have systemic symptoms such as weight loss, fevers, and night sweats. In the case of kidney transplant patients, in a total of 148 cases, skin lesions were found to be the most common manifestation, followed by osteoarticular disease. Patients may present with inflammatory changes in the subcutaneous tissue adjacent to the graft and subsequently invade deeper tissues.[53] MAC can involve primary allograft, and cases of liver and renal allograft involvement have been reported.[54,55]

In a report of 33 heart transplant patients by Abad and colleagues,[56] 39% manifested with skin disease and half of them had dissemination. The most frequent organisms isolated were *M abscessus, M fortuitum,* and *M chelonae.* They cause surgical site infections with disseminated skin involvement that may be associated with non-sterile techniques and contamination of surgical material.[45]

M chelonae has been associated with cosmetic procedures. It can cause localized infection such as cellulitis, abscess, or osteomyelitis. However, disseminated infection can also occur.[57,58] Patients usually have a history of direct inoculation with subsequent appearance of nodules, which are often red to violaceous, lymphadenopathy, and sporotrichoid forms with ascending lymphadenitis.[57]

Diagnosis

The American Thoracic Society (ATS) and Infectious Diseases Society of America (IDSA) have established criteria for diagnosis of pulmonary NTM infection, which include clinical, radiographic, and microbiologic criteria. Imaging findings typically involve nodular, cavitary opacities or findings consistent with bronchiectasis. For extrapulmonary sites of infection, specimens must be obtained from sterile samples, for AFB staining, cultures, and histopathology. The presence of suppurative granulomas, well-formed granulomas, or focal abscesses along with AFB positive staining are sufficient to make the diagnosis of NTM infection; however, granulomatous inflammation may be absent in immunosuppressed patients and AFB staining is not specific of NTM infection. The lack of hallmark histologic findings does not exclude the diagnosis in these patients, thus, less clear signs of inflammatory response in biopsies and tissue cultures must be considered given the complexity of the disease.[59] Mycobacterial blood cultures must be obtained when the disseminated disease is suspected, however, rapid growing mycobacteria may grow in routine blood culture bottles.

Identification of species is important for optimizing therapy. Some species require enriched media, lower temperature, and longer incubation; hence, it is important to have a high suspicion and inform the lab. Molecular methods polymerase chain reaction (PCR) are available for the diagnosis of certain species such as MAC and *M kansasii*. Sequencing analysis of the 16S subunit aids direct detection from clinical samples and matrix-assisted laser desorption ionization time-of-flight mass spectrometry (MALDI-TOF) is useful for rapid identification of isolates from culture. In the study by Toney and colleagues[60] in which the MALDI-TOF MS platform was evaluated to identify 314 isolates of non-tuberculous mycobacteria, it was found that 94% of the isolates could be classified to species level, and in the case of fast-growing mycobacteria, 99% were correctly identified. In a cohort of 448 patients with MAC, sequencing identified 54% of the isolates were *M avium*, 18% *M intracellulare,* and 28% *M chimaera*.[2] Drug susceptibility testing is useful when the in vitro activity correlates with the clinical outcomes. Macrolides for MAC, clarithromycin and rifampin for *M kansasii*, macrolides, and amikacin for *M abscessus spp* are the key drugs that have shown a correlation between in vitro susceptibility testing and clinical outcomes. Some strains of *M abscessus spp* have an erm gene that leads to inducible resistance to macrolides. This can be identified by prolonged incubation for 14 days or by molecular detection of the erm gene.[34]

Treatment

The treatment of NTM infections involves multiple drug regimens for prolonged periods, usually months to years. The duration and regimen depend on the site of infection, severity, net state of immunosuppression, and the NTM species. Adjuvant surgical management must be considered in selected cases such as those with abscesses, necrosis, or infections associated with devices that must be removed.[34,38,45,57]

An empiric drug regimen of two to three drugs is selected initially, based on the species and severity of infection. As the treatment varies according to the species, it would be important to identify the species. Treatment response must be assessed with cultures and imaging, as appropriate. The duration of treatment varies based on the severity, species, and clinical response. Tapering of immunosuppression may be required and must be done carefully to avoid immune reconstitution.

Table 3 lists the drugs that are used for the treatment of common species. The detailed treatment regimens with dosing are listed in IDSA/ATS guidelines and AST Infectious Diseases Community of Practice.

Some of the key issues in the management of these infections are the drug interactions between the rifamycins and calcineurin inhibitors as described above in the TB section. In contrast to rifamycins, macrolides such as clarithromycin and azithromycin are inhibitors of the CYP3A4 enzymes and can increase the levels of calcineurin inhibitors.

Furthermore, treatment may be associated with adverse events. Aminoglycosides can cause nephrotoxicity, and ototoxicity. Rifamycins and isoniazid can cause hepatotoxicity. Macrolides and fluoroquinolones can prolong corrected QT interval (QTc), so electrocardiogram (EKG) should be monitored while on treatment. Fluoroquinolones such as moxifloxacin, levofloxacin, and ciprofloxacin are also alternative agents of treatment of various species of NTM as listed in the table above. The side effects associated with it are hypoglycemia, tendinitis, aortic aneurysm, or dissection. Ethambutol can cause ocular symptoms so regular eye exams are necessary. Many of these agents can also cause gastrointestinal side effects.[38,40] Omadacycline and eravacycline are tetracycline analogs that have in vitro activity against *M abscessus*, and are generally tolerated better than tigecycline.[61] Bedaquiline is also an oral option with activity against the *M abscessus* complex.[62]

Table 3
Treatment regimens for common non-tuberculous bacteria

NTM Species	First Line Drugs	Second Line Drugs
MAC	Azithromycin Rifabutin Ethambutol	Amikacin Rifampin Moxifloxacin
M kansasii	Azithromycin or Isoniazid Rifabutin Ethambutol	Clarithromycin Rifampin Moxifloxacin
M xenopi	Azithromycin or Moxifloxacin Rifabutin Ethambutol	Clarithromycin Rifampin Amikacin
M abscessus	Azithromycin Amikacin Imipenem Cefoxitin Tigecycline	Linezolid Clofazimine Minocycline Clarithromycin Moxifloxacin Omadacycline Eravacycline Bedaquiline
M chelonae	Azithromycin Amikacin Imipenem Tigecycline Linezolid	

Abbreviations: MAC, M. avium complex, NTM; non-tuberculous mycobacteria.

The ATS/IDSA guidelines recommend an initial treatment phase with three active drugs with macrolide as a part of the regimen. This is followed by a continuation phase with two to three drugs. For strains that have inducible macrolide resistance, initial treatment with four drugs with at least two parenteral drugs is recommended.

Surgical management can also be considered in some cases. Three studies that compared medical and surgical management of NTM revealed no significant differences in cure, death, or recurrence. Surgical complications were observed in 7% to 35% of patients. Post-operative mortality of 1% to 9% was reported.[34,63] The duration of treatment is guided by clinical response and patient tolerability. For limited skin and soft tissue infections, treatment duration of 4 to 6 months is recommended. For severe disease with pulmonary or bone involvement and disseminated disease, a minimum duration of 6 to 12 months is recommended. Sputum cultures must be obtained to assess for a microbiologic cure, and treatment should be continued for 12 months after the conversion. For M abscessus, the risk of treatment failure is greater, and the culture conversion rate is 24% to 42%.[64,65] The treatment of M abscessus involves an initial phase of 8 to 12 weeks with three to four parenteral antimicrobials, followed by a continuation phase with two to three oral antimicrobials for 12 months after the sputum cultures turn negative, along with regular imaging monitoring.[64]

SUMMARY

Latent TB diagnosis and management remain a challenge in SOT population. Further randomized controlled trials are needed to evaluate an optimal approach to LTBI diagnosis and management. The efficacy and safety of fluoroquinolones for LTBI in this population also need to be assessed. TB management in SOT population is also challenging given the DDI. The management of NTM is also very difficult due to prolonged treatment of drug toxicities and interactions with immunosuppressants. The newer oral medications such as omadacycline, eravacycline, and bedaquiline are promising oral options for second-line treatment, however, more clinical studies are needed.

CLINICS CARE POINTS

- Isoniazid for 9 months is the first line recommended treatment for latent tuberculosis infection. However, shorter regimens such as rifampin for 4 months, INH+Rifapentine for 12 weeks or INH + rifampin for 3 months can be considered in the pre-transplant setting.

- All patients with latent TB infection who are undergoing organ transplantation must be treated to reduce their risk of TB reactivation. In liver transplant patients, the timing of treatment must be decided based on their liver function. In patients with decompensated cirrhosis, treatment can be deferred to post-transplantation until the normalization of liver enzymes.

- In patients with M abscessus before lung transplantation, the patients must be able to tolerate multidrug therapy and show clinical response, before they proceed with transplant.

DISCLOSURES

The authors have nothing to disclose.

REFERENCES

1. Subramanian AK, Theodoropoulos NM. Infectious Diseases Community of Practice of the American Society of Transplantation. Mycobacterium tuberculosis infections in solid organ transplantation: Guidelines from the infectious diseases community of practice of the American Society of Transplantation. Clin Transplant 2019;33(9):e13513.
2. Abad CL, Razonable RR. Prevention and treatment of tuberculosis in solid organ transplant recipients. Expert Rev Anti Infect Ther 2020;18(1):63–73.
3. Epstein DJ, Subramanian AK. Prevention and Management of Tuberculosis in Solid Organ Transplant Recipients. Infect Dis Clin North Am 2018;32(3):703–18.
4. Torre-Cisneros J, Doblas A, Aguado JM, et al. Tuberculosis after solid-organ transplant: incidence, risk factors, and clinical characteristics in the RESITRA (Spanish Network of Infection in Transplantation) cohort. Clin Infect Dis 2009; 48(12):1657–65.
5. Basiri A, Moghaddam SM, Simforoosh N, et al. Preliminary report of a nationwide case-control study for identifying risk factors of tuberculosis following renal transplantation. Transplant Proc 2005;37(7):3041–4.
6. Kwon DE, Han SH, Han KD, et al. Incidence rate of active tuberculosis in solid organ transplant recipients: Data from a nationwide population cohort in a high-endemic country. Transpl Infect Dis 2021;23(6):e13729.
7. Thitisuriyarax S, Vanichanan J, Udomkarnjananun S, et al. Risk factors and clinical outcomes of tuberculosis among kidney transplant recipients in high endemic country. Transpl Infect Dis 2021;23(3):e13566.
8. Malinis M, La Hoz RM, Vece G, et al. Donor-derived tuberculosis among solid organ transplant recipients in the United States-2008 to 2018. Transpl Infect Dis 2022;24(2):e13800.

9. Maung Myint T, Rogerson TE, Noble K, et al. Tests for latent tuberculosis in candidates for solid organ transplantation: A systematic review and meta-analysis. Clin Transplant 2019;33(8):e13643.

10. Rogerson TE, Chen S, Kok J, et al. Tests for latent tuberculosis in people with ESRD: a systematic review. Am J Kidney Dis 2013;61(1):33–43.

11. Hand J, Sigel K, Huprikar S, et al. Tuberculosis after liver transplantation in a large center in New York City: QuantiFERON® -TB Gold-based pre-transplant screening performance and active tuberculosis post-transplant. Transpl Infect Dis 2018;20(2):e12845.

12. Manuel O, Humar A, Preiksaitis J, et al. Comparison of quantiferon-TB gold with tuberculin skin test for detecting latent tuberculosis infection prior to liver transplantation. Am J Transplant 2007;7(12):2797–801.

13. Lyu J, Lee SG, Hwang S, et al. Chest computed tomography is more likely to show latent tuberculosis foci than simple chest radiography in liver transplant candidates. Liver Transpl 2011;17(8):963–8.

14. Guirao-Arrabal E, Santos F, Redel-Montero J, et al. Risk of tuberculosis after lung transplantation: the value of pretransplant chest computed tomography and the impact of mTOR inhibitors and azathioprine use. Transpl Infect Dis 2016;18(4): 512–9.

15. Morris MI, Daly JS, Blumberg E, et al. Diagnosis and management of tuberculosis in transplant donors: a donor-derived infections consensus conference report [published correction appears in Am J Transplant. 2013 Feb;13(2):528]. Am J Transplant 2012;12(9):2288–300.

16. Schmidt T, Schub D, Wolf M, et al. Comparative analysis of assays for detection of cell-mediated immunity toward cytomegalovirus and M. tuberculosis in samples from deceased organ donors. Am J Transplant 2014;14(9):2159–67.

17. Tabarsi P, Yousefzadeh A, Najafizadeh K, et al. Performance of QuantiFERON TB Gold test in detecting latent tuberculosis infection in brain-dead organ donors in Iran: a brief report. Saudi J Kidney Dis Transpl 2014;25(6):1240–3.

18. Simkins J, Abbo LM, Camargo JF, et al. Twelve-Week Rifapentine Plus Isoniazid Versus 9-Month Isoniazid for the Treatment of Latent Tuberculosis in Renal Transplant Candidates. Transplantation 2017;101(6):1468–72.

19. Abad CLR, Deziel PJ, Razonable RR. Treatment of latent TB Infection and the risk of tuberculosis after solid organ transplantation: Comprehensive review. Transpl Infect Dis 2019;21(6):e13178.

20. Kumar N, Kedarisetty CK, Kumar S, et al. Antitubercular therapy in patients with cirrhosis: challenges and options. World J Gastroenterol 2014;20(19): 5760–72.

21. Holty JE, Gould MK, Meinke L, et al. Tuberculosis in liver transplant recipients: a systematic review and meta-analysis of individual patient data. Liver Transpl 2009;15(8):894–906.

22. Steele MA, Burk RF, DesPrez RM. Toxic hepatitis with isoniazid and rifampin. A meta-analysis. Chest 1991;99(2):465–71.

23. Ghayumi SMA, Shamsaeefar A, Motazedian N, et al. Isoniazid prophylaxis in liver transplant recipient with latent tuberculosis: Is it harmful for transplanted liver? Transpl Infect Dis 2022;24(4):e13849.

24. Torre-Cisneros J, San-Juan R, Rosso-Fernández CM, et al. Tuberculosis prophylaxis with levofloxacin in liver transplant patients is associated with a high incidence of tenosynovitis: safety analysis of a multicenter randomized trial. Clin Infect Dis 2015;60(11):1642–9.

25. Singh N, Paterson DL. Mycobacterium tuberculosis infection in solid-organ transplant recipients: impact and implications for management. Clin Infect Dis 1998; 27(5):1266–77.

26. Sweeney TE, Braviak L, Tato CM, et al. Genome-wide expression for diagnosis of pulmonary tuberculosis: a multicohort analysis. Lancet Respir Med 2016;4(3): 213–24.

27. Warsinske HC, Rao AM, Moreira FMF, et al. Assessment of Validity of a Blood-Based 3-Gene Signature Score for Progression and Diagnosis of Tuberculosis, Disease Severity, and Treatment Response. JAMA Netw Open 2018;1(6): e183779.

28. Baciewicz AM, Chrisman CR, Finch CK, et al. Update on rifampin and rifabutin drug interactions. Am J Med Sci 2008;335(2):126–36.

29. Klatt ME, Eschenauer GA. Review of Pharmacologic Considerations in the Use of Azole Antifungals in Lung Transplant Recipients. J Fungi (Basel) 2021; 7(2):76.

30. Abad CLR, Razonable RR. Mycobacterium tuberculosis after solid organ transplantation: A review of more than 2000 cases. Clin Transplant 2018;32(6): e13259.

31. Asaoka M, Hagiwara E, Etori S, et al. Identification and Characteristics of Co-isolation of Multiple Nontuberculous Mycobacteria. Intern Med 2021;60(20): 3213–9.

32. Boyle DP, Zembower TR, Reddy S, et al. Comparison of Clinical Features, Virulence, and Relapse among Mycobacterium avium Complex Species. Am J Respir Crit Care Med 2015;191(11):1310–7.

33. Mora AD, Giraldo S, Castillo DA, et al. [Clinical behavior of infection and disease caused by non-tuberculous mycobacteria in Latin America: Scoping review]. Rev Peru Med Exp Salud Pública 2021;38(2):318–25.

34. Daley CL, Iaccarino JM, Lange C, et al. Treatment of Nontuberculous Mycobacterial Pulmonary Disease: An Official ATS/ERS/ESCMID/IDSA Clinical Practice Guideline. Clin Infect Dis 2020;71(4):e1–36.

35. Malinis MF. Management of Mycobacterium Other than Tuberculosis in Solid Organ Transplantation. Infect Dis Clin North Am 2018;32(3):719–32.

36. Mejia-Chew C, Carver PL, Rutjanawech S, et al. Risk factors for Nontuberculous Mycobacteria Infections in Solid Organ Transplant recipients: a multinational case-control study [published online ahead of print, 2022 Jul 26]. Clin Infect Dis 2022;76(3):e995–1003.

37. Longworth SA, Blumberg EA, Barton TD, et al. Non-tuberculous mycobacterial infections after solid organ transplantation: a survival analysis. Clin Microbiol Infect 2015;21(1):43–7.

38. Friedman DZP, Doucette K. Mycobacteria: Selection of Transplant Candidates and Post-lung Transplant Outcomes. Semin Respir Crit Care Med 2021;42(3): 460–70.

39. Baker AW, Lewis SS, Alexander BD, et al. Two-Phase Hospital-Associated Outbreak of Mycobacterium abscessus: Investigation and Mitigation. Clin Infect Dis 2017;64(7):902–11.

40. Riccardi N, Monticelli J, Antonello RM, et al. Mycobacterium chimaera infections: An update. J Infect Chemother 2020;26(3):199–205.

41. Rao M, Silveira FP. Non-tuberculous Mycobacterial Infections in Thoracic Transplant Candidates and Recipients. Curr Infect Dis Rep 2018;20(6):14.

42. Huang HC, Weigt SS, Derhovanessian A, et al. Non-tuberculous mycobacterium infection after lung transplantation is associated with increased mortality. J Heart Lung Transplant 2011;30(7):790–8.

43. Ebisu Y, Natori Y, Rosello G, et al. Mycobacterium abscessus Infections in Solid Organ Transplant Recipients: Single-Center Experience in the United States, 2013-2018. Open Forum Infect Dis 2022;9(7):ofac254.

44. Shah SK, McAnally KJ, Seoane L, et al. Analysis of pulmonary non-tuberculous mycobacterial infections after lung transplantation. Transpl Infect Dis 2016; 18(4):585–91.

45. Osmani M, Sotello D, Alvarez S, et al. Mycobacterium abscessus infections in lung transplant recipients: 15-year experience from a single institution. Transpl Infect Dis 2018;20(2):e12835.

46. Longworth SA, Daly JS. Management of infections due to nontuberculous mycobacteria in solid organ transplant recipients-Guidelines from the American Society of Transplantation Infectious Diseases Community of Practice. Clin Transplant 2019;33(9):e13588.

47. Van Ingen J, Turenne CY, Tortoli E, et al. A definition of the Mycobacterium avium complex for taxonomical and clinical purposes, a review. Int J Syst Evol Microbiol 2018;68(11):3666–77.

48. Reed C, von Reyn CF, Chamblee S, et al. Environmental risk factors for infection with Mycobacterium avium complex. Am J Epidemiol 2006;164(1):32–40.

49. Qvist T, Pressler T, Thomsen VO, et al. Nontuberculous mycobacterial disease is not a contraindication to lung transplantation in patients with cystic fibrosis: a retrospective analysis in a Danish patient population. Transplant Proc 2013; 45(1):342–5.

50. Perez AA, Singer JP, Schwartz BS, et al. Management and clinical outcomes after lung transplantation in patients with pre-transplant Mycobacterium abscessus infection: A single center experience. Transpl Infect Dis 2019;21(3):e13084.

51. Lobo LJ, Chang LC, Esther CR Jr, et al. Lung transplant outcomes in cystic fibrosis patients with pre-operative Mycobacterium abscessus respiratory infections. Clin Transplant 2013;27(4):523–9.

52. Pena T, Klesney-Tait J. Mycobacterial Infections in Solid Organ and Hematopoietic Stem Cell Transplantation. Clin Chest Med 2017;38(4):761–70.

53. Ricotta EE, Adjemian J, Blakney RA, et al. Extrapulmonary Nontuberculous Mycobacteria Infections in Hospitalized Patients, United States, 2009-2014. Emerg Infect Dis 2021;27(3):845–52.

54. Rawla MS, Kozak A, Hadley S, et al. Mycobacterium avium-intracellulare-associated acute interstitial nephritis: a rare cause of renal allograft dysfunction. Transpl Infect Dis 2009;11(6):529–33.

55. Singhal A, Gates C, Malhotra N, et al. Successful management of primary nontuberculous mycobacterial infection of hepatic allograft following orthotopic liver transplantation for hepatitis C. Transpl Infect Dis 2011;13(1):47–51.

56. Abad CL, Razonable RR. Non-tuberculous mycobacterial infections in solid organ transplant recipients: An update. J Clin Tuberc Other Mycobact Dis 2016; 4:1–8.

57. Pennington KM, Vu A, Challener D, et al. Approach to the diagnosis and treatment of non-tuberculous mycobacterial disease. J Clin Tuberc Other Mycobact Dis 2021;24:100244.

58. Wallace RJ Jr, Brown BA, Onyi GO. Skin, soft tissue, and bone infections due to Mycobacterium chelonae chelonae: importance of prior corticosteroid therapy,

frequency of disseminated infections, and resistance to oral antimicrobials other than clarithromycin. J Infect Dis 1992;166(2):405–12.

59. Gonzalez-Santiago TM, Drage LA. Nontuberculous Mycobacteria: Skin and Soft Tissue Infections. Dermatol Clin 2015;33(3):563–7.

60. Toney NC, Zhu W, Jensen B, et al. Evaluation of MALDI Biotyper Mycobacteria Library for Identification of Nontuberculous Mycobacteria. J Clin Microbiol 2022;60(9):e0021722.

61. Kaushik A, Ammerman NC, Martins O, et al. *In Vitro* Activity of New Tetracycline Analogs Omadacycline and Eravacycline against Drug-Resistant Clinical Isolates of *Mycobacterium abscessus*. Antimicrob Agents Chemother 2019;63(6): e00470–519.

62. Brown-Elliott BA, Philley JV, Griffith DE, et al. In Vitro Susceptibility Testing of Bedaquiline against Mycobacterium avium Complex. Antimicrob Agents Chemother 2017;61(2):e01798–816.

63. Jarand J, Levin A, Zhang L, et al. Clinical and microbiologic outcomes in patients receiving treatment for Mycobacterium abscessus pulmonary disease. Clin Infect Dis 2011;52(5):565–71.

64. Griffith DE, Daley CL. Treatment of Mycobacterium abscessus Pulmonary Disease. Chest 2022;161(1):64–75.

65. Park J, Cho J, Lee CH, et al. Progression and Treatment Outcomes of Lung Disease Caused by Mycobacterium abscessus and Mycobacterium massiliense. Clin Infect Dis 2017;64(3):301–8.

Emerging Diagnostics and Therapeutics for Invasive Fungal Infections

Daniel Z.P. Friedman, MD, MSc[a], Ilan S. Schwartz, MD, PhD[b],*

KEYWORDS

- Transplant • Mycology • Diagnosis • Diagnostic • Treatment • Antifungal • Olorofim
- Fosmanogepix

KEY POINTS

- The advantages of molecular testing generally include high sensitivity and pathogen specificity, the use of some assays on noninvasive samples (like blood), the detection of resistance-associated mutations, and the potential for rapid turnaround time.
- Disadvantages of molecular testing include cost, delays in turnaround time associated with referral laboratory testing, and the inability to distinguish infection from colonization in non-sterile samples.
- Antifungals in advanced stages of clinical development include agents with novel mechanisms of action (olorofim and fosmanogepix, inhibitors of dihydroorotate dehydrogenase and Gwt1, respectively), as well as new members with advantages over existing antifungals (oteseconazole, opelconazole, rezafungin, ibrexafungerp, encochleated amphotericin B).

INTRODUCTION

The number of patients at risk for fungal infections continues to increase because of improved survival of medically and surgically complex patients, new indications for immunosuppression, and the use of novel immunosuppressing agents.[1] However, the diagnosis and management of fungal infections continue to present major challenges that have lagged compared with advances in other areas of medicine. First, traditional diagnostics have suffered from a lack of sensitivity and/or specificity and may require invasive sampling that is impractical in clinically tenuous patients.[2] Second, treatment is often unsatisfactory, which may stem from intrinsic or acquired

a Section of Infectious Diseases and Global Health, The University of Chicago, 5841 South Maryland Avenue, MC5065, Chicago, IL 60637, USA; b Division of Infectious Diseases, Department of Medicine, Duke University School of Medicine, 315 Trent Drive, Durham, NC 27705, USA
* Corresponding author.
E-mail address: ilan.schwartz@duke.edu

Infect Dis Clin N Am 37 (2023) 593–616
https://doi.org/10.1016/j.idc.2023.05.001
0891-5520/23/© 2023 Elsevier Inc. All rights reserved.

resistance in fungal pathogens, drug–drug interactions, toxicities, unpredictable pharmacokinetics, and inconvenience posed by frequency or route of dosing.[3]

In the past decade, there have been significant advances in the tools available for diagnosing and treating fungal infections.[4] Herein, we review selected recent advances in fungal diagnostics and antifungal therapies that are newly available or in late-stage clinical development, emphasizing their impact on the care of solid organ transplant (SOT) recipients.

RECENT ADVANCES IN FUNGAL DIAGNOSTICS

In 2021, the Fungal Diagnostics Laboratory Consortium published disease-specific and methodology-specific gaps in diagnosing invasive fungal infections.[5] Classically, the gold standard for diagnosing a fungal infection is a culture from a sterile site. However, this approach has some limitations: some pathogens, such as *Pneumocystis jirovecii*, cannot be readily grown in culture; some species require specialized media or extended incubation for growth; and sensitivity can be affected by prior treatments. There is a need for noninvasive markers of invasive fungal infections that are commercially available and have acceptable operating characteristics and actionable turnaround times. The advantages and disadvantages of various diagnostic modalities, including multiplex assays and next-generation sequencing (NGS) in the care of SOT recipients, were recently reviewed in a consensus conference.[6]

Biomarkers

Available biomarkers for invasive fungal infections include 1,3-beta-D-glucan (BDG) and *Aspergillus* galactomannan (GM).[7]

BDG is a cell wall component of many fungal pathogens, and it can be detected in the serum during several fungal infections, including *Pneumocystis* pneumonia (PCP), invasive candidiasis, and aspergillosis. For invasive candidiasis, the sensitivity and specificity are ~75% to 80% and ~60% to 80%, respectively.[7] In PCP, sensitivity was 91% and specificity was 79%.[8] BDG can be falsely positive in several conditions other than fungal disease, including intravenous immunoglobulin, albumin, and sepsis.[7] Recent reviews have been unable to quantify the operating characteristics of BDG for invasive aspergillosis because of the scarcity and heterogeneity of the data.[7,9]

GM is a mannoprotein found in the cell wall of *Aspergillus* spp., in addition to several other pathogens, including some *Fusarium* spp., *Histoplasma capsulatum*, and *Blastomyces spp.*, as well as less pathogenic fungi like *Penicillium* spp. Its detection in bronchoalveolar lavage (BAL) can support a diagnosis of invasive mold infection, but it cannot distinguish invasive disease from airway colonization. Detection of GM in the serum is found in invasive pulmonary aspergillosis (and occasionally other invasive mycoses), but the sensitivity varies according to host characteristics. It is most sensitive in the setting of patients with hematological malignancies or allogeneic stem cell transplantation but is considerably less sensitive in patients with SOT.[7]

In general, the specificity of detection of biomarkers like BDG and GM is improved when multiple samples (ideally collected sequentially) are positive. For example, the positive predictive value of BDG for the diagnosis of invasive fungal infection is improved with 2 consecutive positive tests.[10] These tests may have a role in screening high-risk immunocompromised patients, with detection being a starting point for further clinical, radiographic, and mycological assessment; however, the data are currently insufficient to support this practice.

MOLECULAR DIAGNOSTICS
Polymerase Chain Reaction

Nucleic acid amplification techniques such as polymerase chain reaction (PCR) present a promising diagnostic modality that involves a highly specific test on noninvasive samples with rapid turnaround. Assays have been in development since the late 1990s.[11] PCR tests that are currently available and in clinical use are for the targeted detection of respiratory pathogens like *Pneumocystis*, *Aspergillus*, and Mucorales (**Table 1**).

PANFUNGAL POLYMERASE CHAIN REACTION

Panfungal assays refer to primers that target conserved fungal binding sites that flank barcoding regions, such as internal transcribed spacers (ITS)-1 and ITS-2 and the D1/D2 regions of the 28s rRNA gene. Amplification with such broad-range fungal primers followed by sequencing has been used for the identification of fungi in clinical samples.[12] Although a variety of sample types have been used, the test is best studied for the identification of fungi seen in formalin-fixed paraffin-embedded tissue. The sensitivity is improved by limiting use to tissue samples in which fungal elements are seen on histological examination.[12] These assays can be helpful in situations where species differentiation can contribute to the refinement of management decisions but when cultures are not obtained or are negative.

PNEUMOCYSTIS

Pneumocystis jirovecii, the cause of PCP, does not grow in culture, and the diagnosis was historically made by direct examination of respiratory samples with fungal stains or immunofluorescence. However, while specific, the test lacked sensitivity, leading to unacceptable rates of false negative results.

In many centers, PCR has already supplanted direct examination for the diagnosis of PCP. The main advantage is higher sensitivity, but this comes at the cost of specificity because positive results can also be seen in the setting of colonization. Quantitative PCR (qPCR) can help distinguish colonization from infection.[13] Although BAL represents the optimal sample type, there have been some studies that have explored using less invasive samples, such as nasopharyngeal aspirates, with promising results.[14]

ASPERGILLOSIS

There are several commercially available *Aspergillus* PCR assays available in Europe[12,15] but they are not yet available in North America. It should be noted that most data evaluating *Aspergillus* PCR are derived from neutropenic cohorts, and there are few published data on SOT recipients.[16]

AsperGenius (PathoNostics) and MycoGENIE (Ademtech) are multiplex assays, each with 2 PCR components that can be used directly on patient samples (BAL and serum).[12,15] The first PCR can detect and identify the most common *Aspergillus* species associated with invasive aspergillosis, and the second can detect the presence of major resistance-associated mutations in Cyp51A.

For detection of *Aspergillus* spp. from BAL, AsperGenius has a sensitivity and specificity range from 42% to 84% and 80% to 91%, respectively[15,17–20]; and MycoGENIE has a sensitivity and specificity range of 54% to 93% and 90%, respectively.[21,22] From serum, the sensitivity and specificity of AsperGenius have been reported as ∼80%

Table 1
Molecular diagnostics for invasive fungal infections

Test	Pathogens	Sample Type	Advantages	Disadvantages	Comments
PCR					
Broad-range PCR	Wide range of fungal pathogens	Usually tissue	Can detect most pathogens	Less helpful in samples from non-sterile sites Poor performance in mixed infections Typically send-out	Sensitivity is best when fungi are visible on histopathology Fresh tissue samples have the highest sensitivity
Pathogen-directed PCR assays			Generally more sensitive than culture-based methods May permit an earlier diagnosis	Cost (variable) Difficult to reliably distinguish colonization from infection in airway samples	
	Pneumocystis	BAL, induced sputum, perhaps nasopharyngeal aspirate	Highly sensitive	Will detect colonization and infection	With qPCR, cycle threshold may be able to suggest whether detection represents colonization or infection
	Aspergillus	BAL, serum	More sensitive than culture in BAL Some assays allow the detection of major azole resistance-associated mutations	Unable to distinguish colonization from infection from airway samples	

	Mucorales	BAL, serum	More sensitive than culture Allows for noninvasive testing	Send-out test Turn-around time
	Aspergillus, Mucorales (and *Nocardia*) +/– *Pneumocystis*	BAL	Syndromic testing allows testing of multiple pathogens with clinical overlap	Few published data Appears to have limited sensitivity Unable to distinguish colonization from infection
Metagenomic Next-Generation Sequencing (eg, Karius)	Fungi (and bacteria, protozoa, algae, and DNA viruses)	Serum	Unbiased (agnostic) testing (can detect a pathogen even without a priori suspicion)	Cost (~$2000/test) Turn-around time (several days) Poor specificity (can detect small fragments of organisms, often with unclear significance)

Abbreviation: BAL, bronchoalveolar lavage

and 79% to 91%, respectively[15]; whereas MycoGENIE has a reported sensitivity and specificity of 100% and 85%, respectively.[21]

AsperGenius and MycoGENIE test for the presence of Cyp51A mutations TR34/L98H and TR46/T289A/y121F, the 2 mutations most commonly associated with azole-resistant *A fumigatus*, particularly in Europe.[17,18] Azole-resistant *A fumigatus* is uncommon in North America, and seldom linked to the detected mutations[23]; consequently, a low pretest probability could limit the positive predictive value of resistance-associated mutations in this setting. Moreover, the detection of a resistance-associated mutation does not mean clinical failure on azoles is certain. For example, in a large prospective study of 276 Dutch and Belgian hematology patients with pulmonary infiltrates evaluated with an AsperGenius PCR assay on BAL fluid, 6 patients had azole-resistant *A fumigatus* detected; despite the presence of azole resistance-associated mutations, only 1 failed to improve with azole therapy.[24] Finally, current assays only detect resistance-associated mutations in *A fumigatus*.

Aspergillus PCR assays are likely best used to supplement than supplant routine fungal diagnostics like fungal culture and GM. It is unclear whether the best diagnostic approach is a parallel or stepwise testing strategy when routine fungal tests are negative but high clinical suspicion for aspergillosis persists. Specificity of PCR declines when other tests are negative, as suggested by the finding that among hematology patients with new pulmonary infiltrate, there was an association of 6 week mortality with positive BAL GM as the sole mycological criterion for invasive aspergillosis (ie, when BAL fungal culture and *Aspergillus* PCR were negative) but not positive BAL *Aspergillus* PCR as the sole positive mycological test.[24]

In addition to their use in diagnosing clinical disease, molecular assays using whole blood or serum have been evaluated for routine screening for early/subclinical aspergillosis in immunocompromised patients at high risk of invasive aspergillosis (defined as neutropenic patients with cancer and allogeneic stem cell or SOT recipients). In a systematic review and meta-analysis, the sensitivity and specificity of a single positive sample were determined to be 79.2% and 79.6%, respectively. Alternatively, requiring 2 consecutive positive tests lowered sensitivity to 59.6% and increased specificity to 95.1%. The authors concluded that 2 consecutive positive tests should prompt further workup for clinical, radiological, and/or mycological findings of invasive aspergillosis or can be used to trigger preemptive therapy when the pretest probability is sufficiently high.[25]

MUCORMYCOSIS

A multiplex PCR assay for *Rhizomucor*, *Rhizopus/Mucor*, and *Lichtheimia*-Mucorales fungi most commonly implicated in mucormycosis—is commercially available and can be used on BAL specimens or blood. In BAL samples, qPCR was considerably more sensitive than culture for detecting Mucorales: out of 374 tested immunocompromised patients in France with pneumonia, Mucorales were detected in BAL by qPCR in 24 of whom just 2 of 24 had positive cultures.[26]

Because some high-risk patients (especially those with hematological malignancy, thrombocytopenia, or tenuous respiratory status) cannot tolerate bronchoscopy, it is notable that Mucorales qPCR can also be performed on serum. The MODIMUCOR study prospectively evaluated 232 high-risk patients with suspected invasive mold infection (based on suggestive imaging and clinical symptoms) with twice-weekly serum Mucorales qPCR. This cohort included 20 patients and 7 patients with proven and probable mucormycosis, respectively, among whom 23/27 had positive serum Mucorales qPCR tests. The sensitivity of serum Mucorales qPCR was 85.2%, and the specificity was 89.8%. The positive and negative likelihood ratios were 8.3 and 0.17, respectively.

Importantly, the time to positivity of serum qPCR was earlier (median of 4 days) than histologic or other mycological evidence. The authors also found a negative qPCR within 7 days of initiating liposomal amphotericin B (AMB) was associated with an 85% lower 30 day mortality (adjusted HR 0.15, 95% confidence interval [CI] 0.03–0.73, $P = .02$).[27]

Although the Mucorales qPCR test used by Millon and colleagues has the most robust data to support its use, it is an in-house developed test that is not commercially available. However, there are at least 4 commercially available PCR tests for Mucorales: these include MucorGenius (PathoNostics), MycoGenie Aspergillus species-Mucorales Species (Ademtech), Fungiplex Mucorales PCR (Bruker), and Fungal Plus PCR (Eurofins-Viracor).[28] Data evaluating the performance of these in diagnosing mucormycosis have only been published for the MucorGenius assay,[29–31] which was reported to have a sensitivity of 90% and a specificity exceeding 95%, comparable to the in-house qPCR assay.[32] The Fungal Plus multiplex PCR, which has primers for Aspergillus, Mucorales, and Nocardia, with or without Pneumocystis, has just one published study evaluating its use with just a single case of mucormycosis (which the test failed to detect).[33]

Metagenomic Next-Generation Sequencing

There has been increasing interest in platforms that are agnostic (ie, don't require targeting of specific pathogens) and can diagnose invasive fungal infections from noninvasive samples. The Karius test is a metagenomic NGS platform that can detect cell-free DNA (cfDNA) from plasma to identify over 1250 human pathogens, including bacteria, fungi, and DNA viruses.[34]

The performance of Karius's cfDNA sequencing for the diagnosis of invasive mold infections was evaluated in a retrospective study of 114 hematopoietic stem cell transplant recipients with pneumonia who had stored serum that had been collected within 14 days of invasive mold infection diagnosis or (among those without invasive mold infections) the date of BAL. Among these, 75 had proven or probable mold infections, but cfDNA sequencing identified molds in just 38 (sensitivity 51%, 95% CI 39%–62%). When testing was limited to samples collected within 3 days of the diagnosis of invasive mold infections, or BAL, the sensitivity was modestly improved (61%). The specificity was 95% (95% CI 82%–100%).[35]

Moreno and colleagues evaluated an in-house cfDNA PCR assay for the diagnosis of PCP. Their retrospective cohort included 149 patients clinically suspected to have PCP, including 47% with SOT. In total, 10 patients had proven PCP and 27 had probable PCP. The sensitivity and specificity to detect proven or probable PCP were 48.6% (95% CI 31.9%–65.6%) and 99.1% (95% CI 94.9%–100%), respectively.[36] Further study with large, well-characterized cohorts will be important to confirm the specificity of cfDNA in PCP disease.

The use of cfDNA sequence testing is limited by poor sensitivity in localized infections, uncertain specificity with some results (given that the detection of fragments of cfDNA may not be of clinical consequence), a slow turnaround time (53 hours), and high cost (>$2000 per sample).[37] Karius cfDNA sequence testing is currently only approved for use on plasma, and in general, metagenomic NGS platforms cannot be used on non-sterile samples like BAL. The role of plasma cfDNA sequencing for diagnosing fungal pneumonia in immunocompromised patients in whom routine microbiological diagnostic tests like BAL fungal culture, GM, and PCR are negative is uncertain.

NEW THERAPEUTICS FOR INVASIVE FUNGAL INFECTIONS

The antifungal pipeline is currently the most robust it has been in decades. These include new therapeutics from existing classes of antifungals (azoles, echinocandins, and polyenes) and 3 novel first-in-class antifungals. All of them have distinct advantages in spectrum, side effect profile, drug–drug interactions, frequency, and/or route of administration over existing antifungals in the armamentarium.

NEW DRUGS, OLD CLASSES
Opelconazole

The triazoles—itraconazole, voriconazole, posaconazole, and isavuconazole—remain the cornerstone of prophylaxis and treatment of invasive fungal infections in SOT recipients, especially lung transplant recipients who are at greatest risk of pulmonary mold infections. Though their use is widespread and dates back over 3 decades, these antifungals are associated with significant drug–drug interactions and, sometimes, prohibitive systemic side effects.

Opelconazole is an inhaled topical triazole with an anticipated niche for the prophylaxis and treatment of invasive pulmonary aspergillosis and may overcome obstacles of drug–drug interactions and adverse effects. Early in vitro and in vivo studies demonstrate that opelconazole has favorable activity against most *Aspergillus* species (though notably not *A niger*), reaches adequate drug levels within pulmonary tissues, and has minimal systemic absorption.[38,39] It has activity against *Candida* and *Cryptococcus* spp., and although it did not have any antifungal activity against most Mucorales, opelconazole showed moderate activity against *Rhizopus oryzae*.[38]

Inhaled opelconazole appears to be safe and well tolerated, even by those with mild reactive airway diseases.[40] It is currently being investigated in a phase 2 study for prophylaxis against aspergillosis in lung transplant recipients.[41] Although treatment studies are not yet on the horizon, data from an animal study and case report have demonstrated that the addition of opelconazole to systemic azoles resulted in synergy with the successful treatment of refractory pulmonary and tracheobronchial aspergillosis,[42,43] highlighting a potential indication for future investigation.

Oteseconazole

Oteseconazole is a tetrazole antifungal that is highly specific for the fungal cytochrome P450 51 (CYP51, lanosterol 14-α-demethylase). This high specificity results in 2 unique characteristics: oteseconazole is associated with considerably less toxicity and drug–drug interactions that arise from inhibition of human CYP enzymes (a phenomenon often encountered with other azoles and of special relevance to transplant patients on tacrolimus) and has an extraordinarily long half-life (138 days), a consequence of minimal metabolism by human CYP enzymes.[44] Oteseconazole has broad activity against yeasts, dermatophytes, some mucorales, and some dimorphic fungi.[44] It has an oral route of administration.

Because of concern about teratogenicity in animal studies and in light of the long half-life, oteseconazole is contraindicated for use in women of childbearing potential.[45] Oteseconazole was approved by the Food and Drug Administration (FDA) in July 2022 for the treatment of recurrent vulvovaginal candidiasis in women who are not of childbearing potential. It is unclear what, if any, role this agent will play in the prevention or management of fungal infections in the setting of transplantation. Although the long-half life and dearth of drug–drug interactions are attractive, the lack of activity against most clinically relevant molds and restriction of use to men and women who are postmenopausal and/or without childbearing potential temper enthusiasm for its utility in most patients. It may well become a valuable option in the treatment of recurrent yeast and dermatophyte infections in select patient populations.

Rezafungin

The available echinocandins (micafungin, caspofungin, and anidulafungin) are important agents for the management of invasive candidiasis, particularly infections caused by fluconazole-resistant *Candida* species such as *C glabrata* and *C auris*.[46] Echinocandins are not associated with electrocardiographic QT interval prolongation, drug–drug interactions, hepatotoxicity that limit azoles, or nephrotoxicity of AMB, making them favored options in transplant recipients.[47,48] However, their use has been limited by the need for daily intravenous administration, stemming from poor bioavailability and their pharmacokinetics.

Rezafungin is a new echinocandin that retains similar activity to others in the class; however, its prolonged half-life permits once-weekly dosing, which could facilitate outpatient treatment without the need for central venous access. In addition to convenience, once-weekly dosing enables a high upfront maximum serum concentration that may achieve earlier sterilization of blood and deep-seated infections, potentially reducing the risk of resistance that can develop during prolonged therapy.[49,50] In neutropenic mouse models, rezafungin showed potent activity against *C albicans* and *A fumigatus*,[51] with subsequent in vitro studies showing additional activity against wild-type *C glabrata*, *Cryptococcus tropicalis*, *Cryptococcus krusei*, *Cryptococcus parapsilosis*, *A niger*, *A flavus*, and *A terreus*.[52–54] In vitro and in vivo animal studies have also shown activity against the multidrug-resistant *C auris*.[55–58]

In phase 2 and 3 trials of candidemia and invasive candidiasis, weekly rezafungin was non-inferior to daily caspofungin, followed by an oral step down in all-cause mortality, serious adverse reactions, and blood culture clearance.[59,60] Although *C albicans* was the most frequent cause of infection, about 50% were other non-*albicans* species, with *C glabrata* and *C parapsilosis* accounting for almost 35% combined.

Rezafungin is also being evaluated for prophylaxis against invasive fungal infections and PCP. An ongoing phase 3 trial (ReSPECT) is comparing the use of rezafungin to the combination of fluconazole and trimethoprim–sulfamethoxazole for the prevention of invasive fungal and *Pneumocystis jirovecii* infections in recipients of allogeneic stem cell transplants.[60] These data could provide insights for future studies and similar uses in SOT recipients.

Encochleated Amphotericin B

Amphotericin B is an antifungal with a broad spectrum of activity that includes most fungal pathogens, and even after 60 years, it remains foundational in the management of severe, life-threatening fungal infections. However, bioavailability is poor (<5%) necessitating intravenous administration,[61] and prolonged use is limited by significant adverse reactions, including nephrotoxicity, infusion reactions, and electrolyte abnormalities.

A new oral formulation of AMB is in development and being studied for the management of invasive candidiasis, cryptococcosis, and aspergillosis. The drug is trapped within a cochleate—a spiral sheet of a lipid bilayer and calcium ions—that protects the drug from gastric degradation and permits the uptake and concentration of AMB within phagocytes, which maintains a low serum concentration to reduce toxicities (especially nephrotoxicity).[62] Animal studies of cryptococcal meningoencephalitis, systemic candidiasis, and invasive aspergillosis found that encochleated AMB (cAMB) achieved adequate tissue concentrations (including within the central nervous system) and effectively decreased fungal burden.[63–65] A phase 1 trial showed that cAMB is safe and well tolerated in humans with few instances of electrolyte abnormalities and renal dysfunction,[62] and in a subsequent study, subjects safely tolerated it for up to 8 weeks.[66]

Although early clinical data for the use of cAMB in severe or refractory mucocutaneous candidiasis are conflicting,[66,67] a phase 2 randomized trial comparing cAMB to intravenous AMB as part of a flucytosine-containing treatment regimen in the initial treatment of HIV-associated cryptococcal meningitis showed favorable results. The investigators reported 30 day survival of 97.5% (39/40) in the cAMB arm and 18 week survival of 90% (36/40), comparable to the control arm (87% [26/30]). The cerebrospinal fluid (CSF) early fungicidal activity and CSF sterility at 2 weeks, 2 validated outcomes in cryptococcal meningitis trials, were comparable in both study arms. Fewer grade 3 or higher laboratory adverse effects (like anemia and hypokalemia) were observed in the cAMB arm.[68] Phase 3 trials are keenly anticipated.

If further clinical trials can confirm the efficacy of cAMB in cryptococcosis and other invasive fungal infections, the addition to the armamentarium of an oral drug with the antifungal properties of AMB will be welcomed. We expect that cAMB may play a pivotal role in the management of cryptococcosis, endemic mycoses, and some mold infections in transplant recipients.

FIRST-IN-CLASS DRUGS
Ibrexafungerp

Ibrexafungerp is a novel, first-in-class triterpenoid glucan synthase inhibitor that is a derivative of the naturally occurring echinocandin, emfumafungin.[69,70] Though structurally and mechanistically similar to conventional echinocandins, the bioavailability of ibrexafungerp is such that oral administration is feasible. Ibrexafungerp has few drug–drug interactions and has no effect on the pharmacokinetics of drugs metabolized by cytochrome P450 2C8[71] or 3A4[72] (which includes tacrolimus).

With potent activity against most *Candida* species, ibrexafungerp is a promising candidate drug for the prevention and treatment of invasive candidiasis, especially in species that are azole-resistant or echinocandin-resistant.[73–79] Importantly, ibrexafungerp has excellent activity against *C auris*,[80–86] and has anti-biofilm activity similar to that of micafungin.[87]

Ibrexafungerp has good activity against azole-sensitive and azole-resistant *Aspergillus* species, similar to that of the other echinocandins[73,88–90]; in vitro and in vivo, ibrexafungerp can be synergistic with voriconazole, isavuconazole, or AMB.[89,91] For non-*Aspergillus* molds, ibrexafungerp showed no activity against Mucorales, *Scopulariopsis*, or *Fusarium* but demonstrated high activity against *Paecilomyces variotii* and *Lomentospora prolificans* (against which no echinocandin, azole, or AMB had comparable activity).[92]

Ibrexafungerp has now been approved by the FDA for the treatment of vulvovaginal candidiasis. Beyond this indication, ibrexafungerp will likely be an important option for difficult-to-treat yeasts and may have a role in preventing and treating mold infections. There are several ongoing studies evaluating ibrexafungerp for treating invasive candidiasis and aspergillosis. Phase 2 study data found that ibrexafungerp was comparable in safety and efficacy to the standard of care for non-neutropenic patients with candidemia or invasive candidiasis.[93] Two subsequent phase 3 trials for the treatment of invasive candidiasis, MARIO and CARES (the latter specifically studying *C auris* infections), are ongoing.[94,95] Interim analysis of CARES trial data demonstrated that 89% of patients with *C auris* infections (candidemia, urinary tract infections, or intra-abdominal infections) had stable disease or response whereas on ibrexafungerp.[96]

For *Aspergillus*, the phase 2 SCYNERGIA trial is evaluating the combination of ibrexafungerp and voriconazole to voriconazole monotherapy for the treatment of invasive pulmonary aspergillosis.[97] The phase 3 FURI trial is also in process and is evaluating ibrexafungerp for the management of non-CNS mycoses refractory to standard of care.[98] This trial includes patients with a wide range of diagnoses, including invasive and mucocutaneous candidiasis, invasive and allergic aspergillosis, and dimorphic mycoses. Interim analyses of the data indicate that for invasive candidiasis, the 30 day survival following the start of ibrexafungerp was 94%, and 86% of patients had stable disease, partial response, or complete response[99]; in a small sample of patients with aspergillosis in this trial, 82% had stable disease, partial response, or complete response.[100]

Fosmanogepix

Manogepix has a unique mechanism of action compared with conventional antifungal agents. Through inhibition of the protein, Gwt1, manogepix impedes the fungal glycosylphosphatidyl-inositol anchor synthesis pathway, which is a critical process for the production of cell wall mannoproteins. As a result, the fungal cell is affected by cell wall fragility, reduced germ tube and hyphal formation, endoplasmic reticulum stress, and decreased potential for biofilm formation.[101] The prodrug of manogepix, fosmanogepix, has greater than 90% bioavailability,[102] which makes this an attractive option for outpatient management of challenging fungal infections.

Fosmanogepix has the broadest in vitro spectrum of activity of the novel antifungals (**Table 2**). It has activity against many yeasts, molds, and dimorphic fungi. Fosmanogepix has excellent activity against most *Candida* species, including the azole-resistant strains and *C auris*; *C krusei* is a notable exception. Although mechanisms of resistance have been identified,[103] its barrier to resistance against *Candida* is high in vitro, which makes fosmanogepix a viable option for prolonged management of high inoculum infections (such as endocarditis or intra-abdominal abscesses).[104] Fosmanogepix has in vitro activity against *Cryptococcus neoformans* and *Cryptococcus gattii*.[105] Against molds, fosmanogepix had low minimal inhibitory concentrations (MICs) for most *Aspergillus* species and other difficult-to-treat molds, such as *Fusarium*, *Scedosporium*, and *Lomentospora*.[106–108] The MICs were generally higher for Mucorales fungi.[109]

In animal studies, fosmanogepix shows similarly promising results. Studies show favorable outcomes for the management of *C auris* infections,[110] including *Candida* endophthalmitis and meningoencephalitis,[111] cryptococcal meningitis,[112] pulmonary scedosporiosis,[113] disseminated fusariosis,[113] and pulmonary mucormycosis.[114] Fosmanogepix was synergistic with liposomal AMB in improving survival in animals with aspergillosis, mucormycosis, and fusariosis.[115]

Fosmanogepix has been evaluated in 3 human studies. The first was a single-arm, phase 2 trial of 20 non-neutropenic participants with candidemia, 80% of whom attained treatment success with a mean time for blood culture clearance of 2.4 days.[116] A second phase 2 trial, the APEX trial, evaluated the efficacy of fosmanogepix in managing invasive candidiasis or candidemia with *C auris*.[117] Though the study was terminated early in 2020 because of the ongoing COVID-19 pandemic, no data have been published to date. A third phase 2 trial, the AEGIS trial, investigated the efficacy of fosmanogepix for the management of aspergillosis and other rare mold infections, with the primary outcome being 6 week all-cause mortality. This study completed enrollment in early 2022, and results are pending.[118] A phase 3 study comparing fosmanogepix versus caspofungin followed by fluconazole for the management of candidemia and invasive candidiasis is underway.[119]

Olorofim

Olorofim is an orotomide antifungal that inhibits dihydroorotate dehydrogenase (DHODH), thereby impairing the fungal pyrimidine biosynthesis pathway,[120] and ultimately leading to cell lysis. Olorofim has a unique spectrum of activity owing to phylogenetic and structural differences of DHODH across species; it has excellent in vitro activity against many clinically relevant molds and dimorphic fungi, including

Table 2
Novel antifungals

Drug	Pharmacology	Spectrum of Activity						Phase of Development and Anticipated Indications	Notes
		Candida	Cryptococcus	Aspergillus	Mucorales	Dimorphic Fungi[a]	Others		
Oteseconazole	Class: tetrazole MOA: Inhibition of lanosterol 14-α-demethylase ROA: oral	+	+	-	+ (variable activity against *Rhizopus*)	+	*Trichophyton*	FDA-approved for r/r VVC in women without childbearing potential Anticipated use: treatment of r/r VVC, r/r dermatophytosis	Extremely long half-life (138 d) Once-weekly dosing Teratogenic in animal studies; absolutely contraindicated in women with reproductive potential
Opelconazole	Class: triazole MOA: Inhibition of lanosterol 14-α-demethylase ROA: inhaled	+	+	+	- (some activity against *Rhizopus*)	ND		Phase 2 trials Anticipated use: Prophylaxis of IPA	Limited systemic absorption
Rezafungin	Class: echinocandin MOA: Inhibition of β-D-glucan synthase ROA: intravenous	+ (variable against C *parapsilosis*)	-	+	-	ND	*Fusarium Pneumocystis*	Phase 3 trials Anticipated use: IC (including *C auris*)	Once-weekly dosing
Encochleated amphotericin B	Class: polyene MOA: Binding of ergosterol and formation of pores within the cell membrane ROA: oral	+	+	+	+	+		Phase 2 trials Anticipated use: Induction therapy for cryptococcosis and endemic mycosis, r/r mold infections	Minimal nephrotoxicity

Drug	Characteristics						Notable species	Clinical status	Additional features
Ibrexafungerp	Class: triterpenoid MOA: Inhibition of β-D-glucan synthase ROA: oral	+	ND	+	-	+	L prolificans P variotii Pneumocystis	FDA-approved for r/r VVC, phase 3 trials Anticipated use: Oral step down for IC (including C auris)	Active against most echinocandin-resistant Candida Anti-biofilm
Fosmanogepix	Class: GPI inhibitor MOA: Inhibition of Gwt1 ROA: oral, intravenous	+ (except C krusei)	+	+	+/-	+	Fusarium L prolificans Scedosporium Trichophyton	Phase 3 trials Anticipated use: r/r mold infections	High barrier to resistance Anti-biofilm
Olorofim	Class: orotomide MOA: Inhibition of DHODH ROA: oral, intravenous	-	+	-	+	+	F oxysporum L prolificans Scedosporium T marneffei Trichophyton	Phase 3 trials Anticipated use: r/r aspergillosis and mold infections	.

Abbreviations: DHODH, dihydroorotate dehydrogenase; FDA, Food and Drug Administration; GPI, glycophosphatidylinositol; Gwt1, glycosylphosphatidylinositol-anchored wall protein transfer 1; IC, invasive candidiasis; IPA, invasive pulmonary aspergillosis; MOA, mechanism of action; r/r, resistant or refractory; ROA, route of administration; VVC, vulvovaginal candidiasis.

[a] Includes Coccidioides, Histoplasma, and Blastomyces species.

Aspergillus spp.[121–130] (including azole-resistant strains and the AMB-resistant *A terreus*), *Scedosporium* spp.,[128,129,131–134] *Lomentospora prolificans*,[129,131–135] dimorphic fungi,[136–139] and some *Fusarium* spp.[122,128,140] Notably, olorofim does not have any activity against fungi in the order Mucorales[122,128] or yeasts (particularly *Candida* and *Cryptococcus*) and exhibits no activity against human DHODH.[120] Olorofim is highly bioavailable, facilitating oral administration, and has a large volume of distribution, being able to attain high concentrations within the lungs, kidneys, and plasma.[120,141]

The phase 2 trial, FORMULA-OLS, specifically studied the efficacy of olorofim for patients with invasive mold infections who lacked suitable alternative therapy options.[142] The primary infections included those caused by *Aspergillus* spp., *Lomentospora prolificans*, and *Scedosporium* spp. A phase 3 trial comparing olorofim versus liposomal AMB followed by standard of care for proven/probable invasive aspergillosis (OASIS) is underway.[143]

CONCLUSION AND FUTURE DIRECTIONS

Fungal infections are notoriously difficult to diagnose and manage, particularly in immunocompromised hosts like transplant recipients. Consequently, recent and ongoing advances in the development of new diagnostics and therapeutics are sorely welcomed.

Advances in medical mycology and molecular diagnostics have permitted the detection of fungal antigens, nucleic acids, and biomarkers by noninvasive methods. Supplementing these genomic and proteomic assays, noninvasive metabolomic studies are being developed that could permit the diagnosis and prognostication of invasive fungal infections.[144] A notable example is the profiling of volatile metabolites produced by *Aspergillus* species in exhaled breath, which may permit the early diagnosis of pulmonary aspergillosis.[145,146] This strategy could provide a means for surveillance for invasive pulmonary infections—especially in lung transplant recipients—that would obviate bronchoscopic diagnosis and could substitute widespread prophylactic antifungal use with a noninvasive preemptive approach.

After several decades of a trickling pipeline, the last few years have seen a welcomed surge of clinical studies investigating novel antifungals. Though research into expanding the antifungal armamentarium is essential, it cannot happen in isolation. Improving antifungal stewardship in medicine and agriculture, individualizing prophylaxis and monitoring for immunocompromised patients, and minimizing immunosuppression whenever possible are just several necessary strategies to help mitigate the risk of losing the agents to antifungal resistance.

Finally, the development of better tests and treatments is just the first step in improving outcomes for our patients. As we learn how to best implement these fungal diagnostics and antifungal therapies, we must advocate for these advances to be widely and equitably accessible.

CLINICS CARE POINTS

- Pathogen-directed PCR assays provide more sensitive means of detecting important fungal pathogens. Notably, PCR for Pneumocystis should be performed on BAL samples when possible instead of convential staining or immunofluorescence in high risk patients to decrease the false negative rate.

- Though most newer antifungals are not yet FDA-approved, enrolment into ongoing trials and applying for compassionate use are current options for treating difficult refractory or resistant fungal infections in transplant patients.

DISCLOSURE

The authors have no conflicts to disclose.

REFERENCES

1. Friedman DZP, Schwartz IS. Emerging Fungal Infections: New Patients, New Patterns, and New Pathogens. J Fungi 2019;5(3):67.
2. Terrero-Salcedo D, Powers-Fletcher MV. Updates in Laboratory Diagnostics for Invasive Fungal Infections. J Clin Microbiol 2020;58(6):014877.
3. Schwartz IS, Patterson TF. The emerging threat of antifungal resistance in transplant infectious diseases. Curr Infect Dis Rep 2018;20(3):2.
4. Hoenigl M, Sprute R, Egger M, et al. The Antifungal Pipeline: Fosmanogepix, Ibrexafungerp, Olorofim, Opelconazole, and Rezafungin. Drugs 2021;81(15): 1703–29.
5. Zhang S.X., Babady N.E., Hanson K.E., et al., Recognition of Diagnostic Gaps for Laboratory Diagnosis of Fungal Diseases: Expert Opinion from the Fungal Diagnostics Laboratories Consortium (FDLC). Kraft CS, ed, J Clin Microbiol, 59(7), 2021, e01784-20.
6. Azar MM, Turbett S, Gaston D, et al. A consensus conference to define the utility of advanced infectious disease diagnostics in solid organ transplant recipients. Am J Transplant 2022;22(12):3150–69.
7. Thompson GR, Boulware DR, Bahr NC, et al. Non-invasive Testing and Surrogate Markers in Invasive Fungal Diseases. Open Forum Infect Dis 2022;9(6): ofac112.
8. Del Corpo O, Butler-Laporte G, Sheppard DC, et al. Diagnostic accuracy of serum (1-3)-β-D-glucan for *Pneumocystis jirovecii* pneumonia: a systematic review and meta-analysis. Clin Microbiol Infect 2020;26(9):1137–43.
9. White SK, Schmidt RL, Walker BS, et al. (1→3)-β-D-glucan testing for the detection of invasive fungal infections in immunocompromised or critically ill people. Cochrane Database Syst Rev 2020;7(7):cd009833.
10. Lamoth F, Akan H, Andes D, et al. Assessment of the Role of 1,3-β-d-Glucan Testing for the Diagnosis of Invasive Fungal Infections in Adults. Clin Infect Dis 2021;72(Suppl 2):S102–8.
11. Van Burik JA, Myerson D, Schreckhise RW, et al. Panfungal PCR assay for detection of fungal infection in human blood specimens. J Clin Microbiol 1998;36(5):1169–75.
12. Kidd SE, Chen SCA, Meyer W, et al. A New Age in Molecular Diagnostics for Invasive Fungal Disease: Are We Ready? Front Microbiol 2019;10:2903.
13. Alanio A, Desoubeaux G, Sarfati C, et al. Real-time PCR assay-based strategy for differentiation between active *Pneumocystis jirovecii* pneumonia and colonization in immunocompromised patients. Clin Microbiol Infect 2011;17(10): 1531–7.
14. Senécal J, Smyth E, Del Corpo O, et al. Non-invasive diagnosis of *Pneumocystis jirovecii* pneumonia: a systematic review and meta-analysis. Clin Microbiol Infect 2022;28(1):23–30.
15. White PL. Recent advances and novel approaches in laboratory-based diagnostic mycology. Med Mycol 2019;57(Supplement_3):S259–66.
16. White PL, Bretagne S, Caliendo AM, et al. *Aspergillus* Polymerase Chain Reaction- An Update on Technical Recommendations, Clinical Applications, and Justification for Inclusion in the Second Revision of the EORTC/MSGERC Definitions of Invasive Fungal Disease. Clin Infect Dis 2021;72(Suppl 2):S95–101.

17. Chong GLM, Sande WWJ van de, Dingemans GJH, et al. Validation of a New *Aspergillus* Real-Time PCR Assay for Direct Detection of *Aspergillus* and Azole Resistance of *Aspergillus fumigatus* on Bronchoalveolar Lavage Fluid. J Clin Microbiol 2015;53(3):868–74.

18. Chong GM, van der Beek MT, von dem Borne PA, et al. PCR-based detection of *Aspergillus fumigatus Cyp51A* mutations on bronchoalveolar lavage: a multicentre validation of the AsperGenius assay ® in 201 patients with haematological disease suspected for invasive aspergillosis. J Antimicrob Chemother 2016; 71(12):3528–35.

19. White PL, Barnes RA, Springer J, et al. Clinical Performance of *Aspergillus* PCR for Testing Serum and Plasma: a Study by the European *Aspergillus* PCR Initiative. Warnock DW. J Clin Microbiol 2015;53(9):2832–7.

20. White PL, Posso RB, Barnes RA. Analytical and Clinical Evaluation of the Patho-Nostics AsperGenius Assay for Detection of Invasive Aspergillosis and Resistance to Azole Antifungal Drugs during Testing of Serum Samples. J Clin Microbiol 2015;53(7):2115–21.

21. Dannaoui E, Gabriel F, Gaboyard M, et al. Molecular Diagnosis of Invasive Aspergillosis and Detection of Azole Resistance by a Newly Commercialized PCR Kit. J Clin Microbiol 2017;55(11):3210–8.

22. Guegan H, Robert-Gangneux F, Camus C, et al. Improving the diagnosis of invasive aspergillosis by the detection of *Aspergillus* in broncho-alveolar lavage fluid: Comparison of non-culture-based assays. J Infect 2018;76(2):196–205.

23. Etienne KA, Berkow EL, Gade L, et al. Genomic Diversity of Azole-Resistant *Aspergillus fumigatus* in the United States. mBio 2021;12(4):e01803–21.

24. Huygens S, Dunbar A, Buil JB, et al. Clinical impact of PCR-based Aspergillus and azole resistance detection in invasive aspergillosis. A prospective multicenter study. Clin Infect Dis 2023. https://doi.org/10.1093/cid/ciad141.

25. Cruciani M, Mengoli C, Barnes R, et al. Polymerase chain reaction blood tests for the diagnosis of invasive aspergillosis in immunocompromised people. Cochrane Database Syst Rev 2019;9(9):Cd009551.

26. Scherer E, Iriart X, Bellanger AP, et al. Quantitative PCR (qPCR) Detection of Mucorales DNA in Bronchoalveolar Lavage Fluid To Diagnose Pulmonary Mucormycosis. J Clin Microbiol 2018;56(8):002899.

27. Millon L, Caillot D, Berceanu A, et al. Evaluation of Serum Mucorales Polymerase Chain Reaction (PCR) for the Diagnosis of Mucormycoses: The MODIMUCOR Prospective Trial. Clin Infect Dis 2022;75(5):777–85.

28. Dannaoui E. Recent Developments in the Diagnosis of Mucormycosis. J Fungi 2022;8(5):457.

29. Rocchi S, Scherer E, Mengoli C, et al. Interlaboratory evaluation of Mucorales PCR assays for testing serum specimens: A study by the fungal PCR Initiative and the Modimucor study group. Med Mycol 2021;59(2):126–38.

30. Guegan H, Iriart X, Bougnoux ME, et al. Evaluation of MucorGenius® mucorales PCR assay for the diagnosis of pulmonary mucormycosis. J Infect 2020;81(2): 311–7.

31. Hebart H, Löffler J, Reitze H, et al. Prospective screening by a panfungal polymerase chain reaction assay in patients at risk for fungal infections: implications for the management of febrile neutropenia. Br J Haematol 2000;111(2):635–40.

32. Mercier T, Reynders M, Beuselinck K, et al. Serial Detection of Circulating Mucorales DNA in Invasive Mucormycosis: A Retrospective Multicenter Evaluation. J Fungi 2019;5(4):113.

33. Smith CB, Shi X, Liesman RM, et al. Evaluation of the Diagnostic Accuracy and Clinical Utility of Fungal Profile Plus Polymerase Chain Reaction Assay in Pulmonary Infections. Open Forum Infect Dis 2022;9(12):ofac646.
34. Blauwkamp TA, Thair S, Rosen MJ, et al. Analytical and clinical validation of a microbial cell-free DNA sequencing test for infectious disease. Nat Microbiol 2019;4(4):663–74.
35. Hill JA, Dalai SC, Hong DK, et al. Liquid Biopsy for Invasive Mold Infections in Hematopoietic Cell Transplant Recipients With Pneumonia Through Next-Generation Sequencing of Microbial Cell-Free DNA in Plasma. Clin Infect Dis 2020;73(11):e3876–83.
36. Moreno A, Epstein D, Budvytiene I, et al. Accuracy of *Pneumocystis jirovecii* Plasma Cell-Free DNA PCR for Noninvasive Diagnosis of *Pneumocystis* Pneumonia. J Clin Microbiol 2022;60(5):e0010122.
37. O'Grady J. A powerful, non-invasive test to rule out infection. Nat Microbiol 2019;4(4):554–5.
38. Colley T, Alanio A, Kelly SL, et al. *In Vitro* and *In Vivo* Antifungal Profile of a Novel and Long-Acting Inhaled Azole, PC945, on *Aspergillus fumigatus* Infection. Antimicrob Agents Chemother 2017;61(5):022800.
39. Kimura G, Nakaoki T, Colley T, et al. *In Vivo* Biomarker Analysis of the Effects of Intranasally Dosed PC945, a Novel Antifungal Triazole, on *Aspergillus fumigatus* Infection in Immunocompromised Mice. Antimicrob Agents Chemother 2017; 61(9):001244.
40. Cass L, Murray A, Davis A, et al. Safety and nonclinical and clinical pharmacokinetics of PC945, a novel inhaled triazole antifungal agent. Pharmacol Res Perspect 2021;9(1):e00690.
41. National Library of Medicine (U.S. A Randomized Controlled Open-label Study to Assess the Safety and Tolerability of Nebulized PC945 for Prophylaxis or Preemptive Therapy Against Pulmonary Aspergillosis in Lung Transplant Recipients. ClinicalTrials.gov 2022. Available at: https://clinicaltrials.gov/ct2/show/NCT 05037851. Accessed November 29, 2022.
42. Colley T, Sehra G, Daly L, et al. Antifungal synergy of a topical triazole, PC945, with a systemic triazole against respiratory *Aspergillus fumigatus* infection. Sci Rep 2019;9(1):9482.
43. Pagani N, Armstrong-James D, Reed A. Successful salvage therapy for fungal bronchial anastomotic infection after -lung transplantation with an inhaled triazole anti-fungal PC945. J Heart Lung Transplant 2020;39(12):1505–6.
44. Hoenigl M, Sprute R, Arastehfar A, et al. Invasive candidiasis: investigational drugs in the clinical development pipeline and mechanisms of action. Expert Opin Investig Drugs 2022;31(8):795–812.
45. Sobel JD. New Antifungals for Vulvovaginal Candidiasis: What Is Their Role? Clin Infect Dis 2023;76(5):783–5.
46. Centers for Disease Control and Prevention. Treatment and Management of Infections and Colonization. Candida auris 2021. Available at: https://www.cdc.gov/fungal/candida-auris/c-auris-treatment.html. Accessed December 10, 2022.
47. Winston DJ, Limaye AP, Pelletier S, et al. Randomized, Double-Blind Trial of Anidulafungin Versus Fluconazole for Prophylaxis of Invasive Fungal Infections in High-Risk Liver Transplant Recipients: Antifungal Prophylaxis in Liver Transplants. Am J Transplant 2014;14(12):2758–64.
48. Saliba F, Pascher A, Cointault O, et al. Randomized Trial of Micafungin for the Prevention of Invasive Fungal Infection in High-Risk Liver Transplant Recipients. Clin Infect Dis 2015;60(7):997–1006.

49. Locke JB, Almaguer AL, Zuill DE, et al. Characterization of *In Vitro* Resistance Development to the Novel Echinocandin CD101 in *Candida* Species. Antimicrob Agents Chemother 2016;60(10):6100–7.

50. Bader JC, Lakota EA, Flanagan S, et al. Overcoming the Resistance Hurdle: Pharmacokinetic-Pharmacodynamic Target Attainment Analyses for Rezafungin (CD101) against *Candida albicans* and *Candida glabrata*. Antimicrob Agents Chemother 2018;62(6):e02614–7.

51. Ong V, Hough G, Schlosser M, et al. Preclinical Evaluation of the Stability, Safety, and Efficacy of CD101, a Novel Echinocandin. Antimicrob Agents Chemother 2016;60(11):6872–9.

52. Pfaller MA, Messer SA, Rhomberg PR, et al. Activity of a long-acting echinocandin, CD101, determined using CLSI and EUCAST reference methods, against *Candida* and *Aspergillus* spp., including echinocandin- and azole-resistant isolates. J Antimicrob Chemother 2016;71(10):2868–73.

53. Pfaller MA, Messer SA, Rhomberg PR, et al. Activity of a Long-Acting Echinocandin (CD101) and Seven Comparator Antifungal Agents Tested against a Global Collection of Contemporary Invasive Fungal Isolates in the SENTRY 2014 Antifungal Surveillance Program. Antimicrob Agents Chemother 2017; 61(3):020455.

54. Arendrup MC, Meletiadis J, Zaragoza O, et al. Multicentre determination of rezafungin (CD101) susceptibility of Candida species by the EUCAST method. Clin Microbiol Infect 2018;24(11):1200–4.

55. Berkow EL, Lockhart SR. Activity of CD101, a long-acting echinocandin, against clinical isolates of *Candida auris*. Diagn Microbiol Infect Dis 2018;90(3):196–7.

56. Hager CL, Larkin EL, Long LA, et al. Evaluation of the efficacy of rezafungin, a novel echinocandin, in the treatment of disseminated *Candida auris* infection using an immunocompromised mouse model. J Antimicrob Chemother 2018; 73(8):2085–8.

57. Lepak AJ, Zhao M, Andes DR. Pharmacodynamic Evaluation of Rezafungin (CD101) against *Candida auris* in the Neutropenic Mouse Invasive Candidiasis Model. Antimicrob Agents Chemother 2018;62(11):015722.

58. Helleberg M, Jorgensen KM, Hare RK, et al. Rezafungin *In Vitro* Activity against Contemporary Nordic Clinical *Candida* Isolates and *Candida auris* Determined by the EUCAST Reference Method. Antimicrob Agents Chemother 2020;64(4): 024388.

59. Thompson GR, Soriano A, Skoutelis A, et al. Rezafungin Versus Caspofungin in a Phase 2, Randomized, Double-blind Study for the Treatment of Candidemia and Invasive Candidiasis: The STRIVE Trial. Clin Infect Dis 2021;73(11):e3647–55.

60. National Library of Medicine (U.S. Study of Rezafungin Compared to Standard Antimicrobial Regimen for Prevention of Invasive Fungal Diseases in Adults Undergoing Allogeneic Blood and Marrow Transplantation (ReSPECT). ClinicalTrials.gov 2022. Available at: https://clinicaltrials.gov/ct2/show/NCT04368559. Accessed December 4, 2022.

61. Halde C, Newcomer VD, Wright ET, et al. An Evaluation of Amphotericin B In Vitro and In Vivo in Mice Against *Coccidioides Immitis* and *Candida Albicans*, and Preliminary Observations Concerning the Administration of Amphotericin B to Man. J Invest Dermatol 1957;28(3):217–32.

62. Skipper CP, Atukunda M, Stadelman A, et al. Phase I EnACT Trial of the Safety and Tolerability of a Novel Oral Formulation of Amphotericin B. Antimicrob Agents Chemother 2020;64(10):008388.

63. Lu R, Hollingsworth C, Qiu J, et al. Efficacy of Oral Encochleated Amphotericin B in a Mouse Model of Cryptococcal Meningoencephalitis. mBio 2019;10(3): 007244.

64. Gonzalez-Lara MF, Sifuentes-Osornio J, Ostrosky-Zeichner L. Drugs in Clinical Development for Fungal Infections. Drugs 2017;77(14):1505–18.

65. Delmas G, Park S, Chen ZW, et al. Efficacy of Orally Delivered Cochleates Containing Amphotericin B in a Murine Model of Aspergillosis. Antimicrob Agents Chemother 2002;46(8):2704–7.

66. Freeman A, Stratton P, Swaim D, et al. Oral encochleated amphotericin B (CAMB) in the treatment of chronic azole resistant mucocutaneous candidiasis. New Orleans, LA: Poster presented at: The American Society of Microbiology ASM Microbe; 2017. Available at: https://s3.amazonaws.com/content.stockpr. com/matinasbiopharma/files/pages/matinasbiopharma/db/274/description/NIH+ Poster+ASM+2017-30May2017.pdf. Accessed December 4, 2022.

67. National Library of Medicine (U.S. Safety and Efficacy of Oral Encochleated Amphotericin B (CAMB/MAT2203) in the Treatment of Vulvovaginal Candidiasis (VVC). ClinicalTrials.gov 2018. Available at: https://www.clinicaltrials.gov/ct2/ show/study/NCT02971007?term=NCT02971007. Accessed December 6, 2022.

68. Atukunda M, Kagimu E, Rutakingirwa MK, et al. Oral Encochleated Amphotericin B for Cryptococcal Meningitis: a Phase II Randomized Trial. Open Forum Infect Dis 2022;9(Suppl 2):S40, 869.

69. Hector RF, Bierer DE. New beta-glucan inhibitors as antifungal drugs. Expert Opin Ther Pat 2011;21(10):1597–610.

70. Peláez F, Cabello A, Platas G, et al. The Discovery of Enfumafungin, a Novel Antifungal Compound Produced by an Endophytic *Hormonema* Species Biological Activity and Taxonomy of the Producing Organisms. Syst Appl Microbiol 2000;23(3):333–43.

71. Wring S, Murphy G, Atiee G, et al. Lack of Impact by SCY-078, a First-in-Class Oral Fungicidal Glucan Synthase Inhibitor, on the Pharmacokinetics of Rosiglitazone, a Substrate for CYP450 2C8, Supports the Low Risk for Clinically Relevant Metabolic Drug-Drug Interactions. J Clin Pharmacol 2018;58(10):1305–13.

72. Wring S, Murphy G, Atiee G, et al. Clinical Pharmacokinetics and Drug-Drug Interaction Potential for Coadministered SCY-078, an Oral Fungicidal Glucan Synthase Inhibitor, and Tacrolimus. Clin Pharmacol Drug Dev 2019;8(1):60–9.

73. Jimenez-Ortigosa C, Paderu P, Motyl MR, et al. Enfumafungin derivative MK-3118 shows increased *in vitro* potency against clinical echinocandin-resistant *Candida* Species and *Aspergillus* species isolates. Antimicrob Agents Chemother 2014;58(2):1248–51.

74. Pfaller MA, Messer SA, Motyl MR, et al. Activity of MK-3118, a new oral glucan synthase inhibitor, tested against *Candida* spp. by two international methods (CLSI and EUCAST). J Antimicrob Chemother 2013;68(4):858–63.

75. Pfaller MA, Messer SA, Rhomberg PR, et al. Differential Activity of the Oral Glucan Synthase Inhibitor SCY-078 against Wild-Type and Echinocandin-Resistant Strains of Candida Species. Antimicrob Agents Chemother 2017; 61(8):001611.

76. Schell WA, Jones AM, Borroto-Esoda K, et al. Antifungal Activity of SCY-078 and Standard Antifungal Agents against 178 Clinical Isolates of Resistant and Susceptible *Candida* Species. Antimicrob Agents Chemother 2017;61(11). https:// doi.org/10.1128/AAC.01102-17.

77. Scorneaux B, Angulo D, Borroto-Esoda K, et al. SCY-078 Is Fungicidal against *Candida* Species in Time-Kill Studies. Antimicrob Agents Chemother 2017; 61(3):019611.

78. Wiederhold NP, Najvar LK, Jaramillo R, et al. Oral glucan synthase inhibitor SCY-078 is effective in an experimental murine model of invasive candidiasis caused by WT and echinocandin-resistant *Candida glabrata*. J Antimicrob Chemother 2018;73(2):448–51.

79. Nunnally NS, Etienne KA, Angulo D, et al. *In Vitro* Activity of Ibrexafungerp, a Novel Glucan Synthase Inhibitor against *Candida glabrata* Isolates with FKS Mutations. Antimicrob Agents Chemother 2019;63(11):016922.

80. Arendrup MC, Jorgensen KM, Hare RK, et al. *In Vitro* Activity of Ibrexafungerp (SCY-078) against Candida auris Isolates as Determined by EUCAST Methodology and Comparison with Activity against C. albicans and C. glabrata and with the Activities of Six Comparator Agents. Antimicrob Agents Chemother 2020; 64(3):021366.

81. Berkow EL, Angulo D, Lockhart SR. *In Vitro* Activity of a Novel Glucan Synthase Inhibitor, SCY-078, against Clinical Isolates of *Candida auris*. Antimicrob Agents Chemother 2017;61(7):004355.

82. Larkin E, Hager C, Chandra J, et al. The emerging pathogen *Candida auris*: Growth phenotype, virulence factors, activity of antifungals, and effect of SCY-078, a novel glucan synthesis inhibitor, on growth morphology and biofilm formation. Antimicrob Agents Chemother 2017;61(5):e02396.

83. Gamal A, Chu S, McCormick TS, et al. Ibrexafungerp, a Novel Oral Triterpenoid Antifungal in Development: Overview of Antifungal Activity Against *Candida glabrata*. Front Cell Infect Microbiol 2021;1:642358.

84. Zhu YC, Barat SA, Borroto-Esoda K, et al. Pan-resistant *Candida auris* isolates from the outbreak in New York are susceptible to ibrexafungerp (a glucan synthase inhibitor). Int J Antimicrob Agents 2020;55(4):105922.

85. Ghannoum M, Arendrup MC, Chaturvedi VP, et al. Ibrexafungerp: A Novel Oral Triterpenoid Antifungal in Development for the Treatment of *Candida auris* Infections. Antibiotics 2020;9(9):539.

86. Wiederhold NP, Najvar LK, Olivo M, et al. Ibrexafungerp Demonstrates *In Vitro* Activity against Fluconazole-Resistant *Candida auris* and *In Vivo* Efficacy with Delayed Initiation of Therapy in an Experimental Model of Invasive Candidiasis. Antimicrob Agents Chemother 2021;65(6):e02694.

87. Marcos-Zambrano LJ, Gomez-Perosanz M, Escribano P, et al. The novel oral glucan synthase inhibitor SCY-078 shows in vitro activity against sessile and planktonic *Candida* spp. J Antimicrob Chemother 2017;72(7):1969–76.

88. Pfaller MA, Messer SA, Motyl MR, et al. *In vitro* activity of a new oral glucan synthase inhibitor (MK-3118) tested against *Aspergillus* spp. by CLSI and EUCAST broth microdilution methods. Antimicrob Agents Chemother 2013;57(2):1065–8.

89. Ghannoum M, Long L, Larkin EL, et al. Evaluation of the Antifungal Activity of the Novel Oral Glucan Synthase Inhibitor SCY-078, Singly and in Combination, for the Treatment of Invasive Aspergillosis. Antimicrob Agents Chemother 2018; 62(6):e02444.

90. Rivero-Menendez O, Soto-Debran JC, Cuenca-Estrella M, et al. *In Vitro* Activity of Ibrexafungerp against a Collection of Clinical Isolates of *Aspergillus*, Including Cryptic Species and Cyp51A Mutants, Using EUCAST and CLSI Methodologies. J Fungi 2021;7(3):232.

91. Petraitis V, Petraitiene R, Katragkou A, et al. Combination Therapy with Ibrexafungerp (Formerly SCY-078), a First-in-Class Triterpenoid Inhibitor of (1->3)-beta-d-

Glucan Synthesis, and Isavuconazole for Treatment of Experimental Invasive Pulmonary Aspergillosis. Antimicrob Agents Chemother 2020;64(6):e02429.

92. Lamoth F, Alexander BD. Antifungal activities of SCY-078 (MK-3118) and standard antifungal agents against clinical non-Aspergillus mold isolates. Antimicrob Agents Chemother 2015;59(7):4308–11.

93. Spec A, Pullman J, Thompson GR, et al. MSG-10: a Phase 2 study of oral ibrexafungerp (SCY-078) following initial echinocandin therapy in non-neutropenic patients with invasive candidiasis. J Antimicrob Chemother 2019;74(10):3056–62.

94. National Library of Medicine (U.S. A Phase 3, Multicenter, Prospective, Randomized, Double-blind Study of Two Treatment Regimens for Candidemia and/or Invasive Candidiasis: Intravenous Echinocandin Followed by Oral Ibrexafungerp Versus Intravenous Echinocandin Followed by Oral Fluconazole (MARIO). ClinicalTrials.gov 2022. Available at: https://clinicaltrials.gov/ct2/show/study/NCT05178862. Accessed December 8, 2022.

95. National Library of Medicine (U.S. Open-Label Study to Evaluate the Efficacy, Safety, Tolerability and Pharmacokinetics of Oral Ibrexafungerp (SCY-078) as an Emergency Use Treatment for Patients With Candidiasis, Including Candidemia, Caused by *Candida Auris*. ClinicalTrials.gov 2021. Available at: https://clinicaltrials.gov/ct2/show/study/NCT03363841. Accessed December 8, 2022.

96. Azie N, King T, Chen T, et al. Outcomes of oral ibrexafungerp in the treatment of 18 patients with Candida auris infections, from the CARES study. Albuquerque, New Mexico, USA: Poster presented at: Mycoses Study Group Education & Research Consortium Biennial Meeting; 2022.

97. National Library of Medicine (U.S. A Multicenter, Randomized, Double-Blind Study to Evaluate the Safety and Efficacy of the Coadministration of SCY-078 With Voriconazole in Patients With Invasive Pulmonary Aspergillosis. ClinicalTrials.gov 2022. Available at: https://clinicaltrials.gov/ct2/show/NCT03672292. Accessed December 8, 2022.

98. National Library of Medicine (U.S. Open-Label Study to Evaluate the Efficacy and Safety of SCY-078 (Ibrexafungerp) in Patients With Fungal Diseases That Are Refractory to or Intolerant of Standard Antifungal Treatment (FURI). ClinicalTrials.gov 2022. Available at: https://clinicaltrials.gov/ct2/show/study/NCT03059992. Accessed December 11, 2022.

99. Prattes J, King T, Azie N, et al. All-cause mortality in patients with invasive candidiasis or candidemia from an interim analysis of a phase 3 ibrexafungerp open-label study (FURI). Washington, DC, USA: Poster presented at: Infectious Disease Society of America IDWeek 2022; 2022.

100. Prattes J, King T, Azie N, et al. Oral ibrexafungerp outcomes by fungal disease in patients from an interim analysis of a phase 3 open-label study (FURI). New Delhi, India: Poster presented at: 21st Congress of the International Society of Human and Animal Mycology; 2022.

101. Lima SL, Colombo AL, de Almeida Junior JN. Fungal Cell Wall: Emerging Antifungals and Drug Resistance. Front Microbiol 2019;10(2573):1–9.

102. Hodges MR, Ople E, Shaw KJ, et al. Phase 1 Study to Assess Safety, Tolerability and Pharmacokinetics of Single and Multiple Oral Doses of APX001 and to Investigate the Effect of Food on APX001A Bioavailability. Open Forum Infect Dis 2017;4(S1):S534.

103. Liston SD, Whitesell L, Kapoor M, et al. Enhanced Efflux Pump Expression in *Candida* Mutants Results in Decreased Manogepix Susceptibility. Antimicrob Agents Chemother 2020;64(5):e00261.

104. Kapoor M, Moloney M, Soltow QA, et al. Evaluation of Resistance Development to the Gwt1 Inhibitor Manogepix (APX001A) in *Candida* Species. Antimicrob Agents Chemother 2019;64(1):e01387–419.

105. Trzoss M, Covel JA, Kapoor M, et al. Synthesis of analogs of the Gwt1 inhibitor manogepix (APX001A) and *in vitro* evaluation against *Cryptococcus* spp. Bioorg Med Chem Lett 2019;29(23):126713.

106. Shaheen SK, Juvvadi PR, Allen J, et al. *In Vitro* Activity of APX2041, a New Gwt1 Inhibitor, and *In Vivo* Efficacy of the Prodrug APX2104 against *Aspergillus fumigatus*. Antimicrob Agents Chemother 2021;65(10):e0068221.

107. Miyazaki M, Horii T, Hata K, et al. In Vitro Activity of E1210, a Novel Antifungal, against Clinically Important Yeasts and Molds. Antimicrob Agents Chemother 2011;55(10):4652–8.

108. Pfaller MA, Huband MD, Flamm RK, et al. *In Vitro* Activity of APX001A (Manogepix) and Comparator Agents against 1,706 Fungal Isolates Collected during an International Surveillance Program in 2017. Antimicrob Agents Chemother 2019; 63(8):e00840.

109. Rivero-Menendez O, Cuenca-Estrella M, Alastruey-Izquierdo A. *In vitro* activity of APX001A against rare moulds using EUCAST and CLSI methodologies. J Antimicrob Chemother 2019;74(5):1295–9.

110. Wiederhold NP, Najvar LK, Shaw KJ, et al. Efficacy of Delayed Therapy with Fosmanogepix (APX001) in a Murine Model of *Candida auris* Invasive Candidiasis. Antimicrob Agents Chemother 2019;63(11):e01120.

111. Petraitiene R, Petraitis V, Maung BBW, et al. Efficacy and Pharmacokinetics of Fosmanogepix (APX001) in the Treatment of *Candida* Endophthalmitis and Hematogenous Meningoencephalitis in Nonneutropenic Rabbits. Antimicrob Agents Chemother 2021;65(3):e01795.

112. Gebremariam T, Alkhazraji S, Gu Y, et al. Galactomannan Is a Biomarker of Fosmanogepix (APX001) Efficacy in Treating Experimental Invasive Pulmonary Aspergillosis. Antimicrob Agents Chemother 2019;64(1):e01966.

113. Alkhazraji S, Gebremariam T, Alqarihi A, et al. Fosmanogepix (APX001) Is Effective in the Treatment of Immunocompromised Mice Infected with Invasive Pulmonary Scedosporiosis or Disseminated Fusariosis. Antimicrob Agents Chemother 2020;64(3):017355.

114. Gebremariam T, Alkhazraji S, Alqarihi A, et al. Fosmanogepix (APX001) Is Effective in the Treatment of Pulmonary Murine Mucormycosis Due to *Rhizopus arrhizus*. Antimicrob Agents Chemother 2020;64(6):001788.

115. Gebremariam T, Gu Y, Alkhazraji S, et al. The Combination Treatment of Fosmanogepix and Liposomal Amphotericin B Is Superior to Monotherapy in Treating Experimental Invasive Mold Infections. Antimicrob Agents Chemother 2022; 66(7):e0038022.

116. National Library of Medicine (U.S. An Open-Label Study to Evaluate the Efficacy and Safety of APX001 in Non Neutropenic Patients With Candidemia, With or Without Invasive Candidiasis, Inclusive of Patients With Suspected Resistance to Standard of Care Antifungal Treatment. ClinicalTrials.gov 2021;. https:// clinicaltrials.gov/ct2/show/study/NCT03604705. Accessed December 5, 2022.

117. National Library of Medicine (U.S. An Open-Label Study to Evaluate the Efficacy and Safety of APX001 in Patients With Candidemia and/or Invasive Candidiasis Caused by *Candida Auris*. ClinicalTrials.gov 2022. Available at: https:// clinicaltrials.gov/ct2/show/study/NCT04148287. Accessed December 5, 2022.

118. National Library of Medicine (U.S. A Phase 2, Open-Label Study to Evaluate the Safety and Efficacy of APX001 in the Treatment of Patients With Invasive Mold

Infections Caused by *Aspergillus* Species or Rare Molds. ClinicalTrials.gov 2022. Available at: https://clinicaltrials.gov/ct2/show/study/NCT04240886. Accessed December 5, 2022.
119. National Library of Medicine (U.S. An Interventional Efficacy and Safety Phase 3 Double-Blind, 2-Arm Study to Investigate IV Followed by Oral Fosmanogepix (PF-07842805) Compared With IV Caspofungin Followed by Oral Fluconazole in Adult Participants With Candidemia and/or Invasive Candidiasis. ClinicalTrials.gov 2022;. https://clinicaltrials.gov/ct2/show/NCT05421858. Accessed December 5, 2022.
120. Oliver JD, Sibley GEM, Beckmann N, et al. F901318 represents a novel class of antifungal drug that inhibits dihydroorotate dehydrogenase. Proc Natl Acad Sci U S A 2016;113(45):12809–14.
121. Buil JB, Rijs AJMM, Meis JF, et al. *In vitro* activity of the novel antifungal compound F901318 against difficult-to-treat *Aspergillus* isolates. J Antimicrob Chemother 2017;72(9):2548–52.
122. Jørgensen KM, Astvad KMT, Hare RK, et al. EUCAST Determination of Olorofim (F901318) Susceptibility of Mold Species, Method Validation, and MICs. Antimicrob Agents Chemother 2018;62(8):004877.
123. Lackner M, Birch M, Naschberger V, et al. Dihydroorotate dehydrogenase inhibitor olorofim exhibits promising activity against all clinically relevant species within *Aspergillus* section *Terrei*. J Antimicrob Chemother 2018;73(11):3068–73.
124. du Pré S, Beckmann N, Almeida MC, et al. Effect of the Novel Antifungal Drug F901318 (Olorofim) on Growth and Viability of *Aspergillus fumigatus*. Antimicrob Agents Chemother 2018;62(8):e00231–418.
125. Rivero-Menendez O, Cuenca-Estrella M, Alastruey-Izquierdo A. *In vitro* activity of olorofim (F901318) against clinical isolates of cryptic species of *Aspergillus* by EUCAST and CLSI methodologies. J Antimicrob Chemother 2019;74(6):1586–90.
126. Seyedmousavi S, Chang YC, Law D, et al. Efficacy of Olorofim (F901318) against *Aspergillus fumigatus, A. nidulans*, and *A. tanneri* in Murine Models of Profound Neutropenia and Chronic Granulomatous Disease. Antimicrob Agents Chemother 2019;63(6):e00129.
127. Talbot JJ, Frisvad JC, Meis JF, et al. cyp51A Mutations, Extrolite Profiles, and Antifungal Susceptibility in Clinical and Environmental Isolates of the *Aspergillus viridinutans* Species Complex. Antimicrob Agents Chemother 2019;63(11):e00632.
128. Astvad KMT, Jorgensen KM, Hare RK, et al. Olorofim Susceptibility Testing of 1,423 Danish Mold Isolates Obtained in 2018-2019 Confirms Uniform and Broad-Spectrum Activity. Antimicrob Agents Chemother 2020;65(1):e01527.
129. Kirchhoff L, Dittmer S, Buer J, et al. In vitro activity of olorofim (F901318) against fungi of the genus, *Scedosporium* and *Rasamsonia* as well as against *Lomentospora prolificans, Exophiala dermatitidis* and azole-resistant *Aspergillus fumigatus*. Int J Antimicrob Agents 2020;56(3):106105.
130. Kirchhoff L, Dittmer S, Furnica DT, et al. Inhibition of azole-resistant *Aspergillus fumigatus* biofilm at various formation stages by antifungal drugs, including olorofim. J Antimicrob Chemother 2022;77(6):1645–54.
131. Wiederhold NP, Law D, Birch M. Dihydroorotate dehydrogenase inhibitor F901318 has potent *in vitro* activity against *Scedosporium* species and *Lomentospora prolificans*. J Antimicrob Chemother 2017;72(7):1977–80.
132. Biswas C, Law D, Birch M, et al. *In vitro* activity of the novel antifungal compound F901318 against Australian *Scedosporium* and *Lomentospora* fungi. Med Mycol 2018;56(8):1050–4.

133. Rivero-Menendez O, Cuenca-Estrella M, Alastruey-Izquierdo A. *In vitro* activity of olorofim against clinical isolates of *Scedosporium* species and *Lomentospora prolificans* using EUCAST and CLSI methodologies. J Antimicrob Chemother 2020;75(12):3582–5.
134. Seyedmousavi S, Chang YC, Youn JH, et al. *In Vivo* Efficacy of Olorofim against Systemic Scedosporiosis and Lomentosporiosis. Antimicrob Agents Chemother 2021;65(10):e0043421.
135. Kirchhoff L, Dittmer S, Weisner AK, et al. Antibiofilm activity of antifungal drugs, including the novel drug olorofim, against *Lomentospora prolificans*. J Antimicrob Chemother 2020;75(8):2133–40.
136. Wiederhold NP, Najvar LK, Jaramillo R, et al. The Orotomide Olorofim Is Efficacious in an Experimental Model of Central Nervous System Coccidioidomycosis. Antimicrob Agents Chemother 2018;62(9):e00999.
137. Singh A, Singh P, Meis JF, et al. *In vitro* activity of the novel antifungal olorofim against dermatophytes and opportunistic moulds including *Penicillium* and *Talaromyces* species. J Antimicrob Chemother 2021;76(5):1229–33.
138. Zhang J, Liu H, Xi L, et al. Antifungal Susceptibility Profiles of Olorofim (Formerly F901318) and Currently Available Systemic Antifungals against Mold and Yeast Phases of *Talaromyces marneffei*. Antimicrob Agents Chemother 2021;65(6): e00256.
139. Borba-Santos LP, Rollin-Pinheiro R, da Silva Fontes Y, et al. Screening of Pandemic Response Box Library Reveals the High Activity of Olorofim against Pathogenic *Sporothrix* Species. J Fungi 2022;8(10).
140. Al-Hatmi AM, de Hog GS, Meis JF. Multiresistant *Fusarium* Pathogens on Plants and Humans: Solutions in (from) the Antifungal Pipeline? Infect Drug Resist 2019;12:3727–37.
141. Wiederhold NP. Review of the Novel Investigational Antifungal Olorofim. J Fungi 2020;6(3).
142. National Library of Medicine (U.S. Phase IIb Study of F901318 as Treatment of Invasive Fungal Infections Due to *Lomentospora prolificans, Scedosporium* spp., *Aspergillus* spp., and Other Resistant Fungi in Patients Lacking Suitable Alternative Treatment Options. ClinicalTrials.gov 2022. Available at: https://clinicaltrials.gov/ct2/show/study/NCT03583164. Accessed December 5, 2022.
143. National Library of Medicine (U.S. Phase III, Adjudicator-blinded, Randomised Study to Evaluate Efficacy and Safety of Treatment With Olorofim Versus Treatment With AmBisome® Followed by Standard of Care in Patients With Invasive Fungal Disease Caused by *Aspergillus* Species. ClinicalTrials.gov 2022. Available at: https://clinicaltrials.gov/ct2/show/study/NCT05101187. Accessed December 6, 2022.
144. Wang H, Zhang W, Tang YW. Clinical microbiology in detection and identification of emerging microbial pathogens: past, present and future. Emerg Microbes Infect 2022;11(1):2579–89.
145. Koo S, Thomas HR, Daniels SD, et al. A Breath Fungal Secondary Metabolite Signature to Diagnose Invasive Aspergillosis. Clin Infect Dis 2014;59(12):1733–40.
146. Wei S, sheng Chen Y, Shi Y. Metabolomic profiling of exhaled breath condensate for the diagnosis of pulmonary aspergillosis. Front Cell Infect Microbiol 2022;12: 1008924.

Current Concepts in the Diagnosis and Management of *Pneumocystis* Pneumonia in Solid Organ Transplantation

Paul A. Trubin, MD[a],*, Marwan M. Azar, MD, FAST[b,c]

KEYWORDS

- *Pneumocystis jirovecii* • Pneumonia • PCP • Solid organ transplantation
- Immunocompromised

KEY POINTS

- *Pneumocystis* pneumonia contributes to significant morbidity and mortality in solid organ transplant recipients.
- The risk of infection depends on the net state of immunosuppression and is dynamic over time from transplantation.
- Although effective primary and secondary prophylaxis regimens have reduced the incidence of *Pneumocystis* infection after solid organ transplantation, late-onset infection may occur once prophylaxis has ceased.
- The diagnostic landscape now encompasses molecular testing and less-invasive sampling techniques.
- Effective treatment regimens have reduced the morbidity and mortality from *Pneumocystis* pneumonia in solid organ transplant recipients.

INTRODUCTION

Pneumocystis jirovecii, formerly *Pneumocystis carinii*, has long been known to cause disease in humans, particularly as an opportunistic pathogen of immunocompromised hosts. Much of the contemporary experience involving the recognition, diagnosis, and management of pneumocystosis has its roots in the human immunodeficiency virus (HIV) epidemic, although in the past several decades, *Pneumocystis*-related disease has been increasingly characterized in other immunocompromised populations,

[a] Department of Medicine, Section of Infectious Diseases, Yale School of Medicine, 135 College Street, New Haven, CT 06510, USA; [b] Department of Medicine, Section of Infectious Diseases; [c] Department of Laboratory Medicine; Yale School of Medicine, 135 College Street, New Haven, CT 06510, USA
* Corresponding author. Department of Infectious Diseases, Yale School of Medicine, 135 College Street, New Haven, CT 06510.
E-mail address: paul.trubin@yale.edu

Infect Dis Clin N Am 37 (2023) 617–640
https://doi.org/10.1016/j.idc.2023.03.005
0891-5520/23/© 2023 Elsevier Inc. All rights reserved.

including in solid organ transplant recipients (SOTRs); hematopoietic stem cell transplant recipients and patients living with hematologic malignancies; and patients receiving immunomodulatory treatment for inflammatory conditions. Despite increasing understanding of the pathogen's biologic and epidemiologic characteristics and the implementation of effective preventive and therapeutic strategies in at-risk patient populations, *Pneumocystis jirovecii* pneumonia (PCP) continues to occur in SOTRs in the absence of prophylaxis. This review highlights current understanding of the epidemiology, pathophysiology, clinical presentation, diagnosis, and management of a human disease caused by *Pneumocystis* in the context of solid organ transplantation (SOT).

FEATURES OF THE PATHOGEN AND HOST-PATHOGEN INTERACTION

Pneumocystis' unique characteristics have important implications for its defiance of simple taxonomic classification and its pathogenicity. The organism is difficult to maintain in culture continuously in vitro, limiting morphologic and biochemical descriptions. *Pneumocystis* exists in three principal forms in vivo: the trophozoite, the cyst, and the sporozoite (or intracystic body)[1] with a life cycle that encompasses both sexual and asexual reproduction (**Fig. 1**).

Structure

The cyst cell wall contains multiple carbohydrates as well as cholesterol and phytosterols with notable absence of ergosterol. β-1,3-Glucan, a major component of the cell wall, is an important target of alveolar macrophages in phagocytosis and affords important diagnostic and therapeutic targets.[2] The organism's inability to synthesize certain sterol compounds may explain its lack of susceptibility to antifungal agents including the azoles and polyenes.[3]

Host-Pathogen Interactions

Host immune response is a critical factor in PCP. An immunocompetent response can result in asymptomatic elimination, while an immunocompromised, dysregulated response leads to impaired clearance of the pathogen with resultant interstitial damage.[4] Major surface glycoproteins (Msg) and β-glucans act as pathogen-associated molecular patterns (PAMPs) recognized by pattern-recognition receptors (PRRs), including toll-like receptors (such as TLR2 and TLR4) and C-type lectin receptors, expressed on the surfaces of antigen-presenting cells (APCs), myeloid cells, and alveolar epithelial cells.[5] APCs are activated by interactions between PAMPs and PRRs, resulting in the production of proinflammatory cytokines, particularly through nuclear factor kappa-B; adaptive immunity is engaged via stimulation of dendritic cells.[6,7] The lymphocyte immune response involves rapid increases of both CD4-positive and CD8-positive T lymphocytes in the first week of infection; B lymphocytes and immunoglobulins A and G thereafter increase in the pulmonary compartment, with their presence therein corresponding to decreases in fungal load.[8] T helper cell involvement occurs predominantly through Th2 response.[8] The particular stage of *Pneumocystis* infection in the lungs may differentially influence the immune response.[9] Macrophage phagocytosis is the major mechanism of pathogen clearance via interactions with antigens including Msg and β-glucan.[10,11] Cell-mediated cytotoxicity may also play a role.[12–14]

Immune responses in PCP differ in states of immunocompetence versus immunodeficiency, with a key example being differential macrophage polarization.[15] Overall, the immune response in immunocompetent states seems to depend to a large degree

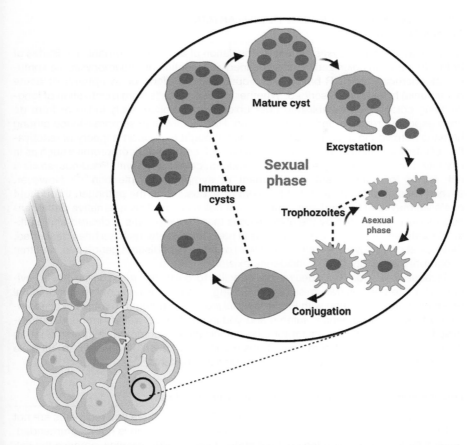

Fig. 1. Life cycle of *Pneumocystis jirovecii*; in the asexual phase, trophic forms containing a mitochondrion and nucleus undergo mitosis; in the sexual phase, haploid trophic forms conjugate to produce a precystic zygote or sporocyte (or immature cyst), followed by meiosis then mitosis yielding eight haploid nuclei (or mature cyst). With maturation of the cyst, inner spores are released from the glycogen spore case. Sporozoites emerge from the cyst and are thought to become trophozoites with the capability of asexual or sexual reproduction to restart the lifecycle. Maintenance of the lifecycle in the host can occur via either trophic (asexual) or sexual reproductive phases. (Created with BioRender.com.)

upon communication between B lymphocytes and CD4-positive T lymphocytes, whereas in immunocompromised states, proinflammatory cells including Th1, CD4-positive T lymphocytes, CD8-positive lymphocytes, and natural killer cells are associated with fungal clearance.[16] Deficiency in cellular immune response is the principal contributing factor to disease susceptibility.[16] Reduction of CD4-positive T lymphocytes in particular increases susceptibility to PCP.[17,18] Host antibody production specifically against *Pneumocystis* antigens may play a relatively minor role in clearing the pathogen.[19] Interactions between B lymphocytes and CD4-positive T lymphocytes appear to hold critical importance.[20,21] Host susceptibility can be broadly characterized as congenital, iatrogenic, acquired in the context of HIV infection, and related to malnutrition.[22]

EPIDEMIOLOGY IN SOLID ORGAN TRANSPLANTATION
General Epidemiology

Acquisition of Pneumocystis occurs via inhalation of aerosolized organisms. States of both infection and colonization (often defined as detection of Pneumocystis via immunohistochemistry or PCR-based techniques without signs or symptoms of acute pneumonia) have been described. Whether infection results from reactivation of long-standing colonization established after ubiquitous exposure early in life or from de novo exposure remains under investigation. Historically, high seroprevalence among humans from young ages into adulthood was thought to support a theory of reactivation of latent infection in the setting of newfound T-cell immunocompromise such as in HIV infection or posttransplantation.[23,24] Indeed, colonization with Pneumocystis is a risk factor for subsequent development of symptomatic infection.[4,25] However, several lines of data suggest that frequent re-exposures to the pathogen throughout one's life may lead to short-lived episodes of colonization. This alternative pathogenesis model is supported by the observations that Pneumocystis is cleared after sufficient treatment, that clustered outbreaks in nosocomial settings have been described, that repeat or de novo infections occur with organisms of distinct genotypes, and that geographic variability of PCP incidence exists.[4,26]

Because Pneumocystis species are specific to particular mammalian hosts, evidence for interspecies transmissibility is lacking, and there is no known environmental reservoir; human infection with Pneumocystis jirovecii is thought to originate predominantly from other humans.[27] Infants and young children as well as immunocompromised patients, in whom asymptomatic colonization is common, may serve as an important reservoir.[28] Interhuman transmission has been suggested in multiple studies in both patients with PCP and in colonized patients.[29,30]

Epidemiology and Risk in the Immunocompromised Host

Baseline rates of Pneumocystis colonization in SOT candidates and recipients are not well characterized, as screening before or after transplantation is not recommended. Several factors influencing the host net state of immunosuppression increase the risk of PCP. Corticosteroid use in particular is a long-known risk factor because of known impacts on T-cell function.[31] In general, a steroid dose and duration of greater than or equal to 20 mg prednisone daily for 1 month raises the risk of PCP sufficiently to warrant prophylaxis.[32–34] When combined with other immunosuppressing states or medications, lower doses of steroids may be sufficient to confer a risk of PCP. In addition to the immunologic status of the host, factors including prior respiratory viral infection, cytomegalovirus (CMV) infection, and underlying lung disease may increase the risk of PCP.[35]

In the context of SOT, the risk of Pneumocystis infection is highest at predictable times after transplantation and correlates generally with the extent of T-cell immunocompromise and its recovery over time. The risk is greatest within the first 6 months after transplantation (when the effect of induction immunosuppression is greatest); during periods of intensification of immunosuppression for treatment of allograft rejection involving the use of corticosteroids or lymphocyte-depleting therapy and following CMV infection.[36] Before the widespread implementation of prophylaxis against PCP, the incidence after SOT ranged from 5% to 15% but has dropped to 0.3%–2.6% in the prophylaxis era.[37,38]

PCP outbreaks among SOTRs in nosocomial settings have been described among various SOT organ types, and a genetic analysis of both aerosolized and clinical specimens points to the occurrence of person-to-person transmission.[39–45]

Late-Onset Infection in Solid Organ Transplantation

In the past two decades, evidence to support a phenomenon of "late-onset" PCP has emerged, with multiple studies describing patients diagnosed with infection more than 1 year after transplantation. Late-onset PCP has been described in association with prophylaxis cessation, intensification of immunosuppression, advanced age (immuno-senescence), nosocomial outbreaks, lower absolute lymphocyte count, mechanistic target of rapamycin inhibitors, and CMV infection.[37,46–51] Higher rates of PCP have been reported among heart, lung, and combined heart-lung transplantation patients than among kidney or liver transplantation patients, likely due to the need for higher levels of immunosuppression.[52] The exact incidence of late-onset PCP varies among different localities and transplantation programs.

CLINICAL PRESENTATIONS IN SOLID ORGAN TRANSPLANTATION

PCP classically presents with shortness of breath (66–68%), nonproductive cough (71–81%), hypoxemia (78–91%), and often fever (81–87%).[22] Hypoxemia may not be present at rest but may be uncovered with ambulatory measurement of oxygen saturation. In contrast to the generally slower progression of disease in persons living with HIV (PWHs), the time course of disease progression is often acute to subacute in SOTRs and may be associated with higher severity of illness.[53,54] Fever may be absent in SOTRs given the effects of immunosuppression.[55] Pneumothorax may complicate PCP spontaneously and is often discovered in the context of acutely worsened short-ness of breath and pleuritic chest pain.[56] The physical examination may include tachypnea and the presence of diffuse crackles.[57]

Extrapulmonary infection may rarely (<1%) occur involving the pleura, vascular sys-tem, liver, spleen, eye, ear, lymph nodes, skin, mastoids, ascitic fluid, omentum and gastrointestinal tract, kidney, bone marrow, pancreas, and adrenal glands.[58]

DIAGNOSTIC METHODS
Radiography

The classical chest imaging appearance is that of a diffuse interstitial pneumonia although a broad spectrum of imaging findings may be encountered depending on the severity of illness, presence of underlying lung disease, and degree of immunosup-pression.[57] The most common imaging finding is of bilateral, symmetric, interstitial reticular, or ground-glass opacities in either a diffuse or perihilar pattern of involve-ment[59] (**Fig. 2**). Reticular or ground-glass opacities often progress radiographically over about 3-5 days to alveolar consolidative opacification[60] (**Fig. 3**). These bilateral, symmetric opacities have been described to have a "butterfly" appearance given their central predominance and sparing of the lungs' periphery (in notable contrast to the typical findings of severe acute respiratory syndrome coronavirus 2 pneumonia which are peripheral-predominant). Chest computed tomography is more sensitive than x-ray for the diagnosis of PCP and may reveal thickened septal lines with more exten-sive consolidation in non-HIV immunocompromised patients.[61]

Alternative radiographic findings such as pulmonary cysts, pneumothoraces, nod-ules, lobar consolidations, unilateral sites of involvement, and effusions may occur. Pul-monary cysts are more common in PWHs but can occur in up to 6% of non-HIV immunocompromised patients with PCP.[62] Cysts are thin-walled, range in size from mil-limeters to several centimeters, are often distributed across multiple lung segments, and can resolve with appropriate treatment[63] (**Fig. 4**). Cyst rupture may lead to pneumo-thorax, which complicates PCP in 5%-20% of cases and is seen more commonly in

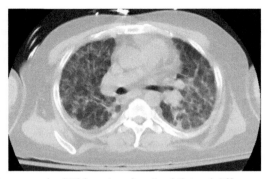

Fig. 2. Computed tomography (CT) imaging showing bilateral diffuse ground glass opacities and septal thickening in a patient with PCP. (*From* Nussbaum E, Azar MM. Pneumocystis Pneumonia. In: Grippi MA, Antin-Ozerkis DE, Dela Cruz CS, Kotloff RM, Kotton C, Pack AI. eds. Fishman's Pulmonary Diseases and Disorders, 6e. McGraw Hill; 2023; with permission.)

PWHs than in SOTRs[60] (**Fig. 5**). Pneumothorax may also develop in the absence of identifiable cystic disease. Rarely, pulmonary nodules are associated with PCP, and their development may imply a granulomatous inflammatory response, which is most commonly reported in patients with hematologic malignancy[64] (**Fig. 6**). Consolidation can develop in more-advanced PCP and is seen more commonly in non-HIV immunocompromised patients.[61] Interstitial fibrosis, honeycombing, cavitation, or calcification can develop after recurrent or extensive disease.[60]

Principles of Microbiologic Diagnosis

Owing to the difficulty in cultivating *Pneumocystis*, culture is not a diagnostic method for PCP. The lower fungal burden in non-HIV immunocompromised patients than that on

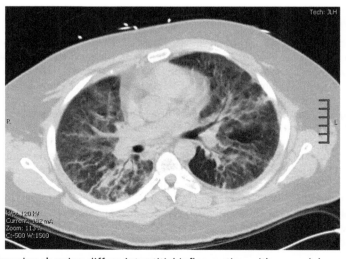

Fig. 3. CT imaging showing diffuse interstitial inflammation with upper-lobe-predominant ground glass opacities and lower-lobe-predominant peribronchovascular consolidation in a patient with PCP. (*From* Nussbaum E, Azar MM. Pneumocystis Pneumonia. In: Grippi MA, Antin-Ozerkis DE, Dela Cruz CS, Kotloff RM, Kotton C, Pack AI. eds. Fishman's Pulmonary Diseases and Disorders, 6e. McGraw Hill; 2023; with permission.)

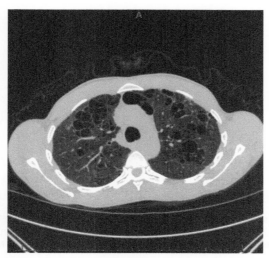

Fig. 4. CT imaging revealing multiple cystic lesions in a patient with PCP. (*From* Nussbaum E, Azar MM. Pneumocystis Pneumonia. In: Grippi MA, Antin-Ozerkis DE, Dela Cruz CS, Kotloff RM, Kotton C, Pack AI. eds. Fishman's Pulmonary Diseases and Disorders, 6e. McGraw Hill; 2023; with permission.)

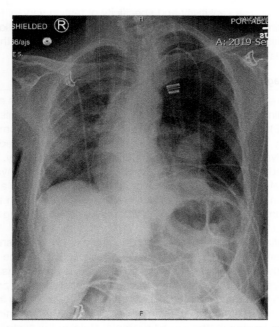

Fig. 5. Chest x-ray demonstrating pneumothorax in a patient with PCP. (*From* Nussbaum E, Azar MM. Pneumocystis Pneumonia. In: Grippi MA, Antin-Ozerkis DE, Dela Cruz CS, Kotloff RM, Kotton C, Pack AI. eds. Fishman's Pulmonary Diseases and Disorders, 6e. McGraw Hill; 2023; with permission.)

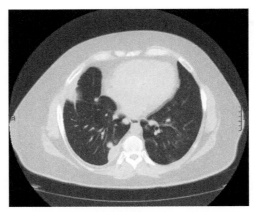

Fig. 6. CT imaging showing nodular lesions in a patient with PCP. (*From* Nussbaum E, Azar MM. Pneumocystis Pneumonia. In: Grippi MA, Antin-Ozerkis DE, Dela Cruz CS, Kotloff RM, Kotton C, Pack AI. eds. Fishman's Pulmonary Diseases and Disorders, 6e. McGraw Hill; 2023; with permission.)

PWHs likely contributes to the difficulty in detecting the pathogen in SOTRs.[65] Several methods are available for PCP diagnosis including histopathology and immunostaining, noninvasive testing with serum $(1 \rightarrow 3)$ β-D-glucan assay (BDG), and molecular testing, now a staple of PCP diagnosis. Diagnostic testing can be applied to multiple specimen types including induced sputum, oral washing, bronchoalveolar lavage (BAL) fluid, and biopsied lung tissue. The sensitivity and specificity of testing vary widely according to the type of specimen and testing, the adequacy of sample collection, specific host immunocompromising condition (particularly whether HIV is present), the use of prophylaxis or recent treatment, and the microbial burden of infection.

Microbiologic Diagnosis: Histopathology and Immunostaining

Hematoxylin and eosin (H&E) staining of infected lung tissue reveals a foamy, eosinophilic exudate filling the alveoli. The foamy exudate contains organisms (themselves unstained by H&E), surface glycoprotein, proteinaceous exudate from the lung tissue, and inflammatory debris. The airspaces may appear honeycombed or vacuolated. Neutrophils and lymphocytes infiltrate the interstitial space. Notably, diseased tissue may be distributed sporadically. Diffuse alveolar damage including hyaline membrane formation within alveoli due to destruction of the alveolar epithelium and the accumulation of debris on the basement membrane has been described in association with PCP.[66] In granulomatous PCP, histology is notable for nonnecrotizing or poorly necrotizing granulomas.[67]

Several specialized stains targeting cell wall, nuclear, or cytoplasmic components bring the organism into sharp relief (**Fig. 7**). These stains can be applied to oral wash, induced sputum, lung fluid, or biopsied lung tissue specimens. Cell wall stains accentuate the cyst form only, and given that trophozoite forms are present in greater numbers (10-fold) during active infection, these stains are relatively insensitive in the setting of low burden of organism such as among SOTRs. Methenamine silver staining (Grocott or Gomori) is a commonly used example, staining the cysts of *Pneumocystis* black against a green background.[68] Additional cell wall stains include toluidine blue, calcofluor, and cresyl echt violet. Nuclear and cytoplasmic stains such as the Giemsa, Wright-Giemsa, and Giemsa-like stains highlight these components of *Pneumocystis*

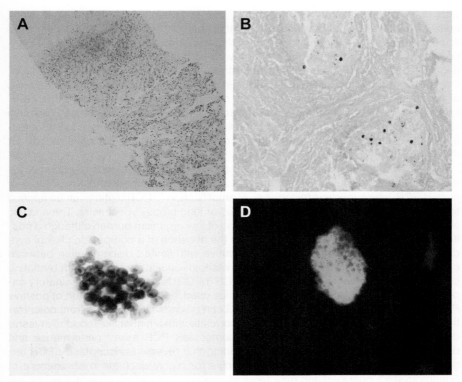

Fig. 7. Histology of *Pneumocystis*; (*A*) tissue necrosis with surrounding histiocytes compatible with necrotizing granulomatous inflammation in a patient with PCP (H&E 100x); (*B*) Grocott or Gomori (GMS) stain (600×) highlighting black appearance of *Pneumocystis* cysts against a green background; (*C*) GMS stain cytology displaying multiple cysts; (*D*) *Pneumocystis* direct immunofluorescence staining. (*From* Nussbaum E, Azar MM. Pneumocystis Pneumonia. In: Grippi MA, Antin-Ozerkis DE, Dela Cruz CS, Kotloff RM, Kotton C, Pack AI. eds. Fishman's Pulmonary Diseases and Disorders, 6e. McGraw Hill; 2023; with permission.)

in all life cycle stages. Nuclei of trophozoite forms appear purple within a blue cytoplasm. The intracystic body nuclei stain deep purple as well. Although distinguishing between aggregates of *Pneumocystis* organisms from nuclei of host cells can prove challenging, the detection of both cysts and trophozoites increases the sensitivity of Giemsa staining.

Immunofluorescence stains use fluorescein-conjugated monoclonal antibodies targeting *Pneumocystis* surface glycoproteins in all life cycle stages and can also be applied to above specimen types. Direct fluorescent antibody involves the binding of a chromophore-associated antibody to *Pneumocystis* target antigens, whereas indirect fluorescent antibody involves the linking of a primary antibody bound to *Pneumocystis* target antigens to a secondary chromophore-associated antibody. In either technique, fluorescence under ultraviolet light reveals bound target antigens in both cysts and trophozoites, yielding higher sensitivity than other stain types.[69]

Microbiologic Diagnosis: (1 → 3) b-D-Glucan and Molecular Testing

Serum BDG assay affords high sensitivity (80–100%) along with a high negative predictive value (≥95%) but lower specificity for PCP.[70–75] Serum BDG levels in patients with PCP are significantly greater than those in patients with colonization, likely because of lower fungal burdens in the latter state.[76,77] BDG may also be elevated in other invasive fungal processes including aspergillosis and candidiasis. False-positive testing may result from infection with nonfungal organisms (such as gram-negative bacteria and *Nocardia*); administration of intravenous immune globulins, therapeutic antibodies, plasmalyte, albumin, and defibrotide; or from the presence of gauze or exposure of blood to dialysis membranes containing unmodified cellulose.[78–81] Higher assay values are associated with an enhanced positive predictive value in patients with high pretest probability.[82] The European Conference on Infections in Leukemia has suggested that a negative serum BDG is sufficient to rule out the diagnosis.[83]

Nucleic acid amplification (NAT) is highly sensitive for the detection of *Pneumocystis*.[84] NAT relies on multicopy gene targeting (eg, for mitochondrial rRNA or Msg) or nested PCR, which involves two rounds of amplification.[85] PCR testing can be applied to induced sputum, oral wash, and BAL fluid or lung biopsy specimens. The analytic sensitivity of PCR assays allows for detection of low organism burden although a positive predictive value for disease is lower in the absence of a compatible clinical syndrome.[4] PCR therefore may be overly sensitive with limited discrimination between colonization and infection.[86] PCR cycle threshold values may aid in differentiating colonization and infection.[87] Quantitative PCR (qPCR) has variable discriminatory capacity depending on the particular cutoff value used.[88,89] The combination of positive *Pneumocystis* PCR and positive serum BDG can discriminate infection from colonization, as quantitatively higher assay results correlate with a higher likelihood of invasive disease.[86,90,91] Efforts to standardize *Pneumocystis* PCR assay performance and diagnostic thresholds continue, with the finding that reverse transcriptase-qPCR targeting the mitochondrial small subunit allows for highly accurate measurement of *Pneumocystis* fungal load and may serve as a reference to which other diagnostic assays are compared.[92] Optimal quantitative diagnostic thresholds for molecular testing continue to be studied, and no standardized quantitative evaluation has been widely recommended to date.

Plasma cell-free DNA (cfDNA) testing, which relies on detection of circulating microbial DNA to make the diagnosis of disseminated or compartmentalized infection, has been recently evaluated for the diagnosis of PCP. In one study, the sensitivity of *P. jirovecii* cfDNA in serum was 100% among proven PCP cases, with lower sensitivities in proven or probable cases (48.6%) and in probable cases (29.6%) while maintaining over 93% specificity. This study also found that cfDNA PCR had similar sensitivity to serum BDG but exhibited higher specificity.[93] Another recent study aiming to assess the clinical impact of a commercially available cfDNA assay found that positive cfDNA testing resulted in changes to the clinical management in about 83% of patients without a preestablished diagnosis of PCP via conventional diagnostics.[94] This noninvasive diagnostic technique remains under further investigation.

Additional Laboratory Testing

Additional nonspecific laboratory indicators can aid in the diagnostic evaluation of PCP. Blood gas analysis, CD4 and absolute lymphocyte count, serum lactate dehydrogenase (LDH), hypercalcemia, angiotensin-converting enzyme (ACE) level, and Krebs von den Lungen antigen (KL-6) have been evaluated in the diagnostic approach to PCP. The blood gas may reveal partial pressure of oxygen (PO_2) less than 60 mm Hg and respiratory alkalosis. An elevated arterial oxygenation gradient is often observed. A gradient over 30 mm Hg signifies a more severe disease, portends higher mortality, and serves as an indication for adjunctive corticosteroid therapy. Serum LDH in PCP is often greater than 300 IU/mL.[95] The ACE level, a nonspecific marker of lung injury, may be elevated in PCP.[96] Serum KL-6, a glycoprotein of pneumocytes and bronchiolar epithelium, may also be detectable in PCP. Hypercalcemia may be observed in PCP, especially in renal transplant recipients, potentially via the activity of 1 α-hydroxylase and granulomatous inflammation.[97] While these laboratory tests lack sufficient specificity, their measurement may support the diagnosis of PCP.[98]

TREATMENT IN SOLID ORGAN TRANSPLANTATION

The management of PCP varies by severity. Severity is defined according to A-a gradient and partial pressure of arterial oxygen while breathing room air, with $PaO_2 >$ 70 mm Hg or PAO_2-PaO_2 gradient < 35 mm Hg indicative of mild disease, PAO_2-PaO_2 35-45 mm Hg indicative of moderate disease, and $PaO_2 < 70$ mm Hg or PAO_2-$PaO_2 > 45$ mm Hg indicative of severe disease.[99] Trimethoprim-sulfamethoxazole (TMP-SMX) is the first-line antimicrobial indicated for the treatment of PCP across the spectrum of disease severity[100] (**Fig. 8**). Sulfamethoxazole interferes with folate metabolism by antagonizing dihydropteroate synthase (DHPS).[101] Several randomized controlled trials demonstrated the efficacy of TMP-SMX to be superior or equivalent to that of intravenous pentamidine in PWH and non-HIV immunocompromised patients.[102–105] These trials also demonstrated common adverse effects with either regimen although TMP-SMX was less likely to be associated with severe adverse

		EFFICACY				
		TMP-SMX	IV Pentamidine	Dapsone + TMP	Clindamycin + Primaquine	Atovaquone
ADVERSE EFFECTS	**TMP-SMX**		TMP-SMX more or equally effective	Equally effective	Equally effective	TMP-SMX more effective
	IV Pentamidine	Less common with TMP-SMX			Clindamycin-Primaquine more effective (salvage therapy)	Equally effective (mild disease)
	Dapsone + TMP	Less common with Dapsone + TMP			Equally effective	
	Clindamycin + Primaquine	Hematologic toxicities with Clindamycin-Primaquine Hepatotoxicity with TMP-SMX	Less common with Clindamycin-Primaquine	Less common with Dapsone + TMP		
	Atovaquone	Less common with Atovaquone	Less common with Atovaquone			

Fig. 8. Efficacy and adverse effects associated with available PCP treatment regimens.

effects such as nephrotoxicity. TMP-SMX was equally effective as clindamycin and primaquine or dapsone-trimethoprim combinations in one randomized controlled trial.[106] Treatment duration is 21 days. Moderate to severe disease is often initially treated with intravenous therapy followed by step-down to oral therapy, whereas mild disease may be treated entirely with oral therapy. Important advantages of TMP-SMX include its widespread availability, relative tolerability, excellent oral bioavailability, and intravenous and oral formulations. Adverse effects range from minor to severe; minor toxicities include gastrointestinal disturbance, rash (mild to severe), hyperkalemia, drug fever, and serum creatinine elevation (although the inhibition of creatinine secretion by trimethoprim is not indicative of a change in glomerular filtration rate).[107] Severe adverse effects that may limit continued use include severe allergic reaction, marked cytopenias, nephritis, pancreatitis, pneumonitis, hepatitis, and central nervous system effects.[57,105] Desensitization in the case of hypersensitivity reactions reduces the likelihood of necessitating treatment discontinuation and future adverse reactions.[108]

Although pentamidine's efficacy for PCP has been well established, its current role is limited because of high rates of severe toxicities (up to 80%).[102–104] Its mechanism of action involves disruption of nucleic acid and protein synthesis but is not fully understood. Adverse effects include nephrotoxicity, hepatitis, pancreatitis, glycemic fluctuations (involving damage to pancreatic β cells, which underpins the rationale against its use in pancreas transplantation to avoid islet cell necrosis), electrolyte disturbances including hypokalemia, hypomagnesemia, and circulatory disturbances including hypotension, tachycardia, and arrhythmias. Pentamidine's long half-life elevates the risk of prolonged toxicity, even beyond discontinuation of therapy. Inhaled pentamidine is not used for treatment owing to limited systemic drug concentrations achievable via that route.

The combination of clindamycin and primaquine is an alternative regimen for treatment of mild to moderate PCP. This combination compares favorably to intravenous pentamidine for mild to moderate disease by retaining high efficacy with a milder adverse effect profile. It also was found to have equivalent clinical efficacy to TMP-SMX and dapsone-TMP although associated with greater toxicity.[106] Posited mechanisms of action include effects on mitochondrial activity for clindamycin and nucleic acid synthesis for primaquine.[109] Clindamycin with primaquine is the preferred salvage regimen for PCP refractory to first-line therapy.[110,111] Primaquine is associated with severe hemolysis in the setting of glucose-6-phosphate dehydrogenase (G6PD) deficiency, so G6PD level should be measured before initiation. Primaquine should be avoided in G6PD deficiency. Adverse effects include gastrointestinal disturbance and rash.

Atovaquone is an alternative option in the treatment of mild to moderate PCP. Atovaquone is thought to interfere with microbial electron transport chain through inhibition of cytochrome b. The principal advantage is a milder adverse effect profile. Atovaquone exhibits inferior efficacy compared with TMP-SMX for treatment of PCP but may be associated with less-frequent adverse effects.[112] Atovaquone is similarly efficacious when compared to intravenous pentamidine for mild to moderate PCP with fewer adverse effects.[113] Adverse effects include drug fever, rash, and gastrointestinal disturbances such as diarrhea and elevated liver function tests. Its bitter taste may limit adherence.

Dapsone and trimethoprim in combination is an alternative treatment option for mild to moderate PCP. Dapsone inhibits folate synthesis. Dapsone-TMP demonstrated equivalent clinical efficacy to TMP-SMX and clindamycin with primaquine.[106] Dapsone can also induce hemolysis in the setting of G6PD deficiency. Adverse effects include hematologic toxicities such as methemoglobinemia and anemia[114] (**Table 1**).

Table 1 Treatment regimens for PCP			
Agent	Route and Dose	Adverse Effects	Clinical Points
TMP-SMX	IV or PO: 15–20 mg/kg/d TMP component	Rash, serum creatinine elevation, cytopenias, hyperkalemia, nephrotoxicity	First-line, most effective Renal function adjustment
Pentamidine	IV: 4 mg/kg/d (300 mg/d maximum)	Nephrotoxicity, hypotension, electrolyte disturbance, cardiac arrhythmia, pancreatitis, hypoglycemia or hyperglycemia, hepatitis	Prolonged half-life, extended adverse effects Infusions over 1–2 hours
Atovaquone	PO: 750 mg BID	Gastrointestinal intolerance, rash, fever, hepatitis, bitter taste	Variable absorption Mild to moderate disease only
Clindamycin & primaquine	Clindamycin: PO: 450–600 mg Q6-8H; IV: 900 mg Q8H Primaquine: 13–30 mg oral base daily	Methemoglobinemia, diarrhea, neutropenia, hemolytic anemia (G6PD deficiency)	Test for G6PD deficiency Mild to moderate disease only Risk of C. difficile colitis
Dapsone & trimethoprim	Dapsone: PO: 100 mg/d TMP: PO/IV: 5 mg/kg/d TMP	Methemoglobinemia, rash, fever, GI intolerance, hemolytic anemia (G6PD deficiency)	Test for G6PD deficiency

Abbreviations: BID, *bis intra diem*; *C. difficile, Clostridium difficile*; GI, gastrointestinal; G6PD, glucose-6-phosphate dehydrogenase; IV, intravenous; PO, *per os*; TMP-SMX, trimethoprim-sulfamethoxazole.

ADJUNCTIVE TREATMENT

Corticosteroids play an important adjunctive role in the treatment of moderate to severe PCP. Steroids reduce the risk of early progression of hypoxemia, respiratory failure, requirement for mechanical ventilation, and death when used with primary antimicrobial therapy in PWH.[115] In non-HIV immunocompromised patients, data are not as clear; one study demonstrated no benefit of adjunctive steroids in this group.[116] Nevertheless, although extrapolation from experience in PWH, steroid use continues to be recommended in moderate to severe PCP for SOTRs.[117] That steroid initiation beyond 72 hours of initiation of anti-*Pneumocystis* antimicrobial therapy is not associated with clinical benefits suggests an early window of therapeutic opportunity.[118] Oral or intravenous regimens may be used.[118] Tapering of the regimen is recommended to avoid a phenomenon of rebound pneumonitis.

EMERGING TREATMENTS

Glucan synthase inhibitors such as echinocandins have also been explored as potential treatment options. Echinocandins noncompetitively inhibit the GSC1 subunit of the enzyme complex responsible for the synthesis of $(1 \rightarrow 3)$ β-D-glucan, abundantly present in cell walls of cystic forms and less so in trophozoite forms. Echinocandins therefore are thought to exert their maximal activity against cystic forms. In animal models, caspofungin was found to primarily active against cystic forms.[119] Other echinocandins including anidulafungin and rezafungin appeared effective against both cyst and trophozoite stages.[120] Echinocandins have also been studied as a part of combination regimens in the setting of concerns regarding activity against trophozoite forms. Caspofungin combined with TMP-SMX eradicated *Pneumocystis* in a pilot study conducted in mice.[121] Echinocandin therapy in human studies has shown efficacy as a salvage agent alone or in combination.[122,123] Monotherapy, however, may be associated with treatment failures.[123,124] The European Conference on Infections in Leukemia proposes echinocandin-containing combination therapy as a salvage therapy option but cautions against echinocandin monotherapy.[100] Novel antifungal agents such as the triterpenoid ibrexafungerp or the newer echinocandin rezafungin have the potential to expand treatment options for PCP.[125–127]

DRUG RESISTANCE

Genetic analyses have revealed polymorphisms or mutations in genes encoding targets of antifungal therapy, such as DHPS or cytochrome b, and suggest the potential for drug resistance.[128] The clinical implications and importance of such genetic variations, however, remain unclear overall. For example, DHPS mutations have been associated only inconsistently with lower survival and higher risk of treatment failure in patients receiving sulfa-based therapy.[129,130] One study noted that a mutation to cytochrome b may have led to prophylaxis failure with atovaquone.[131] The emergence of mutations conferring potential resistance has been noted in the context of prolonged exposure to therapeutic agents.[132] DHPS gene mutations have also been noted in first episodes of PCP, raising the possibility of transmission of resistant strains.[133]

PREVENTION AND MITIGATION IN SOLID ORGAN TRANSPLANTATION

Both primary and secondary prophylaxis strategies are used after SOT. The institution of routine prophylaxis has led to significant reductions (up to 91%) of PCP after SOT along with a substantial decrease of PCP-related mortality.[134] Widespread implementation of prophylaxis has reduced PCP incidence in SOT to 0.3%-2.5% from at least 3% to 5%.[37,38] The ultimate duration of prophylaxis depends on the type of SOT performed and the extent of immunosuppression. PCP prophylaxis is recommended for all SOTRs, generally for at least 6-12 months after transplant.[135] Some SOTRs, including lung or small bowel recipients, undergo lifelong PCP prophylaxis because of the higher risk associated with greater immunosuppression. Secondary prophylaxis to prevent reinfection may also be instituted long-term or lifelong especially if immunosuppression cannot be reduced after the initial infection. Practice across transplantation centers varies, with some programs extending lifelong prophylaxis to cardiac, liver, and renal transplant recipients. Prophylaxis should be considered in the context of intensification of immunosuppression. SOTRs living with HIV often receive lifelong PCP prophylaxis although recent evidence supports the safety of discontinuation of prophylaxis after 6 months.[136]

The drug of choice for PCP prophylaxis is TMP-SMX. Other agents including atovaquone, inhaled pentamidine, and dapsone are second-line owing to less favorable tolerance, cost, and efficacy than TMP-SMX.[55,135] An added benefit of TMP-SMX prophylaxis is its potential to prevent other opportunistic or posttransplant infections through activity against *Toxoplasma gondii*, *Nocardia species*, and some skin, urinary tract, or gastrointestinal tract bacteria. In renal SOTRs, reduced dosing of TMP-SMX prophylaxis with 1 double-strength tablet three times per week reduces the risk of adverse effects and appears of comparable efficacy to a daily dosing strategy[137] (**Table 2**).

FUTURE DIRECTIONS AND UNMET NEEDS

Despite substantial advances in molecular diagnostics, preventive strategies, and the development of tolerable and highly effective treatment regimens, PCP remains a threat to SOTRs. Investigation continues into improved ecologic characterization of *Pneumocystis*, particularly regarding the definition of the environmental reservoir. The assessment of risk for the development of PCP in immunocompromised individuals takes aim at a moving target: The net state of immunosuppression fluctuates after SOT over time and according to iatrogenic, infectious, and other immunologic events. Furthermore, unlike the CD4 count in PWH, no single universal marker of the net state of SOT immunosuppression exists, rendering its appraisal an exercise in approximation. Identifying markers of increased risk of PCP in SOTRs may allow for tailoring of preventive strategies to those at the highest risk. Although molecular diagnostics have offered the opportunity to rule out the diagnosis with a high degree of certainty, the differentiation of colonization from infection continues to pose a substantial clinical challenge. Further study of host-pathogen interaction and of adaptation of the pathogen to host may yield additional therapeutic targets. Novel antifungals with in vitro activity remain to be studied clinically and more widely implemented. Additional compounds with efficacy against *Pneumocystis* continue to be sought at all stages of the drug-development pipeline. One such example is mycosinate, derived from ingredients found naturally in honey.[138] Novel treatment options that maintain high efficacy while minimizing toxicities promise to reshape current treatment paradigms for PCP.

Table 2			
Prophylaxis regimens for PCP			
Agent	**Route and Dose**	**Adverse Effects**	**Clinical Points**
TMP-SMX	PO: 1 single-strength tablet daily or 1 double-strength tablet daily or 1 double-strength tablet 3 times weekly	Serum creatinine elevation, hyperkalemia, bone marrow suppression	First-line, most effective Renal function adjustment
Atovaquone	PO: 1500 mg daily (with food)	Bitter taste, Gastrointestinal intolerance	Failures at doses lower than 1000 mg
Pentamidine	Inhaled: 300 mg monthly	Cough, bronchospasm, hypoglycemia or hyperglycemia, pancreatitis	Higher rates of breakthrough disease (5–20%), especially in lung apices Requires administration by experienced personnel via nebulizer
Dapsone	PO: 50 mg BID or 100 mg daily	Methemoglobinemia, hemolytic anemia (G6PD deficiency), GI intolerance	Test for G6PD deficiency

Abbreviations: GI, gastrointestinal.

CLINICS CARE POINTS

- While PCP foremerly was seen as an earlier compication of solid organ transplantation, with routine prophylaxis a phenomenon of "late-onset" PCP has been observed as infections increasingly have been diagnosed after the first year post-transplantation.

- *Pneumocystis* PCR assays from respiratory samples are sensitive and may detect colonization or infection. Their results should be interpreted in the context of a compatible clinical syndrome.

- The radiographic appearance of PCP in solid organ transplant recipients is variable and ranges from the more commonly observed diffuse ground glass opacification to less commonly observed consolidative, cystic, or nodular lesions.

- The agent considered first-line both prophylaxis against and treatment of PCP is trimethoprim-sulfamethoxazole.

DISCLOSURE

The authors have nothing to disclose.

REFERENCES

1. Kim HK, Hughes WT, Feldman S. Studies of morphology and immunofluorescence of Pneumocystis carinii. Proc Soc Exp Biol Med 1972;141(1):304–9.
2. Kottom TJ, Limper AH. Cell Wall Assembly by Pneumocystis carinii: Evidence for a unique Gsc-1 Subunit Mediating Beta-1,3-Glucan Deposition. J Biol Chem 2000;275(51):40628–34.
3. Furlong ST, Samia JA, Rose RM, et al. Phytosterols are present in Pneumocystis carinii. Antimicrobial Agents Chemother 1994;38(11):2534–40.
4. Morris A, Norris KA. Colonization by Pneumocystis jirovecii and its role in disease. Clin Microbiol Rev 2012;25(2):297–317.
5. Carmona EM, Vassallo R, Vuk-Pavlovic Z, et al. Pneumocystis cell wall beta-glucans induce dendritic cell costimulatory molecule expression and inflammatory activation through a Fas-Fas ligand mechanism. J Immunol 2006;177(1):459–67.
6. Lebron F, Vassallo R, Puri V, et al. Pneumocystis carinii cell wall β-glucans initiate macrophage inflammatory responses through NF-κB activation. J Biol Chem 2003;278(27):25001–8.
7. Limper AH, Lebron F, Evans SE, et al. Pneumocystis carinii: Cell wall β-glucan-mediated pulmonary inflammation. J Eukaryot Microbiol 2003;50(6):646.
8. Shellito JE, Tate C, Ruan S, et al. Murine CD4+ T lymphocyte subsets and host defense against Pneumocystis carinii. JID (J Infect Dis) 2000;181(6):2011–7.
9. Evans HM, Bryant GL III, Garvy BA. The life cycle stages of Pneumocystis murina have opposing effects on the immune response to this opportunistic fungal pathogen. Infect Immun 2016;84(11):3195–205.
10. Ezekowitz R, Williams D, Koziel H, et al. Uptake of Pneumocystis carinii mediated by the macrophage mannose receptor. Nature 1991;351(6322):155–8.
11. Steele C, Marrero L, Swain S, et al. Alveolar macrophage–mediated killing of Pneumocystis carinii f. sp. muris involves molecular recognition by the dectin-1 β-glucan receptor. J Exp Med 2003;198(11):1677–88.
12. Kelly MN, Zheng M, Ruan S, et al. Memory CD4+ T cells are required for optimal NK cell effector functions against the opportunistic fungal pathogen Pneumocystis murina. J Immunol 2013;190(1):285–95.

13. Eddens T, Elsegeiny W, Nelson MP, et al. Eosinophils contribute to early clearance of Pneumocystis murina infection. J Immunol 2015;195(1):185–93.
14. McAllister F, Steele C, Zheng M, et al. In vitro effector activity of Pneumocystis murina-specific T-cytotoxic-1 CD8+ T cells: role of granulocyte-macrophage colony-stimulating factor. Infect Immun 2005;73(11):7450–7.
15. Nandakumar V, Hebrink D, Jenson P, et al. Differential macrophage polarization from pneumocystis in immunocompetent and immunosuppressed hosts: potential adjunctive therapy during pneumonia. Infect Immun 2017;85(3). 009399–16.
16. Charpentier E, Ménard S, Marques C, et al. Immune response in pneumocystis infections according to the host immune system status. J Fungi (Basel) 2021;7(8).
17. Shellito J, Suzara VV, Blumenfeld W, et al. A new model of Pneumocystis carinii infection in mice selectively depleted of helper T lymphocytes. J Clin Invest 1990;85(5):1686–93.
18. Phair J, Muñoz A, Detels R, et al. The risk of Pneumocystis carinii pneumonia among men infected with human immunodeficiency virus type 1. N Engl J Med 1990;322(3):161–5.
19. Lund FE, Schuer K, Hollifield M, et al. Clearance of Pneumocystis carinii in mice is dependent on B cells but not on P. carinii-specific antibody. J Immunol 2003; 171(3):1423–30.
20. Wiley J, Harmsen A. CD40 ligand is required for resolution of Pneumocystis carinii pneumonia in mice. J Immunol 1995;155(7):3525–9.
21. Rong H-M, Li T, Zhang C, et al. IL-10-producing B cells regulate Th1/Th17-cell immune responses in Pneumocystis pneumonia. Am J Physiol Lung Cell Mol Physiol 2019;316(1):L291–301.
22. Fishman JA. Pneumocystis jiroveci. Semin Respir Crit Care Med 2020;41(1): 141–57.
23. Vargas SL, Hughes WT, Santolaya ME, et al. Search for primary infection by Pneumocystis carinii in a cohort of normal, healthy infants. Clin Infect Dis 2001;32(6):855–61.
24. Pifer LL, Hughes WT, Stagno S, et al. Pneumocystis carinii infection: evidence for high prevalence in normal and immunosuppressed children. Pediatrics 1978;61(1):35–41.
25. Le Gal S, Bonnet P, Huguenin A, et al. The shift from pulmonary colonization to Pneumocystis pneumonia. Med Mycol 2021;59(5):510–3.
26. Morris A, Beard CB, Huang L. Update on the epidemiology and transmission of Pneumocystis carinii. Microbes Infect 2002;4(1):95–103.
27. Chabé M, Durand-Joly I, Dei-Cas E. Transmission of Pneumocystis infection in humans. M-S (Med Sci): Méd/Sci 2012;28(6–7):599–604.
28. Gigliotti F, Wright TW. Pneumocystis: where does it live? PLoS Pathog 2012; 8(11):e1003025.
29. Manoloff ES, Francioli P, Taffé P, et al. Risk for Pneumocystis carinii transmission among patients with pneumonia: a molecular epidemiology study. Emerg Infect Dis 2003;9(1):132.
30. Nevez G, Raccurt C, Jounieaux V, et al. Pneumocystosis versus pulmonary Pneumocystis carinii colonization in HIV-negative and HIV-positive patients. AIDS 1999;13(4):535.
31. Yale SH, Limper AH, editors. Pneumocystis carinii pneumonia in patients without acquired immunodeficiency syndrome: associated illnesses and prior corticosteroid therapy. Elsevier; 1996. Mayo Clinic Proceedings.

32. Limper AH, Knox KS, Sarosi GA, et al. An official American Thoracic Society statement: Treatment of fungal infections in adult pulmonary and critical care patients. Am J Respir Crit Care Med 2011;183(1):96–128.

33. Sepkowitz KA. Opportunistic infections in patients with and patients without Acquired Immunodeficiency Syndrome. Clin Infect Dis 2002;34(8):1098–107.

34. Huang L, Morris A, Limper AH, et al. An official ATS workshop summary: recent advances and future directions in pneumocystis pneumonia (PCP). Proc Am Thorac Soc 2006;3(8):655–64.

35. Maini R, Henderson KL, Sheridan EA, et al. Increasing Pneumocystis pneumonia, England, UK, 2000-2010. Emerg Infect Dis 2013;19(3):386–92.

36. Martin S, Fishman J. Pneumocystis pneumonia in solid organ transplant recipients. Am J Transplant 2009;9(s4).

37. de Boer MG, Kroon FP, le Cessie S, et al. Risk factors for Pneumocystis jirovecii pneumonia in kidney transplant recipients and appraisal of strategies for selective use of chemoprophylaxis. Transpl Infect Dis 2011;13(6):559–69.

38. Iriart X, Challan Belval T, Fillaux J, et al. Risk factors of Pneumocystis pneumonia in solid organ recipients in the era of the common use of posttransplantation prophylaxis. Am J Transplant 2015;15(1):190–9.

39. Sassi M, Ripamonti C, Mueller NJ, et al. Outbreaks of Pneumocystis pneumonia in 2 renal transplant centers linked to a single strain of Pneumocystis: implications for transmission and virulence. Clin Infect Dis 2012;54(10):1437–44.

40. Gianella S, Haeberli L, Joos B, et al. Molecular evidence of interhuman transmission in an outbreak of Pneumocystis jirovecii pneumonia among renal transplant recipients. Transpl Infect Dis 2010;12(1):1–10.

41. Le Gal S, Toubas D, Totet A, et al. Pneumocystis infection outbreaks in organ transplantation units in France: a nation-wide survey. Clin Infect Dis 2020; 70(10):2216–20.

42. Yiannakis E, Boswell T. Systematic review of outbreaks of Pneumocystis jirovecii pneumonia: evidence that P. jirovecii is a transmissible organism and the implications for healthcare infection control. J Hosp Infect 2016;93(1):1–8.

43. Azar MM, Cohen E, Ma L, et al. Genetic and epidemiologic analyses of an outbreak of pneumocystis jirovecii pneumonia among kidney transplant recipients in the United States. Clin Infect Dis 2022;74(4):639–47.

44. Vindrios W, Argy N, Le Gal S, et al. Outbreak of Pneumocystis jirovecii infection among heart transplant recipients: molecular investigation and management of an interhuman transmission. Clin Infect Dis 2017;65(7):1120–6.

45. de Boer MG, de Fijter JW, Kroon FP. Outbreaks and clustering of Pneumocystis pneumonia in kidney transplant recipients: a systematic review. Med Mycol 2011;49(7):673–80.

46. Kaminski H, Belliere J, Burguet L, et al. Identification of predictive markers and outcomes of late-onset pneumocystis jirovecii pneumonia in kidney transplant recipients. Clin Infect Dis 2020;73(7):e1456–63.

47. Hosseini-Moghaddam S, Shokoohi M, Singh G, et al. A multicenter case-control study of the effect of acute rejection and cytomegalovirus infection on pneumocystis pneumonia in solid organ transplant recipients. Clin Infect Dis 2019;68(8):1320–6.

48. Ghadimi M, Mohammadpour Z, Dashti-Khavidaki S, et al. m-TOR inhibitors and risk of Pneumocystis pneumonia after solid organ transplantation: a systematic review and meta-analysis. Eur J Clin Pharmacol 2019;75(11):1471–80.

49. Werbel W, Ison M, Angarone M, et al. Lymphopenia is associated with late onset Pneumocystis jirovecii pneumonia in solid organ transplantation. Transpl Infect Dis 2018;20(3):e12876.
50. Perez-Ordoño L, Hoyo I, Sanclemente G, et al. Late-onset Pneumocystis jirovecii pneumonia in solid organ transplant recipients. Transpl Infect Dis 2014;16(2): 324–8.
51. Neofytos D, Hirzel C, Boely E, et al. Pneumocystis jirovecii pneumonia in solid organ transplant recipients: a descriptive analysis for the Swiss Transplant Cohort. Transpl Infect Dis 2018;20(6):e12984.
52. Iriart X, Bouar ML, Kamar N, et al. Pneumocystis pneumonia in solid-organ transplant recipients. Journal of Fungi 2015;1(3):293–331.
53. Russian DA, Levine SJ. Pneumocystis carinii pneumonia in patients without HIV infection. Am J Med Sci 2001;321(1):56–65.
54. Ewig S, Bauer T, Schneider C, et al. Clinical characteristics and outcome of Pneumocystis carinii pneumonia in HIV-infected and otherwise immunosuppressed patients. Eur Respir J 1995;8(9):1548–53.
55. Martin S, Fishman J. Practice AIDCo. Pneumocystis pneumonia in solid organ transplantation. Am J Transplant 2013;13(s4):272–9.
56. Terzi E, Zarogoulidis K, Kougioumtzi I, et al. Human immunodeficiency virus infection and pneumothorax. J Thorac Dis 2014;6(Suppl 4):S377–82.
57. Kovacs JA, Hiemenz JW, Macher AM, et al. Pneumocystis carinii pneumonia: a comparison between patients with the acquired immunodeficiency syndrome and patients with other immunodeficiencies. Ann Intern Med 1984;100(5): 663–71.
58. Ng VL, Yajko DM, Hadley WK. Extrapulmonary pneumocystosis. Clin Microbiol Rev 1997;10(3):401–18.
59. DeLorenzo LJ, Huang CT, Maguire GP, et al. Roentgenographic patterns of Pneumocystis carinii pneumonia in 104 patients with AIDS. Chest 1987;91(3): 323–7.
60. Boiselle PM, Crans C Jr, Kaplan MA. The changing face of Pneumocystis carinii pneumonia in AIDS patients. AJR Am J Roentgenol 1999;172(5):1301–9.
61. Kanne JP, Yandow DR, Meyer CA. Pneumocystis jiroveci pneumonia: high-resolution CT findings in patients with and without HIV infection. AJR-American Journal of Roentgenology 2012;198(6):W555.
62. Vogel M, Vatlach M, Weissgerber P, et al. HRCT-features of Pneumocystis jiroveci pneumonia and their evolution before and after treatment in non-HIV immunocompromised patients. Eur J Radiol 2012;81(6):1315–20.
63. Lu CL, Hung CC. Reversible cystic lesions of Pneumocystis jirovecii pneumonia. Am J Respir Crit Care Med 2012;185(6):e7–8.
64. Dako F, Kako B, Nirag J, et al. High-resolution CT, histopathologic, and clinical features of granulomatous pneumocystis jiroveci pneumonia. Radiol Case Rep 2019;14(6):746–9.
65. Thomas J, Limper AH, editors. Pneumocystis pneumonia: clinical presentation and diagnosis in patients with and without acquired immune deficiency syndrome. Seminars in respiratory infections. WB Saunders Ltd; 1998.
66. Askin FB, Katzenstein AL. Pneumocystis infection masquerading as diffuse alveolar damage: a potential source of diagnostic error. Chest 1981;79(4): 420–2.
67. Hartel PH, Shilo K, Klassen-Fischer M, et al. Granulomatous reaction to pneumocystis jirovecii: clinicopathologic review of 20 cases. Am J Surg Pathol 2010; 34(5):730–4.

68. Chandra P, Delaney MD, Tuazon CU. Role of special stains in the diagnosis of Pneumocystis carinii infection from bronchial washing specimens in patients with the acquired immune deficiency syndrome. Acta Cytol 1988;32(1):105–8.

69. Lim SK, Eveland WC, Porter RJ. Direct fluorescent-antibody method for the diagnosis of Pneumocystis carinii pneumonitis from sputa or tracheal aspirates from humans. Appl Microbiol 1974;27(1):144–9.

70. Costa JM, Botterel F, Cabaret O, et al. Association between circulating DNA, serum (1->3)-β-D-glucan, and pulmonary fungal burden in Pneumocystis pneumonia. Clin Infect Dis 2012;55(2):e5–8.

71. Damiani C, Le Gal S, Goin N, et al. Usefulness of (1,3) ß-D-glucan detection in bronchoalveolar lavage samples in Pneumocystis pneumonia and Pneumocystis pulmonary colonization. J Mycol Med 2015;25(1):36–43.

72. Karageorgopoulos DE, Qu JM, Korbila IP, et al. Accuracy of β-D-glucan for the diagnosis of Pneumocystis jirovecii pneumonia: a meta-analysis. Clin Microbiol Infect 2013;19(1):39–49.

73. Yasuoka A, Tachikawa N, Shimada K, et al. (1->3) beta-D-glucan as a quantitative serological marker for Pneumocystis carinii pneumonia. Clin Diagn Lab Immunol 1996;3(2):197–9.

74. Li WJ, Guo YL, Liu TJ, et al. Diagnosis of pneumocystis pneumonia using serum (1-3)-β-D-Glucan: a bivariate meta-analysis and systematic review. J Thorac Dis 2015;7(12):2214–25.

75. Onishi A, Sugiyama D, Kogata Y, et al. Diagnostic accuracy of serum 1, 3-β-D-glucan for Pneumocystis jiroveci pneumonia, invasive candidiasis, and invasive aspergillosis: systematic review and meta-analysis. J Clin Microbiol 2012; 50(1):7–15.

76. Tasaka S, Kobayashi S, Yagi K, et al. Serum (1→ 3) β-D-glucan assay for discrimination between Pneumocystis jirovecii pneumonia and colonization. J Infect Chemother 2014;20(11):678–81.

77. Matsumura Y, Ito Y, Iinuma Y, et al. Quantitative real-time PCR and the (1→ 3)-β-D-glucan assay for differentiation between Pneumocystis jirovecii pneumonia and colonization. Clin Microbiol Infect 2012;18(6):591–7.

78. Alosaimy S, Nauffal M, Soiffer R, et al. Defibrotide formulations contain (1→3)-β-D-glucan that could influence clinical diagnostic testing. Bone Marrow Transplant 2020;55(10):2045–6.

79. Marty FM, Lowry CM, Lempitski SJ, et al. Reactivity of (1->3)-beta-d-glucan assay with commonly used intravenous antimicrobials. Antimicrobial Agents Chemother 2006;50(10):3450–3.

80. Egger M, Prüller F, Raggam R, et al. False positive serum levels of (1-3)-ß-D-Glucan after infusion of intravenous immunoglobulins and time to normalisation. J Infect 2017;76.

81. Tschopp J, Brunel AS, Spertini O, et al. High false-positive rate of (1,3)-β-D-Glucan in Onco-hematological patients receiving immunoglobulins and therapeutic antibodies. Clin Infect Dis 2022;75(2):330–3.

82. Morjaria S, Frame J, Franco-Garcia A, et al. Clinical Performance of (1,3) Beta-D Glucan for the Diagnosis of Pneumocystis Pneumonia (PCP) in Cancer Patients Tested With PCP Polymerase Chain Reaction. Clin Infect Dis 2019;69(8):1303–9.

83. Alanio A, Hauser PM, Lagrou K, et al. ECIL guidelines for the diagnosis of Pneumocystis jirovecii pneumonia in patients with haematological malignancies and stem cell transplant recipients. J Antimicrob Chemother 2016;71(9):2386–96.

84. Flori P, Bellete B, Durand F, et al. Comparison between real-time PCR, conventional PCR and different staining techniques for diagnosing Pneumocystis

jiroveci pneumonia from bronchoalveolar lavage specimens. J Med Microbiol 2004;53(7):603–7.

85. Reid AB, Chen SC-A, Worth LJ. Pneumocystis jirovecii pneumonia in non-HIV-infected patients: new risks and diagnostic tools. Curr Opin Infect Dis 2011; 24(6):534–44.

86. Sasso M, Chastang-Dumas E, Bastide S, et al. Performances of Four Real-Time PCR Assays for Diagnosis of Pneumocystis jirovecii Pneumonia. J Clin Microbiol 2016;54(3):625–30.

87. Fauchier T, Hasseine L, Gari-Toussaint M, et al. Detection of pneumocystis jirovecii by quantitative PCR to differentiate colonization and pneumonia in immunocompromised HIV-positive and HIV-negative patients. J Clin Microbiol 2016; 54(6):1487–95.

88. Alanio A, Desoubeaux G, Sarfati C, et al. Real-time PCR assay-based strategy for differentiation between active Pneumocystis jirovecii pneumonia and colonization in immunocompromised patients. Clin Microbiol Infect 2011;17(10): 1531–7.

89. Botterel F, Cabaret O, Foulet F, et al. Clinical significance of quantifying Pneumocystis jirovecii DNA by using real-time PCR in bronchoalveolar lavage fluid from immunocompromised patients. J Clin Microbiol 2012;50(2):227–31.

90. Morjaria S, Frame J, Franco-Garcia A, et al. Clinical Performance of (1,3) Beta-D glucan for the diagnosis of pneumocystis pneumonia (PCP) in cancer patients tested with PCP polymerase chain reaction. Clin Infect Dis 2018;69(8):1303–9.

91. Damiani C, Le Gal S, Da Costa C, et al. Combined quantification of pulmonary Pneumocystis jirovecii DNA and serum (1->3)-β-D-glucan for differential diagnosis of pneumocystis pneumonia and Pneumocystis colonization. J Clin Microbiol 2013;51(10):3380–8.

92. Gits-Muselli M, White PL, Mengoli C, et al. The Fungal PCR Initiative's evaluation of in-house and commercial Pneumocystis jirovecii qPCR assays: Toward a standard for a diagnostics assay. Med Mycol 2019;58(6):779–88.

93. Moreno A, Epstein D, Budvytiene I, et al. Accuracy of pneumocystis jirovecii plasma cell-free DNA PCR for noninvasive diagnosis of pneumocystis pneumonia. J Clin Microbiol 2022;60(5):e0010122.

94. Foong KS, Mabayoje M, AlMajali A. Clinical impact of noninvasive plasma microbial cell-free deoxyribonucleic acid sequencing for the diagnosis and management of pneumocystis jirovecii pneumonia: a single-center retrospective study. Open Forum Infect Dis 2022;9(12).

95. Vogel M, Weissgerber P, Goeppert B, et al. Accuracy of serum LDH elevation for the diagnosis of Pneumocystis jiroveci pneumonia. Swiss Med Wkly 2011;141: w13184.

96. Singer F, Talavera W, Zumoff B. Elevated levels of angiotensin-converting enzyme in Pneumocystis carinii pneumonia. Chest 1989;95(4):803–6.

97. Hamroun A, Lenain R, Bui Nguyen L, et al. Hypercalcemia is common during Pneumocystis pneumonia in kidney transplant recipients. Sci Rep 2019;9(1): 12508.

98. Esteves F, Calé SS, Badura R, et al. Diagnosis of Pneumocystis pneumonia: evaluation of four serologic biomarkers. Clin Microbiol Infect 2015;21(4). 379.e1-10.

99. Bennett JE, Dolin R, Blaser MJ. Mandell, douglas, and bennett's principles and practice of infectious diseases E-book. Elsevier Health Sciences; 2019.

100. Maschmeyer G, Helweg-Larsen J, Pagano L, et al. ECIL guidelines for treatment of Pneumocystis jirovecii pneumonia in non-HIV-infected haematology patients. J Antimicrob Chemother 2016;71(9):2405–13.

101. Walzer PD, Foy J, Steele P, et al. Activities of antifolate, antiviral, and other drugs in an immunosuppressed rat model of Pneumocystis carinii pneumonia. Antimicrobial Agents Chemother 1992;36(9):1935–42.

102. Young LS. Trimethoprim-sulfamethoxazole in the treatment of adults with pneumonia due to Pneumocystis carinii. Rev Infect Dis 1982;4(2):608–13.

103. Sattler FR, Cowan R, Nielsen DM, et al. Trimethoprim-sulfamethoxazole compared with pentamidine for treatment of Pneumocystis carinii pneumonia in the acquired immunodeficiency syndrome. A prospective, noncrossover study. Ann Intern Med 1988;109(4):280–7.

104. Klein NC, Duncanson FP, Lenox TH, et al. Trimethoprim-sulfamethoxazole versus pentamidine for Pneumocystis carinii pneumonia in AIDS patients: results of a large prospective randomized treatment trial. AIDS 1992;6(3):301–5.

105. Wharton JM, Coleman DL, Wofsy CB, et al. Trimethoprim-sulfamethoxazole or pentamidine for Pneumocystis carinii pneumonia in the acquired immunodeficiency syndrome. A prospective randomized trial. Ann Intern Med 1986; 105(1):37–44.

106. Safrin S, Finkelstein DM, Feinberg J, et al. Comparison of three regimens for treatment of mild to moderate Pneumocystis carinii pneumonia in patients with AIDS. A double-blind, randomized, trial of oral trimethoprim-sulfamethoxazole, dapsone-trimethoprim, and clindamycin-primaquine. ACTG 108 Study Group. Ann Intern Med 1996;124(9):792–802.

107. Jick H. Adverse reactions to trimethoprim-sulfamethoxazole in hospitalized patients. Rev Infect Dis 1982;4(2):426–8.

108. Lin D, Li WK, Rieder MJ. Cotrimoxazole for prophylaxis or treatment of opportunistic infections of HIV/AIDS in patients with previous history of hypersensitivity to cotrimoxazole. Cochrane Database Syst Rev 2007;(2).

109. Queener SF, Bartlett MS, Richardson JD, et al. Activity of clindamycin with primaquine against Pneumocystis carinii in vitro and in vivo. Antimicrobial Agents Chemother 1988;32(6):807–13.

110. Smego RA Jr, Nagar S, Maloba B, et al. A meta-analysis of salvage therapy for Pneumocystis carinii pneumonia. Arch Intern Med 2001;161(12):1529–33.

111. Benfield T, Atzori C, Miller RF, et al. Second-line salvage treatment of AIDS-associated Pneumocystis jirovecii pneumonia: a case series and systematic review. J Acquir Immune Defic Syndr 2008;48(1):63–7.

112. Hughes W, Leoung G, Kramer F, et al. Comparison of Atovaquone (566C80) with Trimethoprim-Sulfamethoxazole to Treat Pneumocystis carinii Pneumonia in Patients with AIDS. N Engl J Med 1993;328(21):1521–7.

113. Dohn MN, Weinberg WG, Torres RA, et al. Oral atovaquone compared with intravenous pentamidine for Pneumocystis carinii pneumonia in patients with AIDS. Atovaquone Study Group. Ann Intern Med 1994;121(3):174–80.

114. Barclay JA, Ziemba SE, Ibrahim RB. Dapsone-induced methemoglobinemia: a primer for clinicians. Ann Pharmacother 2011;45(9):1103–15.

115. Wang LI, Liang H, Ye LI, et al. Adjunctive corticosteroids for the treatment of Pneumocystis jiroveci pneumonia in patients with HIV: A meta-analysis. Exp Ther Med 2016;11(2):683–7.

116. Injean P, Eells SJ, Wu H, et al. A Systematic Review and meta-analysis of the data behind current recommendations for corticosteroids in Non-HIV-Related

PCP: knowing when you are on shaky foundations. Transplant Direct 2017;3(3): e137.

117. Fishman JA, Gans H. Pneumocystis jiroveci in solid organ transplantation: Guidelines from the American Society of Transplantation Infectious Diseases Community of Practice. Clin Transplant 2019;33(9):e13587.

118. Consensus statement on the use of corticosteroids as adjunctive therapy for pneumocystis pneumonia in the acquired immunodeficiency syndrome. N Engl J Med 1990;323(21):1500–4.

119. Cushion MT, Linke MJ, Ashbaugh A, et al. Echinocandin treatment of pneumocystis pneumonia in rodent models depletes cysts leaving trophic burdens that cannot transmit the infection. PLoS One 2010;5(1):e8524.

120. Bartlett MS, Current WL, Goheen MP, et al. Semisynthetic echinocandins affect cell wall deposition of Pneumocystis carinii in vitro and in vivo. Antimicrobial Agents Chemother 1996;40(8):1811–6.

121. Lobo ML, Esteves F, de Sousa B, et al. Therapeutic potential of caspofungin combined with trimethoprim-sulfamethoxazole for pneumocystis pneumonia: a pilot study in mice. PLoS One 2013;8(8):e70619.

122. Huang YS, Liu CE, Lin SP, et al. Echinocandins as alternative treatment for HIV-infected patients with Pneumocystis pneumonia. AIDS 2019;33(8):1345–51.

123. Chen PY, Yu CJ, Chien JY, et al. Anidulafungin as an alternative treatment for Pneumocystis jirovecii pneumonia in patients who cannot tolerate trimethoprim/sulfamethoxazole. Int J Antimicrob Agents 2020;55(1):105820.

124. Nevez G, Le Gal S. Caspofungin and pneumocystis pneumonia: it is time to go ahead. Antimicrobial Agents Chemother 2019;63(10).

125. Cushion M, Ashbaugh A, Borroto-Esoda K, et al. SCY-078 demonstrates anti-fungal activity against Pneumocystis in a prophylactic murine model of Pneumocystis pneumonia. ASM Microbe Online 2018. 00244–18.

126. Cushion MT, Ashbaugh A. The long-acting echinocandin, rezafungin, prevents pneumocystis pneumonia and eliminates pneumocystis from the lungs in prophylaxis and murine treatment models. J Fungi 2021;7(9):747.

127. Rauseo AM, Coler-Reilly A, Larson L, et al. Hope on the horizon: novel fungal treatments in development. Open Forum Infect Dis 2020;7(2):ofaa016.

128. Zhu M, Ye N, Xu J. Clinical characteristics and prevalence of dihydropteroate synthase gene mutations in Pneumocystis jirovecii-infected AIDS patients from low endemic areas of China. PLoS One 2020;15(9):e0238184.

129. Huang L, Beard CB, Creasman J, et al. Sulfa or sulfone prophylaxis and geographic region predict mutations in the Pneumocystis carinii dihydropteroate synthase gene. J Infect Dis 2000;182(4):1192–8.

130. Navin TR, Beard CB, Huang L, et al. Effect of mutations in Pneumocystis carinii dihydropteroate synthase gene on outcome of P carinii pneumonia in patients with HIV-1: a prospective study. Lancet 2001;358(9281):545–9.

131. Argy N, Le Gal S, Coppée R, et al. Pneumocystis cytochrome b mutants associated with atovaquone prophylaxis failure as the cause of Pneumocystis infection outbreak among heart transplant recipients. Clin Infect Dis 2018;67(6): 913–9.

132. Kazanjian P, Armstrong W, Hossler PA, et al. Pneumocystis carinii cytochrome b mutations are associated with atovaquone exposure in patients with AIDS. J Infect Dis 2001;183(5):819–22.

133. Ponce CA, Chabé M, George C, et al. High prevalence of pneumocystis jirovecii dihydropteroate synthase gene mutations in patients with a first episode of

pneumocystis pneumonia in santiago, chile, and clinical response to trimethoprim-sulfamethoxazole therapy. Antimicrobial Agents Chemother 2017;61(2).

134. Green H, Paul M, Vidal L, et al. Prophylaxis of Pneumocystis pneumonia in immunocompromised non-HIV-infected patients: systematic review and meta-analysis of randomized controlled trials. Mayo Clin Proc 2007;82(9):1052–9.

135. Fishman JA, Gans H. Practice tAIDCo. Pneumocystis jiroveci in solid organ transplantation: guidelines from the American Society of Transplantation Infectious Diseases Community of Practice. Clin Transplant 2019;33(9):e13587.

136. Mejia CD, Malat GE, Boyle SM, et al. Experience with a six-month regimen of Pneumocystis pneumonia prophylaxis in 122 HIV-positive kidney transplant recipients. Transpl Infect Dis 2021;23(3):e13511.

137. Prasad GVR, Beckley J, Mathur M, et al. Safety and efficacy of prophylaxis for Pneumocystis jirovecii pneumonia involving trimethoprim-sulfamethoxazole dose reduction in kidney transplantation. BMC Infect Dis 2019;19(1):311.

138. Wiederhold NP, Patterson TF, Rebholz S, et al. The antifungal and anti-pneumocystis activities of the novel compound A3IS (Mycosinate). Antimicrobial Agents Chemother 2022;66(8):e0052122.

Organ Donors with Human Immunodeficiency Virus and Hepatitis C Virus

Expanding the Donor Pool

Jordan Salas, BS[a,b], Kaitlyn Storm, BS[a],
Christine M. Durand, MD[a,*]

KEYWORDS

- Direct-acting antiviral agents • Hepatitis C virus • Solid organ transplantation
- Deceased donor transplantation • HIV Organ Policy Equity Act
- Antiretroviral therapy • HIV transplantation

KEY POINTS

- As the HIV Organ Policy Equity Act legalized transplantation using organs from donors with HIV for recipients with HIV (HIV D+/R+), pilot clinical trials of HIV D+/R+ kidney and liver transplantation have shown excellent short-term outcomes.
- The scope of HIV D+/R+ transplantation and the number of donors with HIV can be optimized by increasing donor education and registration, maximizing donor evaluation and organ recovery, and increasing awareness of HIV D+/R+ transplantation among transplant centers and candidates.
- Owing to the efficacy of direct-acting antivirals, transplantation of organs from donors with hepatitis C virus (HCV) to recipients without HCV (HCV D+/R−) has been safe and effective.
- With HCV D+/R− transplantation, debate remains over whether to give direct-acting antivirals as prophylaxis, before transplant or to give direct-acting antivirals as treatment posttransplant, after HCV transmission with pros and cons for each approach.

INTRODUCTION

People living with human immunodeficiency virus (PLWH) have been living longer and developing more comorbidities with age, such as end-stage liver disease and end-stage renal disease.[1] These conditions have made solid organ transplantation more common and necessary to extend the lifespan and improve the quality of life of PLWH.

[a] Department of Medicine, Johns Hopkins University School of Medicine, 2000 East Monument Street, Baltimore, MD 21205, USA; [b] Department of Medicine, Oregon Health & Science University School of Medicine, 3181 Southwest Sam Jackson Park Road, Portland, OR, USA
* Corresponding author. 2000 East Monument Street, Baltimore, MD 21205.
E-mail address: christinedurand@jhmi.edu

Infect Dis Clin N Am 37 (2023) 641–658
https://doi.org/10.1016/j.idc.2023.04.003
0891-5520/23/© 2023 Elsevier Inc. All rights reserved.
id.theclinics.com

Although transplantation research is continually developing novel ways of improving access to organs, in 2022, approximately 106,000 people were on transplant waiting lists in the United States.[2] Furthermore, roughly 8000 people die annually waiting for an organ.[2] The organ shortage especially impacts PLWH as they have decreased access to transplantation[3] and increased waitlist mortality.[4]

Using organs from donors with treatable infections is one strategy to increase the quality and number of organs available. The use of organs from donors with human immunodeficiency virus for recipients with human immunodeficiency virus (HIV D+/R+) was made possible by the human immunodeficiency virus Organ Policy Equity (HOPE) Act passed in 2013, which allows HIV D+/R+ transplantation under research protocols.[5] The use of organs from donors with Hepatitis C virus (HCV) infection has always been legal; however, in practice, their use has recently been expanded to recipients without HCV (HCV D+/R−) with the emergence of safe, highly effective direct-acting antivirals (DAAs), which are effective and well-tolerated in transplant recipients.[6–9]

In this article, the authors review the historical context and increasing body of evidence showing promising HIV D+/R+ kidney and liver transplantation outcomes. The authors also discuss the historical context and outcomes of HCV D+/R− kidney, liver, heart, and lung transplantation. Finally, the authors examine the challenges of implementation, potential complications of these innovative practices, and the next steps in further improving outcomes.

Historical Context of HIV and Solid Organ Transplantation

Starting in the 1980s, before the development of antiretroviral therapy (ART), transplantation was not standard therapy for transplant candidates living with human immunodeficiency virus (HIV). The literature was limited to the cases where HIV was unintentionally transmitted to transplant recipients or discovered after transplant, in which case outcomes were poor with 6-month mortality rates around 50% for kidney and liver recipients.[10] In the late 1990s, ART reduced opportunistic infections and mortality rates in PLWH. Owing to these advancements, Stock and colleagues conducted the national institutes of health-funded HIV Transplant Recipient (HIVTR) Study from 2003 to 2009 at 19 US transplant centers.[11] In this observational study, 150 kidney and 125 liver transplant recipients with HIV received organs from donors without HIV (HIV D−/R+).[11–13] Participants in HIVTR had good outcomes, and this study paved the way for a growing experience of HIV D−/R+ transplants in the United States with a survival benefit for both kidney[14] and liver[12] transplantation compared to remaining on the waitlist.[12,14] As such, there was a growing need for organs for PLWH in need of a transplant.

In parallel, in South Africa, PLWH and end-stage renal disease did not have dialysis access, and the urgency for novel donor sources was even greater. Renal transplant surgeon Dr. Elmi Muller pioneered the first HIV D+/R+ kidney transplants, providing proof of concept that this was a safe and feasible option.[15] However, this practice was not feasible in the United States due to a 1988 amendment of the National Organ Transplant Act (NOTA), which banned the use of organs from donors with HIV to prevent unintentional transmission by transplantation. Researchers in the United States explored the potential impact of reversing the NOTA amendment and examined several national registries, estimating 500 to 600 potential deceased donors with HIV per year, providing a compelling argument for HIV D+/R+ transplantation.[16] The early experience from South Africa, coupled with the significant number of potential donors with HIV in the United States and support from dozens of medical, transplant, and advocacy organizations, led to the passage of the HOPE Act in 2013.[17]

The HOPE Act reversed the prior ban on the use of organs from donors with HIV and allowed HIV D+/R+ transplantation under research protocols.[5] In 2015, the National Institutes of Health published HOPE Safeguards and Research criteria to regulate HIV D+/R+ transplantation and ensure the safety of transplant recipients, healthcare workers, and the public.[5,18] Theoretical risks to transplant recipients included HIV breakthrough viremia due to donor-to-recipient HIV superinfection, increased risk of allograft rejection, opportunistic infections, and HIV-related organ disease in the allograft.[19]

HIV ORGAN POLICY EQUITY ACT SAFEGUARDS AND RESEARCH REQUIREMENTS

To promote successful outcomes of HIV D+/R+ transplantation, centers should have knowledge and expertise in transplantation for PLWH, which requires effective multidisciplinary collaboration between transplant medicine, infectious diseases, and pharmacists. For example, teams need to understand drug interactions between antiretrovirals and transplant immunosuppressants. Historically, these have been complex, as antiretroviral drugs that strongly induce or inhibit CYP3A4 (eg, etravirine, ritonavir, cobicistat) impact levels of calcineurin inhibitors, such as tacrolimus, which are essential to preventing rejection and have toxicity when levels are too high. Fortunately, this is becoming less of a challenge with the advent of integrase strand transferase inhibitors which do not have significant interactions and allow clinicians to avoid other antiretrovirals.[20] Specifically, the HOPE Act Safeguard and Research Criteria require that the centers meet the minimum experience criteria, and teams must have experience with five HIV D−/R+ transplants of the specific organ type before they are allowed to open a protocol of HIV D+/R+ transplantation of that organ.[18] Although there is no evidence that a specific threshold of center-level experience is associated with better outcomes of HIV D−/R+,[21] these safeguards were developed to ensure teams had some experience and knowledge.

Another important consideration is communication between the transplant center team and the Organ Procurement Organizations (OPOs), the nonprofit organizations contracted to evaluate deceased organ donors. OPOs need to gather a comprehensive infectious disease history of potential donors. The primary goal is to exclude donors with active acquired immune deficiency syndrome-defining opportunistic infections, such as cryptococcal meningitis, as their organs cannot be used under the current HOPE Act regulations.[18] In addition, efforts to gather any ART treatment history and history of resistance are to identify donors with multidrug-resistant HIV, which may increase the risk of HIV superinfection and breakthrough with a resistant strain of virus. Transplant teams can elect to use donors with detectable viral loads, treated or untreated, including donors with a history of ART resistance, as long as they can define posttransplant antiretroviral regimens for the recipients that are safe, tolerable, and effective. In practice, challenges may arise in obtaining complete medical histories for potential donors, especially with limited information available and/or known at the time of donor evaluation.

EARLY OUTCOMES OF THE HIV ORGAN POLICY EQUITY ACT IN KIDNEY TRANSPLANTATION

The first prospective multicenter pilot study of HIV D+/R+ deceased donor kidney transplants under HOPE in the United States was conducted at 14 transplant centers from March 2016 to July 2019.[22] Investigators compared outcomes in 25 HIV D+/R+ kidney transplants with 50 HIV D−/R+ kidney transplants. Results in recipients were encouraging, with no deaths, no differences in 1-year graft survival (91% D+ vs 92%

D−), HIV breakthrough (4% D+ vs 6% D−), infectious hospitalizations (28% D+ vs 26% D−), or opportunistic infections (16% D+ vs 12% D−).[22] Of note, 60% of HIV D+ in this study were ART-experienced in contrast to the earlier South African studies,[23] in which 92% of HIV D+ were ART-naïve. Despite an ART-experienced donor pool in the study population, no episodes of HIV superinfection were observed even after an in-depth virologic analysis.[24] The pilot study observed that rejection was common, and there was a trend toward a higher rate in HIV D+/R+ versus HIV D−/R+ (50% vs 29% D−, $P = .13$), which merits further investigation.[22]

OUTCOMES OF THE HIV ORGAN POLICY EQUITY ACT IN LIVER TRANSPLANTATION

In parallel with the HOPE kidney pilot, the first prospective multicenter pilot study of HIV D+/R+ deceased donor liver transplantation under HOPE was conducted at nine transplant centers from March 2016 to July 2019.[25] It included 45 transplants, 24 HIV D+/R+ compared with 21 HIV D−/R+. In contrast to the HOPE kidney transplant pilot study, HIV D+/R+ liver transplant recipients had higher mortality; however, 1-year survival was good in both groups (HIV D+/R+ 83% vs HIV D−/R+ 100%)[25] and better than in historical cohorts such as HIVTR which had a 1-year patient survival of 76%.[13] Moreover, there were no significant differences in 1-year graft survival (96% D+ vs 100% D−), allograft rejection (10.8% D+ vs 18.2% D−), HIV breakthrough (8% D+ vs 10% D−), or serious adverse events (SAEs) (all $P > .05$).[25] In a weighted analysis, HIV D+/R+ were more likely to have an opportunistic infection; however, these were primarily cytomegalovirus (CMV) viremia, which is one of the most common opportunistic infections posttransplant.[26] The weighted analysis also found a shorter time to incident cancer among HIV D+/R+, primarily viral-associated malignancies, including three cases of human herpes virus 8-related cancer.[25] Thus, although HIV D+/R+ liver transplantation was associated with good short-term patient and graft survival, further investigation of post-transplant infections and malignancies is needed.

HIV FALSE-POSITIVE HOPE DONORS

An unexpected benefit of the HOPE Act was the discovery of another novel donor source, termed false-positive (FP) donors. FP donors are donors with no known history of HIV who have discordant HIV screening tests, which include either a positive anti-HIV antibody or an HIV nucleic acid test (NAT). Organs from FP donors were mainly discarded before the HOPE Act due to potential concerns of a true positive test and lack of confirmatory testing. However, the utilization of HIV D+ for recipients with HIV under HOPE has circumvented these concerns. Based on the annual number of donors screened in the United States and the FP rates of HIV screening assays, the potential FP donor pool was estimated to be approximately 50 to 100 HIV FP donors annually.[27] Although this is a small increase in donors compared with the current waitlist, maximizing every organ is critical, particularly for recipients with HIV, who already face disparities in organ access and waitlist mortality. Of note, the national registry does not collect data to distinguish FP donors from true D+.[28] Thus, studies that rely only on the OPTN database will not be able to accurately measure the impact of biological HIV infection in donors on transplant outcomes.[28,29]

HOPE DONOR CLINICAL, IMMUNOLOGIC, AND VIROLOGIC PROFILES

In a national HOPE donor landscape study by Werbel and colleagues, clinical, virologic, and immunologic characteristics of 92 deceased donors under the Hope Act were examined between March 2016 and March 2020, including 58 true D+ and 34 HIV FP donors.[30] In this study, D+ had a median age of 36 years, 27% were Black, 22% were White, and 76% were male. Most D+ (71%) had a known HIV diagnosis, but 29% were discovered to have HIV upon their death. Of those with known HIV, 90% were prescribed ART. Overall, the median HIV viral load was 882, and the median CD4 count was 194. Investigators in this study were particularly interested in ART drug-resistance mutations in individuals, and genotype results were successfully obtained in 47 donors. Major ART drug-resistance mutations were frequent (42%), but integrase strand transfer inhibitors (4%) and multiclass mutations (%13) were rare.[30] Overall, this was reassuring of a low risk of HIV breakthrough due to resistant virus as most transplant recipients are on integrase strand transfer inhibitor-based ART to avoid drug–drug interactions with transplant immunosuppressants.[31,32]

BARRIERS TO MAXIMIZING THE POTENTIAL OF THE HIV ORGAN POLICY EQUITY ACT

In the first 4 years of HOPE, 92 deceased D+ had organs recovered for a transplant which is below the estimated donor pool.[30] Many factors likely contribute to the gap between potential and actual donors, including attitudes and beliefs of PLWH regarding donation, slow assimilation of new medical practices by the OPOs who evaluate donors and transplant centers, and transplant recipients' willingness to accept D+ organs. To better understand the gap in predicted and actual HOPE donors, the authors discuss the factors that might affect HIV D+/R+ transplantation at various levels of the transplant system, highlighted in **Fig. 1**.

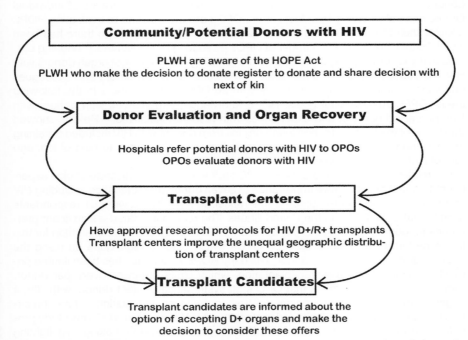

Fig. 1. Factors impacting HIV D+/R+ transplantation are complex and multifaceted, involving several aspects of the transplantation process.

Potential Donors with HIV

The decision to donate by PLWH is a cornerstone of HIV D+/R+ transplantation. In a 2018 study by Nguyen and colleagues, 114 PLWH were surveyed regarding their knowledge, attitudes, and beliefs about organ donation and transplantation at an urban academic HIV clinic in Baltimore, MD.[33] Most respondents were willing to become deceased donors (79.8%) or living donors (62.3%), and 80.7% were aware of the US organ shortage. However, only 24.6% knew about the HOPE Act, and only 21.1% were registered donors. This is very low compared with the registration rate in people without HIV, as reports in 2019 suggested that approximately 58% of the US general population are registered donors.[34] Improving knowledge in this population and increasing the number of registered HOPE donors is an important first step.[33]

A 2022 study by Haidar and colleagues addressed this discrepancy between the supply and demand of organs in this population by designing an intervention to increase the number of registered donors among PLWH at the University of Pittsburgh Medical Centers' Ryan White-funded HIV clinic.[35] In partnership with their local OPO, between July 2018 and April 2019, 856 PLWH completed donor registration cards. Before the intervention, only 11.4% (98/856) of PLWH were registered donors; after the intervention, the proportion increased to 46.7% (400/856). These promising results show how providing education and an opportunity for donor registration can impact potential donors with HIV.

Role of Organ Procurement Organizations in the HIV Organ Policy Equity Act

OPOs are nonprofit organizations contracted by the federal government to evaluate donors and recover organs for transplant in the United States. There are 58 individual OPOs, generally serving their local state. OPOs are the frontline to evaluating HOPE donors; therefore, maximizing their engagement is critical. Although there has been a significant increase in the number of OPOs evaluating HOPE donors,[36] ongoing barriers at the OPO level may contribute to the relatively low number of organ donors with HIV. To better understand these issues, in a 2022 study, Predmore and colleagues conducted semi-structured interviews with 20 OPO staff members in the following areas: OPO organizational goals, HOPE knowledge, experiences with donors with HIV, perceived barriers, and experiences with research initiatives.[37] Results showed that some of the barriers to recovering organs from donors with HIV included obtaining authorization for donation, concerns about disclosing HIV status to next of kin, and fear of HIV infection in those involved in organ recovery.

In a related study, Predmore asked OPO staff to complete a discrete choice experiment to quantify the relative importance of seven donor characteristics, including HIV status, on the decision to pursue a theoretical donor.[38] There were 51 respondents from 36 out of 58 OPOs in the United States. The results indicated a significant preference for donors without HIV over donors with HIV. One potential explanation for this is the performance metrics used by OPOs which place a high value on using the largest number of organs per donor. The early HOPE experience has been limited primarily to kidney and liver transplantation, which limits organ recovery per donor. Although this does not mean that OPO staff systematically reject donors with HIV, it suggests that these two groups are not treated the same. In situations where the capacity to pursue donors is limited, donors without HIV are preferred.[38] This study provides insight into the processes of OPO triage and decision-making, highlighting another step in the transplant process that could be addressed to increase the D+ pool (see **Fig. 1**).

TRANSPLANT CENTER INVOLVEMENT IN THE HIV ORGAN POLICY EQUITY ACT

Successful implementation of HIV D+/R+ transplantation requires that transplant centers are appropriately informed and prepared for this practice. A study in 2018 by Van Pilsum Rasmussen and colleagues surveyed 209 transplant centers and 114 responded.[39] Of the 114 responding centers, 50 had planned HIV D+/R+ protocols and were primarily located in the eastern United States. Centers planning HIV D+/R+ protocols were large volume programs, historically had more transplant recipients with HIV, and were located in areas with increased HIV prevalence ($P < .01$). Centers not planning HIV D+/R+ protocols were more likely to believe that transplant candidates with HIV would not accept organs from D+ ($P < .001$). Barriers at the transplant center level shown in this study include the relatively low proportion of centers planning HIV D+/R+ transplantation, geographic clustering on the coasts, and provider concerns that transplant candidates with HIV would not be willing to accept organs from D+.

Effective execution of the HOPE Act protocol in HIV D+/R+ transplantation requires a collaborative effort that involves various medical disciplines working together. It necessitates an in-depth understanding of drug interactions, as patients living with HIV may be on multiple medications, both for their HIV and any other underlying health conditions. Hence, a thorough knowledge of how these drugs may interact with one another, as well as with the immunosuppressive drugs required for transplantation, is crucial for successful implantation. In addition, a clear understanding of the critical components involved in the transplantation process, such as the evaluation of the donor and recipient with HIV, the surgical procedure itself, and postoperative care, is also vital to ensure positive outcomes. These elements must all be taken into consideration to provide the best possible care for patients undergoing HIV D+/R+ transplantation.

Transplant Recipients' Willingness to Accept Organs from Donors with HIV

Although increasing the D+ pool could mitigate the reduced access to transplantation and increaed waitlist mortality in PLWH, this depends on whether transplant candidates with HIV are willing to accept D+ organs. In a 2020 study by Seaman and colleagues, investigators surveyed transplant candidates living with HIV from nine transplant centers in the United States to understand this better.[40] There were 116 respondents; the median age was 55 years, 68% were male, and 78% were Black. Contrary to the perceptions of transplant centers discussed above, 84% of transplant candidates were willing to accept organs from deceased donors with HIV. Although some candidates had concerns about HIV superinfection (30%) and inferior organ function (16%), the majority were willing to accept a D+ organ and believed this would reduce their waiting time. This study suggests that for transplant candidates, the novel practice of HIV D+/R+ transplantation is acceptable despite potential risks.

Historical Context of Hepatitis C Virus D+/R− Transplantation

In the United States, Hepatitis C virus (HCV) is the most common blood-borne infection and is responsible for more deaths than any other blood-borne infectious disease.[41] The most efficient route of transmission is exposure to blood, and in the United States, the primary risk factor for infection is injection drug use.[42] With the ongoing opioid and injection drug use epidemic, there has been an increase in donors who died of drug overdose and donors with HCV. One national study showed that in 2000, only 1.1% of organ donors had died of a drug overdose, but by 2017, this proportion rose to over 13.4%.[43] Over the same period, HCV seropositivity in these donors rose from 7.8% to 30.0%.[43]

In parallel, the treatment of HCV dramatically changed. Before 2014, HCV infection had to be treated with interferon- and ribavirin-based regimens, which were associated with poor efficacy and low tolerability.[44] However, in 2014, interferon and ribavirin-free direct-acting antiviral (DAA) regimens were approved by the FDA and have been highly effective, achieving sustained virological response (SVR) or HCV cure in nearly 100% of patients.[45] DAAs were quickly integrated into the transplant community and facilitated the expansion of organ transplants from donors with HCV to recipients without HCV (HCV D+/R−). The authors discuss studies supporting the safety of this practice across organ types and trends in this practice in transplantation.

OUTCOMES OF HEPATITIS C VIRUS D+/R− TRANSPLANTATION

One of the first pilot trials of HCV D+/R− kidney transplant was Transplanting Hepatitis C Kidneys into Negative Kidney Recipients (THINKER), published in 2018. The trial included 20 HCV D+/R− kidney transplant recipients from donors with HCV genotype 1.[46] Recipients were tested for HCV starting day 3 posttransplant, and a DAA combination of grazoprevir and elbasvir (GZR/EBR) was given for 12 weeks if virus was detected, which occurred in all participants. Primary outcomes were SVR and adverse events related to HCV or DAAs in the first-year posttransplant.[46] All 20 participants achieved SVR.[46] Five participants exhibited transient elevations in aminotransferase levels; no other HCV infection or treatment-related SAEs were observed, and all 20 recipients exhibited excellent renal function.[46] The median number of days from activation for allografts with HCV to transplant was 57 (interquartile range [IQR] 12–91).[46]

In parallel, the Exploring Renal Transplants Using Hepatitis C Infected Donors for HCV Negative Recipients (EXPANDER) trial was conducted and included 10 HCV D+/R− kidney transplants.[47] In contrast to THINKER, recipients were treated prophylactically with GZR/EBR started immediately before transplantation.[46,47] In addition, donors with genotype 2 or 3 HCV were included, and recipients of organs from these donors were given another DAA, sofosbuvir, in addition to GZR/EBR.[47] HCV prophylaxis was continued for 12 to 16 weeks (depending on genotype). Consistent with THINKER, none of the participants developed chronic HCV infection or experienced rejection, graft loss, or death.[46,47] Before study enrollment, participants had been on the transplant waitlist for a median of 4.2 months (IQR 0.9–18.3) but after enrollment had a median time to transplant of 1 month (IQR 0.7–2).[47]

To better understand the generalizability of HCV D+/R− kidney transplantation, the Multi-center Study to Transplant Hepatitis-C Infected Kidneys (MYTHIC) trial explored this practice at seven centers beginning in 2019. There were 30 HCV D+/R− kidney transplants from donors with HCV-viremia.[48] A pangenotypic DAA regimen of glecaprevir and pibrentasvir (GLE/PIB) was started on day 3 posttransplant and continued for 8 weeks.[48] All 30 participants achieved SVR.[48] Recipients were followed for 25 to 50 weeks posttransplant, during which one participant died of sepsis 4 months post-SVR; three recipients had acute cellular rejection, and three recipients developed polyomavirus (BK) viremia near or greater than 10,000 copies/mL that resolved after immunosuppression reduction.[48] No SAEs were deemed related to HCV infection or treatment.[48] At 1-year posttransplant, there were no cases of liver disease or HCV-related kidney injury.[49] One year survival was 93%, and 1-year graft function was excellent (median creatinine 1.17, IQR 1.02–1.38 mg/dL).[48,49] There were four cases of CMV viremia among 10 recipients without prior CMV who had received transplants from donors with CMV.[49] Moving beyond single-center experiences, MYTHIC confirmed the safety of HCV D+/R− kidney transplantation and found that participants had a 3.5-fold higher cumulative probability of transplant within 1 year versus matched waitlist comparators who did not accept kidneys from donors with HCV.[48,49]

Along with kidney transplants, similar successes have been found with other HCV D+/R− solid organ transplant types. The Using Hepatitis c positive hearts for nEgative Recipients (USHER) trial involved 10 HCV D+/R− heart transplants from donors with HCV genotype 1, followed by treatment with GZR/EBR starting day 3 posttransplant.[50] One recipient died on day 79 posttransplant after experiencing antibody-mediated rejection and multiorgan failure, deemed unrelated to HCV.[50] All of the other nine recipients achieved SVR.[50] Throughout the 18-month study, no SAEs occurred from HCV infection or treatment.[50] The median time from activation to receive HCV D+ hearts to transplant was 39 days.[50]

The Donors of Hepatitis C NAT [nucleic acid amplification test] Positive Thoracic Allografts for Transplantation Evaluation in Non-HCV Recipients (DONATE HCV) study investigated 36 lung and 8 heart HCV D+/R− transplants.[51] All recipients were preemptively treated with sofosbuvir and velpatasvir (SOF/VEL), a pangenotypic DAA regimen, within hours posttransplant for 4 weeks.[51] Although 95% of participants (42 of 44) had a detectable HCV viral load immediately following transplantation, with this postexposure prophylactic regimen, all participants became HCV undetectable approximately 2 weeks posttransplant.[51] Of the first 35 patients that had completed 6 months of follow-up, all had excellent graft function and achieved SVR.[51] No HCV treatment-related SAEs were identified.[51] Although more cases of acute cellular rejection occurred in HCV D+/R− lung transplant recipients compared with recipients of lungs from donors without HCV (HCV D−/R−), the difference was not significant after adjustment for confounding factors.[51] The DONATE study demonstrated the potential for safe HCV + donor to HCV− recipient lung transplantation and illustrated the effectiveness of a shorter DAA regimen when given immediately after transplant.[51]

Although the previously mentioned studies focused primarily on outcomes within 1-year posttransplant, a recent national registry study analyzed 5-year outcomes of HCV D+/R− kidney transplant from July 2016 to December 2021.[52] The study included 4407 HCV D+/R− recipients and 71,498 HCV D−/R−recipients at 217 different centers.[52] After controlling for confounding factors in both donors and recipients, no significant difference was found in 5-year allograft survival between HCV D+/R− and HCV D−/R− groups (72% vs 69%, respective, $P = .47$).[52]

Challenges of Implementing Hepatitis C Virus D+/R− Transplantation

Several barriers impede the success and implementation of HCV D+/R−transplantation. Key among these is the difficulty in securing DAA treatment for recipients promptly. Indeed, DAAs continue to be expensive, and at times, insurance approval remains difficult to obtain; in a study of 28 HCV D+/R− transplants, including 17 kidneys and 11 livers, even after documentation of HCV viremia posttransplant, 35% of initial insurance requests in kidney recipients and 10% of initial insurance requests in liver recipients were rejected and required appeal.[53] One kidney recipient was denied benefit entirely.[53] The median time from submission to insurance approval was 2 days if the initial request was accepted (range 0–35) and 28 days if an appeal was required (range 3–58).[53]

There have been only a handful of documented cases of spontaneous HCV clearance in transplant recipients. However, the likelihood of such clearance in highly immunosuppressed patients is exceedingly low.[54] For the vast majority of transplant recipients, the lengthy approval processes and potential lack of coverage lead to delays in DAA treatment that may be detrimental. A nonindustry-funded study that commenced in July 2018 demonstrated these real-world difficulties with study staff attempting to secure insurance approval for DAA treatments for 14 patients who received livers with HCV.[55] The group found that each patient required a substantial amount of work with time to approval ranging from 24 hours to 10 days.[55] Although ultimately successful in securing DAA treatment for all participants, the group acknowledged that this effort was likely not universal practice and advocated for a system in which insurance preapproves DAA coverage for transplant candidates who receive an organ from a donor with HCV.[55]

Timing of Direct-Acting Antivirals Treatment Strategy in Hepatitis C Virus D+/R− Transplantation

One debate surrounding HCV D+/R− transplantation involves the duration and timing of DAAs. Several studies have explored DAA prophylaxis, beginning before transplant (**Table 1**). The other approach involves a transmit-and-treat approach: starting DAAs after surgery when transmission has occurred. Both methods have potential benefits and unique considerations (**Table 2**). Prophylactic treatment may prevent HCV infection but treating after transmission may be more realistic with insurance requirements and approval timelines.[56]

Although EXPANDER was the first prophylaxis study, more recent studies (see **Table 2**) have supported shorter-duration prophylaxis. The Renal transplants in hepatitis C negative recipients with RNA-positive donors (REHANNA) trial investigated 10 HCV D+/R− kidney transplants with prophylactic GLE/PIB for 4 weeks instead of the full 8-week course.[57] HCV RNA was undetectable in all 10 recipients after 7 days posttransplant, and no SAEs were found to be associated with HCV or DAAs.[57] There were no rejection episodes or deaths, but one graft failed on day 261 posttransplant due to venous thrombosis unrelated to HCV or DAAs.[57] Further shortening the DAA duration, REHANNA-2 (Renal Transplants in Hepatitis C Negative Recipients with Nucleic Acid Positive Donors Using Two Weeks of DAA Prophylaxis) involved 10 HCV D+/R− kidney transplants whose recipients were treated with 2 weeks of GLE/PIB prophylaxis.[58] No participants had evidence of persistent HCV, and there were no SAEs. These

Table 1
Pros and cons of prophylaxis versus transmit-and-treat in hepatitis C virus D+/R− transplantation

Prophylaxis (DAAs Pre- and Posttransplant)	Transmit-and-Treat (DAAs Posttransplant)
Pros:	Pros:
• Reduces or prevents HCV transmission to recipients	• Allows time for insurance approval of DAA regimen
• Allows DAA regimens to be shortened (less costly)	• Allows time for recipients to be extubated and administration of DAA by mouth (PO)
• May lower risk of kidney or liver injury	Cons:
• May lower risk of rejection	• HCV transmission occurs in 100% of cases
Cons:	• Requires full DAA regimen (more costly)
• Requires obtaining insurance approval for treatment in advance of transplant and transmission	• Increases risk of fibrosing cholestatic hepatitis, liver enzyme elevation, HCV-related glomerulonephritis
• The optimal treatment duration is unknown	• May increase risk of posttransplant CMV and BK infections
• HCV transmission may occur if the DAA regimen is too short and may lead to development of DAA resistance	• May increase risk of rejection

Table 2
Hepatitis C virus D+/R− transplantation direct-acting antiviral prophylaxis trials

Author	Study Name	Center	Transplant Recipients (n)	DAA Therapy, Duration (n)	SVR or Transmission Prevention (n, %)
Durand et al,[47] 2018	EXPANDER	Johns Hopkins University	Kidney (10)	Elbasvir/grazoprevir, 12 wk (7)	7/7 (100%)
				Elbasvir/grazoprevir/ sofosbuvir, 12 wk (3)	3/3 (100%)
Gupta et al,[61] 2019	DaPPER	Virginia Commonwealth University	Kidney (50)	Sofosbuvir/velpatasvir, 2 d (10)	7/10 (70%)
				Sofosbuvir/velpatasvir, 4 d (40)	37/40 (93%)
Feld et al,[63] 2020	ASTRAL-1	University of Toledo	Lung (13) Kidney (10) Heart (6) Kidney-pancreas (1)	Ezetimibe and glecaprevir/pibrentasvir, 8 d (30)	30/30 (100%)
Durand et al,[57] 2021	REHANNA	Johns Hopkins University	Kidney (10)	Glecaprevir/pibrentasvir, 4 wk (10)	10/10 (100%)
Ramirez-Sanchez et al,[64] 2022	N/A	University of California, San Diego	Lung (1) Kidney (6) Heart (2) Heart-kidney (1)	Glecaprevir/pibrentasvir, 1 wk (10)	10/10 (100%)
Desai et al,[58] 2022	REHANNA 2	Johns Hopkins University	Kidney (10)	Glecaprevir/pibrentasvir, 2 wk (10)	10/10 (100%)

results suggest that shortened DAA regimens can prevent recipient infection and lower the expense of HCV D+/R− transplantation.[57,58]

Although prophylactic treatment can prevent HCV transmission, there have been several concerns raised about this approach. One is the need to crush and administer DAA tablets through a nasogastric tube (NGT) if transplant recipients remain intubated for days beyond their transplant. Data on administering DAAs this way are limited but have been successful in published reports.[59,60] The need for prolonged intubation is more common with thoracic transplant, and in trials of HCV D+/R− heart and lung transplant, DAAs were given via NGT if needed.[51] Another potential issue with prophylaxis is that if the duration is too short and transmission occurs, the acquired HCV may be more difficult to eradicate due to DAA resistance.[61–64] The DaPPER (Ultra-Short Direct Acting Antiviral Prophylaxis to Prevent Virus Transmission from Hepatitis C Viremic Donors to Hepatitis C Negative Kidney Transplant Recipients) investigated ultrashort SOF/VEL prophylaxis.[61] The study used a two-dose DAA course in 10 recipients, which resulted in 30% transmission, and a four-dose DAA course in 40 patients, which resulted in 7.5% transmission.[61] Recipients with HCV acquisition required retreatment with a 12-week DAA regimen, but only 83% achieved SVR.[61] The same group then explored a 7-day DAA course in 102 recipients, where they still found HCV transmission in 9% of recipients.[62] A separate trial examined an 8-day course of GLE/PIB plus ezetimibe, a lipid-lowering medication that blocks the receptor HCV uses for entry, and found no HCV transmission in 13 lung, 10 kidney, 6 heart, and 1 kidney-pancreas HCV D+/R− transplant recipients when this regimen was given prophylactically.[63] In 2022, another study investigated 7-day GLE/PIB prophylaxis in 10 HCV D+/R− transplants (two hearts, one lung, six kidneys, and one heart-kidney) with no evidence of transmission.[64]

With a transmit-and-treat approach, HCV transmission is universal, as demonstrated by the early trials (THINKER and USHER). With very early treatment, there are few, if any, clinical complications. However, in some real-world trials, where DAAs are delayed on the order of weeks to months, there may be complications. Fibrosing cholestatic hepatitis is a rare but potentially fatal complication of posttransplant acute HCV that has been reported in 1% to 2% of HCV D+/R− transplant cases when DAAs are delayed.[65–67] Liver enzyme elevation is another concern with one transmit-and-treat study finding that 20% of HCV D+/R− recipients experienced clinically significant increases (>3 times higher than the upper limit of the normal value) in aminotransferase levels.[63] Regarding kidney injury, HCV-associated glomerulonephritis has been reported in at least two instances of HCV D+/R− liver transplants with delayed DAA administration.[68,69] Another potential concern with delaying DAA treatment until the transmission is the potential for rejection which has been hypothesized as a result of acute hepatitis C and immune activation.[67,70] A study of recipients of hearts from donors both with and without HCV found that 64% of the HCV D+/R− cases developed acute cellular rejection during the viremia period (defined as <56 days posttreatment initiation which occurred on day 7 posttransplant, on average) compared with 18% of HCV D−/R− cases (P = .001).[70] These negative effects were still observed at 180 days posttransplant when 77% of HCV D+/R− cases experienced rejection versus only 43% of HCV D−/R− cases (P = .02).[70] The researchers concluded that even transient levels of viremia may contribute to increased rates of acute cellular rejection.[70] HCV viremia may also be linked to posttransplant infectious complications, such as CMV and BK infections. Indeed, in a study of 53 patients in the Methodist University Hospital in Tennessee, 34% of HCV D+/R− kidney recipients developed BK viremia, and 60% developed CMV.[66] Another concern is HCV exposure for caregivers in the period before treatment begins. In a study of 90 HCV D+/R− transplant recipients awaiting DAA approval, three caregivers were exposed via accidental needlesticks and required monitoring to ensure they did not become viremic themselves.[56] Finally, the prophylaxis approach is likely more cost-effective. One cost-effective analysis found that DAA prophylaxis with either a 7-day course of SOF/VEL, an 8-day course of GLE/PIB, or a 4-week course of SOF/VEl was more cost-effective than a transmit-and-treat approach with an 8-week course of GLE/PIB.[71]

To further compare prophylaxis versus the transmit-and-treat approach, the Prophylaxis with Direct-acting Antivirals for Kidney Transplantation from Hepatitis C Virus-Infected Donors to Uninfected Recipients: A Randomized Controlled Trial (PREVENT) study with clinical trial number NCT05653232 will begin in 2023 and will involve randomization of these DAA approaches.

SUMMARY

The current literature has shown excellent outcomes for transplant recipients with HIV who received organs from donors with HIV and transplant recipients without HCV receiving organs from donors with HCV. With the current organ shortage, using organs from donors with treatable infections is a novel and productive strategy to increase the quality and number of organs available to people living with and without HIV. Given waitlist mortality, we believe that current evidence supports both practices becoming standard clinical practice with future studies necessary to determine long-term outcomes and reduce potential complications. Finally, addressing barriers to implementation is critical to maximizing the benefit of both novel practices.

CLINICS CARE POINTS

- Using organs from donors with treatable infections can increase the quality and number of available organs and therefore may reduce waitlist mortality.
- Early data demonstrate that people living with HIV can safely receive kidney and liver transplants from donors with HIV under research protocols.
- The most common complication of HIV D+/R+ kidney transplantation has been rejection. The most common complication of HIV D+/R+ liver transplantation has been viral opportunistic infections and virally mediated cancers.
- Direct-acting antiviral therapy for Hepatitis C virus (HCV) is safe and highly effective in transplant recipients, allowing patients without HCV to receive organs from donors with HCV.
- Giving direct-acting antiviral (DAA) therapy prophylactically, before transplant, may reduce costs by shortening the DAA course. More studies are needed to determine whether DAA prophylaxis might reduce associated complications such as liver inflammation, viral infections, and rejection.

FUNDING

National Institutes of Health, National Institute of Allergy and Infectious Diseases: U01AI134591; U01AI138897; U01AI157931.

REFERENCES

1. Althoff KN, Gebo KA, Moore RD, et al. Contributions of traditional and HIV-related risk factors on non-AIDS-defining cancer, myocardial infarction, and end-stage

liver and renal diseases in adults with HIV in the USA and Canada: a collaboration of cohort studies. Lancet HIV 2019;6(2):e93–104.

2. Organ Procurement and Transplantation Network. Current United States Waiting List by Organ. Available at: https://optn.transplant.hrsa.gov/data/view-data-reports/national-data/# Accessed November 7, 2022.

3. Sawinski D, Wyatt CM, Casagrande L, et al. Factors Associated with Failure to List HIV-Positive Kidney Transplant Candidates. Am J Transplant 2009;9(6): 1467–71.

4. Locke JE, Mehta S, Sawinski D, et al. Access to Kidney Transplantation among HIV-Infected Waitlist Candidates. Clin J Am Soc Nephrol 2017;12(3):467–75.

5. Health Resources and Services Administration (HRSA), Department of Health and Human Services(HHS). Organ procurement and transplantation: implementation of the HIV Organ Policy Equity Act. Final rule. Fed Regist 2015;80(89): 26464–7.

6. Roth D, Nelson DR, Bruchfeld A, et al. Grazoprevir plus elbasvir in treatment-naive and treatment-experienced patients with hepatitis C virus genotype 1 infection and stage 4-5 chronic kidney disease (the C-SURFER study): a combination phase 3 study. Lancet 2015;386(10003):1537–45.

7. Feld JJ, Jacobson IM, Hézode C, et al. Sofosbuvir and Velpatasvir for HCV Genotype 1, 2, 4, 5, and 6 Infection. N Engl J Med 2015;373(27):2599–607.

8. Reau N, Kwo PY, Rhee S, et al. LBO-03 - MAGELLAN-2: safety and efficacy of glecaprevir/pibrentasvir in liver or renal transplant adults with chronic hepatitis C genotype 1-6 infection. J Hepatol 2017;66(1, Supplement):S90–1.

9. Nangia G, Borges K, Reddy KR. Use of HCV-infected organs in solid organ transplantation: An ethical challenge but plausible option. J Viral Hepat 2019;26(12): 1362–71.

10. Dummer JS, Erb S, Breinig MK, et al. Infection with human immunodeficiency virus in the Pittsburgh transplant population. A study of 583 donors and 1043 recipients, 1981-1986. Transplantation 1989;47(1):134–40.

11. Stock PG, Barin B, Murphy B, et al. Outcomes of Kidney Transplantation in HIV-Infected Recipients. N Engl J Med 2010;363(21):2004–14.

12. Roland ME, Barin B, Huprikar S, et al. Survival in HIV-positive transplant recipients compared with transplant candidates and with HIV-negative controls. AIDS 2015;30(3):435–44.

13. Terrault NA, Roland ME, Schiano T, et al. Outcomes of liver transplant recipients with hepatitis C and human immunodeficiency virus coinfection. Liver Transpl 2012;18(6):716–26.

14. Locke JE, Gustafson S, Mehta S, et al. Survival Benefit of Kidney Transplantation in HIV-infected Patients. Ann Surg 2017;265(3):604–8.

15. Muller E, Kahn D, Mendelson M. Renal Transplantation between HIV-Positive Donors and Recipients. N Engl J Med 2010;362(24):2336–7.

16. Boyarsky BJ, Hall EC, Singer AL, et al. Estimating the potential pool of HIV-infected deceased organ donors in the United States. Am J Transplant 2011; 11(6):1209–17.

17. Boyarsky BJ, Segev DL. From Bench to Bill: How a Transplant Nuance Became 1 of Only 57 Laws Passed in 2013. Ann Surg 2016;263(3):430–3.

18. Health Resources and Services Administration (HRSA). Department of Health and Human Services (HHS). Final Human Immunodeficiency Virus Organ Policy Equity (HOPE) Act safeguards and research criteria for transplantation of organs infected with HIV. Fed Regist 2015;80(227):73785–96.

19. Boyarsky BJ, Durand CM, Palella FJ Jr, et al. Challenges and Clinical Decision-Making in HIV-to-HIV Transplantation: Insights From the HIV Literature. Am J Transplant 2015;15(8):2023–30.

20. Spagnuolo V, Uberti-Foppa C, Castagna A. Pharmacotherapeutic management of HIV in transplant patients. Expert Opin Pharmacother 2019;20(10):1235–50.

21. Locke JE, Reed RD, Mehta SG, et al. Center-Level Experience and Kidney Transplant Outcomes in HIV-Infected Recipients. Am J Transplant 2015;15(8):2096–104.

22. Durand CM, Zhang W, Brown DM, et al. A prospective multicenter pilot study of HIV-positive deceased donor to HIV-positive recipient kidney transplantation: HOPE in action. Am J Transplant 2021;21(5):1754–64.

23. Muller E, Barday Z. HIV-Positive Kidney Donor Selection for HIV-Positive Transplant Recipients. J Am Soc Nephrol 2018;29(4):1090–5.

24. Bonny TS, Kirby C, Martens C, et al. Outcomes of donor-derived superinfection screening in HIV-positive to HIV-positive kidney and liver transplantation: a multicentre, prospective, observational study. Lancet HIV 2020;7(9):e611–9.

25. Durand CM, Florman S, Motter JD, et al. HOPE in action: A prospective multicenter pilot study of liver transplantation from donors with HIV to recipients with HIV. Am J Transplant 2022;22(3):853–64.

26. Razonable RR, Humar A. Cytomegalovirus in solid organ transplant recipients-Guidelines of the American Society of Transplantation Infectious Diseases Community of Practice. Clin Transplant 2019;33(9):e13512.

27. Durand CM, Halpern SE, Bowring MG, et al. Organs from deceased donors with false-positive HIV screening tests: An unexpected benefit of the HOPE act. Am J Transplant 2018;18(10):2579–86.

28. Durand CM, Werbel W, Doby B, et al. Clarifying the HOPE Act landscape: The challenge of donors with false-positive HIV results. Am J Transplant 2020;20(2):617–9.

29. Wilk AR, Hunter RA, McBride MA, et al. National landscape of HIV+ to HIV+ kidney and liver transplantation in the United States. Am J Transplant 2019;19(9):2594–605.

30. Werbel WA, Brown DM, Kusemiju OT, et al. National Landscape of Human Immunodeficiency Virus-Positive Deceased Organ Donors in the United States. Clin Infect Dis 2022;74(11):2010–9.

31. Azar MM, Malinis MF, Moss J, et al. Integrase strand transferase inhibitors: the preferred antiretroviral regimen in HIV-positive renal transplantation. Int J STD AIDS 2017;28(5):447–58.

32. Waldman G, Rawlings SA, Kerr J, et al. Successful optimization of antiretroviral regimens in treatment-experienced people living with HIV undergoing liver transplantation. Transpl Infect Dis 2019;21(6):e13174.

33. Nguyen AQ, Anjum SK, Halpern SE, et al. Willingness to Donate Organs Among People Living With HIV. J Acquir Immune Defic Syndr 2018;79(1):e30–6.

34. Donate Life America and the Organ Procurement and Transplantation Network. 2019 Donation and Transplantation Statistics. Available at: https://www.donatelife.net/wp-content/uploads/2016/06/2019-NDLM-Donation-and-Transplantation-Statistics-FINAL-Jan2019.pdf. Published January 16, 2019. Accessed 18 February, 2023.

35. Haidar G, Bhamidipati D, Despines L, et al. An initiative to increase organ donor registration among persons with HIV. Am J Transplant 2022;22(12):3186–7.

36. Doby BL, Tobian AAR, Segev DL, et al. Moving from the HIV Organ Policy Equity Act to HIV Organ Policy Equity in action: changing practice and challenging stigma. Curr Opin Organ Transplant 2018;23(2):271–8.

37. Predmore Z, Doby B, Bozzi DG, et al. Barriers experienced by organ procurement organizations in implementing the HOPE act and HIV-positive organ donation. AIDS Care 2022;34(9):1144–50.

38. Predmore Z, Doby B, Durand CM, et al. Potential donor characteristics and decisions made by organ procurement organization staff: Results of a discrete choice experiment. Transpl Infect Dis 2021;23(5):e13721.

39. Van Pilsum Rasmussen SE, Bowring MG, Shaffer AA, et al. Knowledge, attitudes, and planned practice of HIV-positive to HIV-positive transplantation in US transplant centers. Clin Transplant 2018;32(10):e13365.

40. Seaman SM, Van Pilsum Rasmussen SE, Nguyen AQ, et al. Brief Report: Willingness to Accept HIV-Infected and Increased Infectious Risk Donor Organs Among Transplant Candidates Living With HIV. J Acquir Immune Defic Syndr 2020;85(1): 88–92.

41. Ly KN, Hughes EM, Jiles RB, et al. Rising Mortality Associated With Hepatitis C Virus in the United States, 2003–2013. Clin Infect Dis 2016;62(10):1287–8.

42. Zibbell JE, Asher AK, Patel RC, et al. Increases in Acute Hepatitis C Virus Infection Related to a Growing Opioid Epidemic and Associated Injection Drug Use, United States, 2004 to 2014. Am J Public Health 2018;108(2):175–81.

43. Durand CM, Bowring MG, Thomas AG, et al. The Drug Overdose Epidemic and Deceased-Donor Transplantation in the United States: A National Registry Study. Ann Intern Med 2018;168(10):702–11.

44. Axelrod DA, Schnitzler MA, Alhamad T, et al. The impact of direct-acting antiviral agents on liver and kidney transplant costs and outcomes. Am J Transplant 2018; 18(10):2473–82.

45. Afdhal N, Reddy KR, Nelson DR, et al. Ledipasvir and sofosbuvir for previously treated HCV genotype 1 infection. N Engl J Med 2014;370(16):1483–93.

46. Reese PP, Abt PL, Blumberg EA, et al. Twelve-Month Outcomes After Transplant of Hepatitis C-Infected Kidneys Into Uninfected Recipients: A Single-Group Trial. Ann Intern Med 2018;169(5):273–81.

47. Durand CM, Bowring MG, Brown DM, et al. Direct-Acting Antiviral Prophylaxis in Kidney Transplantation From Hepatitis C Virus-Infected Donors to Noninfected Recipients: An Open-Label Nonrandomized Trial. Ann Intern Med 2018;168(8): 533–40.

48. Sise ME, Goldberg DS, Kort JJ, et al. Multicenter Study to Transplant Hepatitis C–Infected Kidneys (MYTHIC): An Open-Label Study of Combined Glecaprevir and Pibrentasvir to Treat Recipients of Transplanted Kidneys from Deceased Donors with Hepatitis C Virus Infection. J Am Soc Nephrol 2020;31(11):2678–87.

49. Sise ME, Goldberg DS, Schaubel DE, et al. One-Year Outcomes of the Multi-Center StudY to Transplant Hepatitis C-InfeCted kidneys (MYTHIC) Trial. Kidney International Reports 2022;7(2):241–50.

50. McLean RC, Reese PP, Acker M, et al. Transplanting hepatitis C virus–infected hearts into uninfected recipients: A single-arm trial. Am J Transplant 2019; 19(9):2533–42.

51. Woolley AE, Singh SK, Goldberg HJ, et al. Heart and Lung Transplants from HCV-Infected Donors to Uninfected Recipients. N Engl J Med 2019;380(17):1606–17.

52. Schaubel DE, Tran AH, Abt PL, et al. Five-Year Allograft Survival for Recipients of Kidney Transplants From Hepatitis C Virus Infected vs Uninfected Deceased Donors in the Direct-Acting Antiviral Therapy Era. JAMA 2022;328(11):1102–4.

53. Holscher CM, Durand CM, Desai NM. Expanding the Use of Organs From Hepatitis C-Viremic Donors: The Evidence Continues to Build. Transplantation 2018; 102(4):546–7.

54. Haque M, Hashim A, Greanya ED, et al. Spontaneous clearance of hepatitis C infection post-liver transplant: A rare but real phenomenon? A case report and review of the literature. Ann Hepatol 2010;9(2):202–6.

55. Bethea E, Arvind A, Gustafson J, et al. Immediate administration of antiviral therapy after transplantation of hepatitis C-infected livers into uninfected recipients: Implications for therapeutic planning. Am J Transplant 2020;20(6):1619–28.

56. Stewart ZA, Stern J, Ali NM, et al. Clinical and Financial Implications of 2 Treatment Strategies for Donor-derived Hepatitis C Infections. Transplant Direct 2021;7(10):e762.

57. Durand CM, Barnaba B, Yu S, et al. Four-Week Direct-Acting Antiviral Prophylaxis for Kidney Transplantation From Hepatitis C-Viremic Donors to Hepatitis C-Negative Recipients: An Open-Label Nonrandomized Study. Ann Intern Med 2021; 174(1):137–8.

58. Desai NMLS, Motter J, Naqvi F, et al. Renal Transplants In Hepatitis C Negative Recipients With Nucleic Acid Positive Donors Using Two Weeks Of DAA Prophylaxis (Rehanna – 2) [abstract]. Am J Transplant 2022. Available at: https://atcmeetingabstracts.com/abstract/renal-transplants-in-hepatitis-c-negative-recipients-with-nucleic-acid-positive-donors-using-two-weeks-of-daa-prophylaxis-rehanna-2/. Accessed 30 November, 2022.

59. Whelchel K, Zuckerman AD, Koren DE, et al. Crushing and Splitting Direct-Acting Antivirals for Hepatitis C Virus Treatment: A Case Series and Literature Review. Open Forum Infect Dis 2021;8(11):ofab525.

60. Shah RB, Garrett KL, Brotherton AL, et al. Elbasvir/grazoprevir administered for 12 weeks via percutaneous endoscopic gastrostomy tube achieves sustained virologic response: A case report and a review of the literature. Pharmacotherapy 2021;41(7):634–40.

61. Gupta G, Yakubu I, Bhati CS, et al. Ultra-short duration direct acting antiviral prophylaxis to prevent virus transmission from hepatitis C viremic donors to hepatitis C negative kidney transplant recipients. Am J Transplant 2020;20(3):739–51.

62. Gupta G, Yakubu I, Zhang Y, et al. Outcomes of short-duration antiviral prophylaxis for hepatitis C positive donor kidney transplants. Am J Transplant 2021; 21(11):3734–42.

63. Feld JJ, Cypel M, Kumar D, et al. Short-course, direct-acting antivirals and ezetimibe to prevent HCV infection in recipients of organs from HCV-infected donors: a phase 3, single-centre, open-label study. Lancet Gastroenterol Hepatol 2020; 5(7):649–57.

64. Ramirez-Sanchez C, Kozuch J, Shah MM, et al. A Pilot Trial for Prevention of Hepatitis C Virus Transmission From Donor to Organ Transplant Recipient With Short-Course Glecaprevir/Pibrentasvir. Open Forum Infect Dis 2022;9(11):ofac550.

65. Cypel M, Feld JJ, Galasso M, et al. Prevention of viral transmission during lung transplantation with hepatitis C-viraemic donors: an open-label, single-centre, pilot trial. Lancet Respir Med 2020;8(2):192–201.

66. Molnar MZ, Nair S, Cseprekal O, et al. Transplantation of kidneys from hepatitis C–infected donors to hepatitis C–negative recipients: Single center experience. Am J Transplant 2019;19(11):3046–57.

67. Kapila N, Al-Khalloufi K, Bejarano PA, et al. Fibrosing cholestatic hepatitis after kidney transplantation from HCV-viremic donors to HCV-negative recipients: A unique complication in the DAA era. Am J Transplant 2020;20(2):600–5.

68. Bohorquez H, Velez JCQ, Lusco M, et al. Hepatitis C–associated focal proliferative glomerulonephritis in an aviremic recipient of a hepatitis C–positive antibody donor liver. Am J Transplant 2021;21(8):2895–9.

69. Aqel B, Wijarnpreecha K, Pungpapong S, et al. Outcomes following liver transplantation from HCV-seropositive donors to HCV-seronegative recipients. J Hepatol 2021;74(4):873–80.

70. Gidea CG, Narula N, Reyentovich A, et al. Increased early acute cellular rejection events in hepatitis C-positive heart transplantation. J Heart Lung Transplant 2020; 39(11):1199–207.

71. Yakubu IZY, Ijioma S, Carroll NV, et al. Cost-Effectiveness Analysis of Short-Duration Anti-Viral Prophylaxis for Hepatitis C Positive Donor Kidney Transplants [abstract]. Am J Transplant 2021;21(suppl 3). Available at: https://atcmeetingabstracts.com/abstract/cost-effectiveness-analysis-of-short-duration-anti-viral-prophylaxis-for-hepatitis-c-positive-donor-kidney-transplants/. Accessed 19 December, 2022.

Printed and bound by CPI Group (UK) Ltd, Croydon, CR0 4YY

08/05/2025

01864750-0002